Older Adults and COVID-19

The COVID-19 pandemic has impacted the lives of people throughout the world, either directly, due to exposure to the virus, or indirectly, due to measures taken to mitigate the virus' effects. Older adults have been particularly hard hit, dying in disproportionately higher numbers, especially in long-term care facilities. Local, regional, and national government actions taken to mitigate the spread of COVID-19 have thus served, in part, to shield older adults from the virus, though not without adverse side effects, including increased social isolation, enhanced economic risk, revealed ageism, delayed medical treatment, and challenges getting basic needs met. This book explores the myriad ways in which the COVID-19 pandemic has affected older adults and their families, caregivers, and communities. It proposes policies and strategies for protecting and improving the lives of older people during the pandemic. It draws lessons for aging policy and practice more generally, given underlying challenges brought to the fore by government, provider, community, and individual responses to the pandemic.

This book was originally published as a special issue of the *Journal of Aging & Social Policy*.

Edward Alan Miller is a Professor of Gerontology & Public Policy and Fellow, Gerontology Institute, at the John W. McCormack Graduate School of Policy & Global Studies, University of Massachusetts Boston, USA, and Adjunct Professor of Health Services, Policy & Practice at the School of Public Health, Brown University, Providence, USA. His research focuses on understanding the determinants and effects of public policies and practices affecting older adults in need of long-term services and supports. He is the author/co-author/editor/co-editor of more than 125 journal articles, 15 book chapters, and 5 books. He is the Editor-in-Chief of the *Journal of Aging & Social Policy*, and Fellow within the Gerontological Society of America.

Older Adults and COVID-19

Implications for Aging Policy and Practice

Edited by
Edward Alan Miller

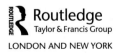
Routledge
Taylor & Francis Group

LONDON AND NEW YORK

First published 2021
by Routledge
2 Park Square, Milton Park, Abingdon, Oxon, OX14 4RN

and by Routledge
52 Vanderbilt Avenue, New York, NY 10017

Routledge is an imprint of the Taylor & Francis Group, an informa business

© 2021 Taylor & Francis

British Library Cataloguing-in-Publication Data
A catalogue record for this book is available from the British Library

ISBN13: 978-0-367-63299-1

Typeset in Minion Pro
by codeMantra

Publisher's Note
The publisher accepts responsibility for any inconsistencies that may have arisen during the conversion of this book from journal articles to book chapters, namely the inclusion of journal terminology.

Disclaimer
Every effort has been made to contact copyright holders for their permission to reprint material in this book. The publishers would be grateful to hear from any copyright holder who is not here acknowledged and will undertake to rectify any errors or omissions in future editions of this book.

This volume is dedicated to my wife, Jessica, and children, Noah, Dina, and Anabelle, the lights of my life even in the darkest of times.

Contents

Local and Community Responses 151

Economic Risks to Older Workers and Retirees 193

Documenting and Combating Ageism 223

Recovery 253

Citation Information

The chapters in this book were originally published in the *Journal of Aging & Social Policy*, volume 32, issue 4–5 (2020). When citing this material, please use the original page numbering for each article, as follows:

For any permission-related enquiries please visit:
http://www.tandfonline.com/page/help/permissions

Contributors

Odichinma Akosionu, MPH Research Assistant, Division of Health Policy and Management, School of Public Health, University of Minnesota, Minneapolis, USA.

Laura D. Allen Doctoral Researcher, Louis and Gabi Weisfeld School of Social Work, Faculty of Social Sciences, Bar-Ilan University, Ramat Gan, Israel.

Beth Almeida, MA Principal, Cove Research, Beverly, USA.

Jacqueline L. Angel, PhD Professor of Sociology and Public Affairs, LBJ School of Public Affairs, The University of Texas at Austin, USA.

Nicholas Bagley, JD Professor, School of Law, University of Michigan, Ann Arbor, USA.

Liza L. Behrens, PhD, RN Postdoctoral Research Fellow, NewCourtland Center for Transitions and Health, University of Pennsylvania School of Nursing, Philadelphia, USA.

Daniel Béland, PhD James McGill Professor and Director of the McGill Institute for the Study of Canada (MISC), Department of Political Science, McGill University, Montreal, Canada.

Lynn A. Blewett, MA, PhD Professor of Health Policy and Director, State Health Access Data Assistance Center (SHADAC), School of Public Health, Division of Health Policy and Management, University of Minnesota, Minneapolis, USA.

Kathrin Boerner, PhD Associate Professor, Department of Gerontology, John W. McCormack Graduate School of Policy and Global Studies, University of Massachusetts Boston, USA.

John R. Bowblis, PhD Professor of Economics, Farmer School of Business, Miami University, Oxford, USA.

Amanda L. Brewster, PhD Assistant Professor, Health Policy and Management, University of California, Berkeley School of Public Health, USA.

Julie P. W. Bynum, MD, PhD Division of Geriatric & Palliative Medicine, University of Michigan School of Medicine, Ann Arbor, USA.

Deborah Carr, PhD Professor and Chair, Department of Sociology, Boston University, USA.

Neil Charness William G. Chase Psychology Department, Florida State University, Tallahassee, USA.

Marc A. Cohen Professor and Co-Director, LeadingAge LTSS Center, McCormack Graduate School of Policy and Global Studies, University of Massachusetts Boston, USA. Center for Consumer Engagement in Health Innovation, Community Catalyst, Boston, USA.

Marc A. Cohen, PhD Professor and Co-Director, Department of Gerontology, LeadingAge LTSS Center, McCormack Graduate School of Policy and Global Studies, University of Massachusetts Boston, USA. Research Director, Center for Consumer Engagement in Health Innovation, Community Catalyst, Boston, USA.

Adelina Comas-Herrera, MSc Assistant Professorial Research Fellow, Care Policy and Evaluation Centre, London School of Economics and Political Science, UK.

Debra Dobbs, PhD Associate Professor, School of Aging Studies, Florida Policy Exchange Center on Aging, University of South Florida, Tampa, USA.

Yinfei Duan, MSN Research Assistant, School of Public Health, University of Minnesota, Minneapolis, USA.

Hans-Joerg Ehni, PhD Professor, Institute for Ethics and the History of Medicine, University of Tuebingen, Germany.

Aida Farmand, MA Department of Economics, The New School for Social Research, USA.

Judy Feder, PhD McCourt School of Public Policy, USA; Georgetown University, Washington, District of Columbia, USA.

Lynn Friss Feinberg, MSW Senior Strategic Policy Advisor, AARP Public Policy Institute, Washington, District of Columbia, USA.

Jose-Luis Fernandez, MSc, PhD Associate Professorial Research Fellow, Care Policy and Evaluation Centre, London School of Economics and Political Science, UK.

Karen Fingerman Professor, Department of Human Development & Family Sciences, The University of Texas at Austin, USA.

Natalie Galucia, MSW Center Manager, Harvey A. Friedman Center for Aging, Washington University, St. Louis, USA.

William Gardner, PhD Professor, School of Epidemiology and Public Health, Child and Adolescent Psychiatry, University of Ottawa, Ontario, Canada.

Teresa Ghilarducci, PhD Bernard L. and Irene Schwartz Professor, Department of Economics, The New School for Social Research, USA. Director, Schwartz Center for Economic Policy Analysis (SCEPA), The New School for Social Research, USA.

Edem Hado, MPH Policy Research Senior Analyst, AARP Public Policy Institute, Washington, District of Columbia, USA.

Ruth Hancock, MSc Professor, Economics of Health and Welfare, Health Economics Group, Norwich Medical School, University of East Anglia, Norwich, UK. Occasional Professorial Research Fellow, Care Policy and Evaluation Centre, London School of Economics and Political Science, UK.

Chris Hatton, PhD Professor of Public Health and Disability, Centre for Disability Research, Lancaster University, UK.

Carrie Henning-Smith, PhD, MPH, MSW Division of Health Policy and Management, Minneapolis, USA. University of Minnesota Rural Health Research Center, Minneapolis, USA. University of Minnesota School of Public Health, Minneapolis, USA.

Robert Hest, MPP Research Fellow, State Health Access Data Assistance Center (SHADAC), School of Public Health, Division of Health Policy and Management, University of Minnesota, Minneapolis, USA.

Karen B. Hirschman, PhD, MSW Research Associate Professor, NewCourtland Term Chair in Health Transitions Research, NewCourtland Center for Transitions and Health, University of Pennsylvania School of Nursing, Philadelphia, USA.

Geoffrey J. Hoffman, PhD Assistant Professor, Department of Systems, Populations and Leadership, University of Michigan School of Nursing, Ann Arbor, USA. Institute for Healthcare Policy and Innovation, University of Michigan, Ann Arbor, USA.

Kathryn Hyer, PhD Professor, School of Aging Studies, Florida Policy Exchange Center on Aging, University of South Florida, Tampa, USA.

Jeffrey Kaye Layton Professor, Neurology and Biomedical Engineering, Oregon Health & Science University and Portland Veterans Affairs Medical Center, Portland, USA.

Anjum Khurshid Assistant Professor, Department of Population Health, Dell Medical School, The University of Texas at Austin, USA.

Miyong T. Kim La Quinta Centennial Endowed Professor, School of Nursing, The University of Texas at Austin, USA.

Martin Knapp, MSc, PhD Professor of Health and Care Policy, Care Policy and Evaluation Centre, Department of Health Policy, London School of Economics and Political Science, UK.

Suzanne R. Kunkel, PhD Executive Director, Scripps Gerontology Center, and University Distinguished Professor, Department of Sociology & Gerontology, Miami University, Oxford, USA.

Yang Li, DBA, MS PhD Candidate, Department of Gerontology, Center for Social & Demographic Research on Aging, Gerontology Institute, John W. McCormack Graduate School of Policy and Global Studies, University of Massachusetts Boston, USA.

Terry Lum, PhD, MSW Professor, Department of Social Work and Social Administration, and Associate Director, Sau Po Center on Aging, The University of Hong Kong, China.

Juliette Malley, PhD, MPhil, MA Assistant Professorial Research Fellow, Care Policy and Evaluation Centre, London School of Economics and Political Science, UK.

Patrik Marier, PhD Professor and Concordia University Research Chair in Aging and Public Policy, Scientific Director, Centre de recherche et d'expertise en gérontologie sociale (CREGÉS), Department of Political Science, Concordia University, Montreal, Canada.

Kathleen McCauley, PhD, RN, FAAN, FAHA Professor of Cardiovascular Nursing, NewCourtland Center for Transitions and Health, University of Pennsylvania School of Nursing, Philadelphia, USA.

David McDaid, MSc Associate Professorial Research Fellow, Care Policy and Evaluation Centre, London School of Economics and Political Science, UK.

Edward Alan Miller, PhD, MPA Professor, Department of Gerontology, and Fellow, Gerontology Institute, John W. McCormack Graduate School of Policy Studies, University of Massachusetts Boston, USA. Adjunct Professor, Department of Health Services, Policy and Practice, School of Public Health, Brown University, Providence, USA.

Sara Moorman, PhD Associate Professor, Department of Sociology, Boston College, USA.

Nancy Morrow-Howell, MSW, PhD Bettie Bofinger Brown Distinguished Professor of Social Policy, Brown School, Washington University, St. Louis, USA. Director, Harvey A. Friedman Center for Aging, Washington University, St. Louis, USA.

Stipica Mudrazija, PhD Senior Research Associate, Income and Benefits Policy Center, Urban Institute, Washington, District of Columbia, USA.

Jan E Mutchler, PhD Professor, Department of Gerontology, Center for Social & Demographic Research on Aging, Gerontology Institute, John W. McCormack Graduate School of Policy and Global Studies, University of Massachusetts Boston, USA.

Mary D. Naylor, PhD, RN, FAAN Marian S. Ware Professor in Gerontology, Director of the NewCourtland Center for Transitions and Health, University of Pennsylvania, Philadelphia, USA.

Weiwen Ng, MPH Research Assistant, Division of Health Policy and Management, School of Public Health, University of Minnesota, Minneapolis, USA.

Sarah E. Patterson, PhD National Institute on Aging Postdoctoral Fellow, Population Studies Center, Institute for Social Research, University of Michigan, Ann Arbor, USA.

Lindsay Peterson, PhD Research Assistant Professor, School of Aging Studies, Florida Policy Exchange Center on Aging, University of South Florida, Tampa, USA.

Federica Previtali, MSc Doctoral Researcher, Social Sciences and Gerontology Research Centre, Tampere University, Finland.

Laurinda Reynolds, MA Professor, Department Chair and Career Education Program Coordinator, Gerontology Department, American River College, Sacramento, USA.

Marisa Scala-Foley, MGS Director, Aging and Disability Business Institute, National Association of Area Agencies on Aging, Washington, District of Columbia, USA.

Cheng Shi, PhD Postdoctoral Fellow, Department of Social Work and Social Administration, The University of Hong Kong, China.

Tetyana P. Shippee, PhD Associate Professor, Division of Health Policy and Management, School of Public Health, University of Minnesota, Minneapolis, USA.

David States, MD, PhD Angstrom Bio, Ann Arbor, USA.

Jeffrey E. Stokes, PhD Assistant Professor, Department of Gerontology, McCormack Graduate School of Policy & Global Studies, University of Massachusetts Boston, USA.

Robyn I. Stone, Dr. PH Senior Vice President for Research, Department of Gerontology, LeadingAge LTSS Center, Washington, District of Columbia, USA. Co-Director, LeadingAge LTSS Center, Washington, District of Columbia, USA.

Emma Swinford, MSW, MPH Program Coordinator, Harvey A. Friedman Center for Aging, Washington University, St. Louis, USA.

Anna-Marie Tabor, JD Director, Pension Action Center, Gerontology Institute, John W. McCormack Graduate School of Policy and Global Studies, University of Massachusetts Boston, USA.

Jane Tavares Research Fellow, LeadingAge LTSS Center, University of Massachusetts Boston, USA.

Mai See Thao, PhD Postdoctoral Fellow in Primary Care Research, Department of Family and Community Medicine, Medical College of Wisconsin, Milwaukee, USA.

Maria Varlamova, MSc Doctoral Researcher, Institute of the Sociology, Jagiellonian University, Krakow, Poland.

Hans-Werner Wahl, PhD Professor, Network of Aging Research, Heidelberg University, Germany.

Noah J. Webster, PhD Assistant Research Scientist, Institute for Social Research, University of Michigan, Ann Arbor, USA.

Christian E. Weller, PhD Professor, Department of Public Policy and Public Affairs, University of Massachusetts Boston, USA. Senior Fellow, Center for American Progress, Washington, District of Columbia, USA.

Traci L. Wilson, DPhil Research Scholar, Scripps Gerontology Center, Miami University, Oxford, USA.

Gerald Wistow, M. Soc. Sci., PGCE Visiting Professor, Care Policy and Evaluation Centre, London School of Economics and Political Science, UK.

Raphael Wittenberg, MSc Associate Professorial Research Fellow, Care Policy and Evaluation Centre, London School of Economics and Political Science, UK.

Gloria Wong, PhD Assistant Professor, Department of Social Work and Social Administration, The University of Hong Kong, China.

Kayla Wong, B. Soc. Sci. Research Assistant, Department of Social Work and Social Administration, The University of Hong Kong, China.

Mark Woodhouse, BA Database Manager, School of Public Health, University of Minnesota, Minneapolis, USA.

Bo Xie School of Nursing, The University of Texas at Austin, USA. School of Information, The University of Texas at Austin, USA.

Introduction: Protecting and Improving the Lives of Older Adults in the COVID-19 Era

Edward Alan Miller

ABSTRACT

The COVID-19 pandemic has impacted the lives of people throughout the world, either directly, due to exposure to the virus, or indirectly, due to measures taken to mitigate the virus' effects. Older adults have been particularly hard hit, dying in disproportionately higher numbers, especially in long-term care facilities. Local, regional, and national government actions taken to mitigate the spread of COVID-19 have thus served, in part, to shield older adults from the virus, though not without adverse side effects, including increased social isolation, enhanced economic risk, revealed ageism, delayed medical treatment, and challenges getting basic needs met. This special issue of the *Journal of Aging & Social Policy* explores the myriad ways in which the COVID-19 pandemic has affected older adults and their families, caregivers, and communities. It proposes policies and strategies for protecting and improving the lives of older people during the pandemic. It draws lessons for aging policy and practice more generally, given underlying challenges brought to the fore by government, provider, community, and individual responses to the pandemic.

Introduction

It would be an understatement to say that the COVID-19 pandemic has impacted the lives of people throughout the world, either directly, due to exposure to the virus, or indirectly, due to measures taken to mitigate the virus' health and economic effects. As May 2020 draws to a close, confirmed COVID-19 infections approach nearly 6,000,000 globally with close to 400,000 deaths worldwide (Johns Hopkins University School of Medicine, 2020). No nation has been spared but some countries have been hit particularly hard by the virus. Although just 4.3% of the world population (U.S. Census Bureau, 2020), the United States constitutes 29.5% of COVID-19 infections and 28.2% of COVID-19-related deaths (Johns Hopkins University School of Medicine, 2020). Other countries experiencing disproportionate impact, whether measured in terms of numbers of infections or deaths, include the United Kingdom, Italy, France, Spain, Brazil, Mexico, and Germany. Unprecedented actions have been taken to stem the tide of coronavirus infection. These actions include state of emergency declarations, shelter-in-place orders, travel bans, school and non-essential business closures, mandated use of face masks, visitor bans (in hospitals and long-term care facilities), and mass testing and distribution of personnel protective equipment (PPE).

The spread and response to COVID-19 has devastated national economies, pushing many into recession. A Brookings Institution analysis of 20 wealthy democracies found that by May 2020 5.7%, or 38 million of 660 million total workers, had filed for unemployment insurance since the pandemic began (Rothwell, 2020). In all, there have been more than 40 million initial unemployment claims in the U.S. since mid-March 2020 (Reiniche, 2020). At 13%, a higher proportion of workers in the U.S. than in other countries are currently receiving unemployment insurance (Rothwell, 2020), with four countries – Canada, Israel, Ireland, and the U.S. – witnessing double digit increase in unemployment insurance claims during this time. Cross-national variation in unemployment reflects, in part, the relative mix of strategies used to mitigate the negative economic consequences of the virus (Rothwell, 2020). Some countries have weighted intervention more heavily toward enhanced unemployment and other individual or household financial support. Other countries have weighted intervention toward subsidizing businesses and stimulating the broader economy to head off large-scale layoffs. Still other countries have employed a relatively balanced mix of these two approaches.

Notably, the intensity of the health and economic pain brought on by the COVID-19 pandemic has been stronger in some segments of the population than others. Exacerbating existing disparities, people from Native American, Hispanic and African American communities, as well as individuals with low incomes and those residing in urban areas, have been disproportionately impacted (Raifman & Raifman, 2020; Webb Hopper et al., 2020). A Harvard University analysis found that during the early weeks of the COVID-19 pandemic "deaths surged higher in Massachusetts cities, towns, and ZIP codes with larger concentrations of poverty, economic segregation, people of color, and crowded housing" (Ryan & Lazard, 2020). According to a May 2020 Kaiser Family Foundation survey, black and Hispanic respondents were more than twice as likely (at 48% and 46%, respectively) as non-Hispanic white respondents (at 23%) to report having trouble affording food, housing, utilities, credit card bills or health expenses due to COVID-19. Respondents with annual incomes below 40,000 USD were more than three times as likely to report having trouble with these expenses than respondents with annual incomes over 90,000 USD (47% v. 14%) (Kaiser Family Foundation, 2020).

Older adults have been especially hard hit by COVID-19. In 2015, people aged 65 years and older constituted 15% of the population in the U.S.; people aged 85 years and older 1.96% (Federal Interagency Forum on Aging-Related Statistics, 2016). Yet, 22% of all COVID-19 cases and 81% of all COVID-19 deaths have occurred among older adults (Center for Disease Control and Prevention, 2020a, 2020b). Deaths per million from COVID-19 rises dramatically with age, increasing from 23.6, 66.6, and 159.1, respectively, among individuals aged 33–44, 45–54, and 55–64 years, to 377.9 and 969.8 among individuals aged 65–74 and 75–84 years, and an astonishing 2,670.6 for individuals 85 years and older (Girvan, 2020).

A large proportion of COVID-19 deaths has occurred in long-term care facilities that care for older adults with physical and cognitive impairments in need of assistance with basic activities of daily living such eating, bathing, and toileting. Just 2.1 million people accounting for 0.62% of the U.S. population reside in a nursing home or assisted living facility, yet, as of May 22, 2020, this population constituted 42% of all COVID-19 deaths (54% when excluding New York, which may be under reporting nursing home fatalities from the virus) (Girvan, 2020). Several states well exceed these national totals. In Massachusetts, for example, 62% of 6,547 COVID-19 deaths have been in long-term care facilities (Wasser, 2020). All but 33 of the state's 319 nursing homes and rest homes reported deaths from COVID-19, including 80 facilities with at least 20 deaths and 19 facilities with 30 or more. These figures are consistent with data reported in other countries where, for example, more than 50% of COVID-19-related deaths have taken place in care homes in France (51%), Belgium (53%), Norway (60%), Ireland (60%), and Canada (62%) (Comas-Herrera et al., 2020).

Local, regional, and national government actions taken to mitigate the spread of the virus have served, in part, to shield older adults from COVID-19, though not without increased social isolation, enhanced economic risk, revealed ageism, delayed medical treatment, and challenges getting basic needs met. These negative effects crosscut with vulnerabilities grounded in the social determinants of health to place older adults, families, and caregivers belonging to racial and ethnic minority and economically disadvantage populations at especially high risk for adverse outcomes. Specific vulnerabilities include underlying comorbidities (such as chronic lung and heart disease, diabetes, cancer and other immunocompromising conditions/treatments), inadequate housing, income and savings, resource scarcity, population density, poor health care access and quality, disproportionate employment in essential or forward-facing occupations, and structural racism and sexism (Raifman & Raifman, 2020; Webb Hopper et al., 2020).

This special double issue of the *Journal of Aging & Social Policy*, "Older Adults and COVID-19: Implications for Aging Policy & Practice," explores the myriad ways in which the COVID-19 pandemic has affected older adults and their families, caregivers, and communities. It proposes policies and strategies for protecting and improving the lives of older individuals during the pandemic. It draws lessons for aging policy and practice more generally, given underlying challenges brought to the fore by government, provider, community, and individual responses to the pandemic.

Issue content

The articles included in this issue, authored by leading scholars in their respective fields, focus on one of eight main areas affected by COVID-19: (1) delivering long-term services and supports (LTSS) in the U.S. (Gardner, States & Bagley; Behrens & Naylor; Shippee et al.; Dobbs, Peterson & Hyer), (2) financing LTSS in the U.S. (Feder; Blewett & Hest), (3) LTSS in other contexts (Béland & Marier; Comas-Herrera et al.; Lum, Shi, Wong & Wong); (4) high risk older adults in communities (Cohen & Tavares; Naylor, Hirschman & McCauley; Henning-Smith), (5) families and caregivers of older adults (Almeida, Cohen, Stone, & Weller; Hedo & Feinberg; Stokes & Patterson; Carr, Boerner & Moorman), (6) local government and community responses (Wilson, Scala-Foley; Kunkel & Brewster; Angel & Mudrazija; Hoffman, Webster & Bynum; Xie et al.), (7) economic risks for older workers and retirees (Ghilarducci & Farmand; Li & Mutchler; Tabor), and (8) documenting and combating ageism (Reynolds; Previtali, Allen & Variamova; Ehni & Wahl). A final, concluding article addresses the post-COVID-19 recovery (Morrow-Howell, Galucia & Swinford).

Delivering long-term services and supports in the U.S

Four U.S.-based articles focus on the delivery of LTSS during the COVID-19 pandemic, primarily in nursing homes but also in assisted living facilities and home and community-based services settings. Gardner, States & Bagely document heightened risk for older adults in long-term care facilities, both directly from COVID-19 and indirectly due to increased isolation and potential for abuse and neglect. The need for enhanced testing, infection control, staffing supports, and supervision in the context of the crisis are noted.

Informed by discussions with nursing home leaders, Behrens & Naylor propose a framework to facilitate decision making and collective action to address the COVID-19 crisis within the nursing home sector. The framework outlines the resources essential to mitigate COVID-19 as facilities seek to maintain or improve operations depending on their current stage of operations: standard, contingency, crisis, or catastrophic.

Shippee and colleagues point to marked racial and ethnic disparities in the quality of LTSS that have worsened during the COVID-19 pandemic. Recommended near term actions in recognition of these disparities include enhanced reporting of COVID-19 by race/ethnicity and prioritizing high proportion minority facilities for testing, PPE, and other supports. Long-term actions to address prevailing disparities affecting residents and frontline workers are suggested as well.

Finally, Dobbs, Peterson & Hyer focus on the challenges faced by assisted living facilities due to COVID-19, including with respect to family visitation, use of third-party providers as essential workers, staffing guidelines, transfer policies, and rural hospitalization. Recommendations include increased use of digital technology, limits on multi-facility visits by home health care workers, enhanced staffing through extension of the personal care attendant program to assisted living, hazard pay for direct care staff, and implementation of comprehensive emergency management plans.

Financing long-term services and supports in the U.S

Two U.S.-based articles focus on the financing of health care and LTSS in the context of Medicaid during the COVID-19 pandemic. Both articles deem Medicaid, the joint federal-state health insurance program for low income Americans, essential to state responses in light of the growing demand for coverage and services. Blewett and Hest observe that states have taken advantage of new authority granted to them by the federal government to streamline and increase the flexibility of Medicaid LTSS eligibility to help facilitate enrollment and prevent disenrollment. They caution, however, against subsequent cutbacks in Medicaid LTSS eligibility and services during this time of great need due to forthcoming budget shortfalls generated by the COVID-19 induced economic crisis.

Feder also cautions against funding reductions but views increasing the federal share of Medicaid spending during the economic crisis as only part of the solution due to the inadequate and inequitable nature of Medicaid LTSS funding across states. Recognizing these extant limitations, Feder suggests that Medicaid LTSS financing should be modified to either adjust federal matching funds by the age of each state's population, or fully federalizing the funding of long-term care expenses for dually eligible beneficiaries (i.e., Medicaid beneficiaries who are also eligible for Medicare).

Long-term services and supports in other contexts

Three additional articles examine LTSS-specific responses to COVID-19 but outside of the U.S., in Canada, England, and Hong Kong. Béland & Marier point to similar challenges and risks posed to long-term care facilities in Canada as the U.S. They argue that the devasting consequences of COVID-19 for long-term care facilities is a "focusing event" that draws attention to the issue, in light of existing policy legacies underlying devolution of funding and oversight to the provinces and a public-private dichotomy in ownership and oversight. Should a resulting "policy window" open up, a first step toward reform suggested by the authors would be to increase provincial and, potentially, federal funding for this highly stressed sector.

Comas-Herrera and colleagues describe challenges to the quality and availability of social care posed by COVID-19 in England, and policy responses made in light of those challenges. Responses noted include a successful call for volunteers in health and social care and measures to promote the financial viability of care providers. They also include provisions aimed at removing barriers to effective coordination between health and social care to provide services, facilitate transfers, monitor infection rates and deaths, distribute PPE, conduct testing, and bolster the provider workforce. The importance of achieving well-co-coordinated response across the central and local government, health services, and private and voluntary sectors is highlighted.

Lum, Shi, Wong & Wong report on Hong Kong's successful effort to manage and contain COVID-19, informed, in part, by lessons drawn from the 2003 SARS epidemic. Home and community-based services were severely restricted. The provision of resources to fund PPE and to pay for additional cleaning staff helped to contain the spread of COVID-19 in long-term care facilities. So too did the adoption of hygiene practices (e.g., remote family visitation, temperature checks, face mask use, and keeping residents in their rooms), combined with population-level behavioral changes.

High risk older adults in communities

Three articles examine the implications of the COVID-19 pandemic for high risk populations, including community-based seniors with respiratory disorders, older adults with COVID-19 transferring back to the community, and older individuals residing in rural communities. Cohen & Tavares document the large number of seniors living in the community with chronic respiratory issues. This already precarious position is further exacerbated by multiple additional health and social risks, including a greater likelihood of being unmarried or living alone, being in fair or poor health or depressed, having multiple chronic conditions and LTSS needs, and living below the poverty line. The authors conclude that current approaches to protecting this population from COVID-19 are inadequate; what is needed is improved testing, better assessment, increased social supports, assurance that basic needs are being met, and protection for home care workers.

Naylor, Hirschman & McCauley draw attention to the transitional care needs of older adults discharged from the hospital to the community with COVID-19. They argue that elements of the evidence-based Transitional Care Model could be put into action now to help these individuals as specific knowledge of the needs of COVID-19 survivors develops over time. Particularly important for implementation of the model are policies targeting training and support for key workforce members (e.g., nurses, social workers, community health workers, family caregivers) and coordinated local efforts to address barriers to transitions.

Henning-Smith examines the unique risks of COVID-19 for older adults living in rural areas who tend to be older, have more underlying health conditions and fewer economic resources, and who experience more limited health care capacity and online connectivity, than their urban counterparts. The author argues that measures are needed to address the devasting economic impact of the pandemic for rural older adults and to overcome the difficulties in meeting their health, social, and emotional needs that place them at heightened risk of illness and isolation.

Families and caregivers of older adults

Four articles emphasize families and caregivers of older adults, specifically in relation to direct care staff, family caregivers, intergenerational relationships, and bereavement. Almeida, Cohen, Stone & Weller describe the economic characteristics and financial and demographic vulnerabilities of the nation's 3.5 million direct care staff who, despite substantial qualifications to perform their work in long-term care facilities and people's homes, face substantial risks during the COVID-19 pandemic. Low wages, limited benefits, and few financial resources make direct care staff especially vulnerable should they fall ill and can no longer work; most have children within the house, placing their families at risk should they contract the virus.

Hado and Feinberg point to the critical role that family members play in looking after and caring for residents of long-term care facilities, and thus to the potential adverse consequences of strict visiting restrictions adopted due to the COVID-19 pandemic on residents' health and well-being. Given this key role, the authors stress how important it is that government officials and providers strengthen communication channels, both between facility staff and families and between families and residents; continue to convene family councils; and mobilize gerontological social work students and other trainees to assist with maintaining communication and providing social support.

Stokes & Patterson highlight how families and intergenerational relationships can serve as a basis of risk for COVID-19, both as a potential source of transmission and through the cessation of key resources and supports should someone become ill. This risk, which may be heightened in multigenerational households where one or more individuals work outside the home, could be alleviated through policies that help family members to balance work and caregiving responsibilities, including paid family and sick leave, direct payments to caregivers, and broad-based income supports.

Last, Carr, Boerner & Moorman argue that in many ways COVID-19 deaths exemplify "bad deaths," distinguished by physical discomfort, difficulty breathing, psychological distress, and care discordant with patients' preferences. These attributes, in turn, exacerbate bereaved survivors' symptoms of depression, anxiety, and anger, compounded by such factors as social isolation, uncertainty, lack of routine, and loss of in-person mourning rituals. The authors conclude that enhanced advanced care planning, as well as virtual funeral services, remote counseling, telephone support groups, and other innovations, are needed to help bereaved older adults and families to adapt to loss during the pandemic.

Local and community responses

Four articles focus on local and community response to COVID-19, including in relation to Area Agencies on Aging (AAAs), municipal government, age-friendly services and supports, and digital connectivity. Wilson, Scala-Foley, Kunkel & Brewster report that AAAs instituted rapid and significant adjustments to service delivery models to meet the basic needs of local seniors during the COVID-19 pandemic. This response, according to the authors, was enabled by the infusion of federal funding and AAAs' expertise in assessing and meeting community needs and in forging partnerships with health care and social service organizations. Looking forward, the authors argue that AAAs can play a key role in ensuring continuity of care in a transformed heath care system, particularly in facilitating transitions from hospital or nursing facility to home.

Angel & Mudrazija highlight the important role that local government can play in helping vulnerable seniors remain at home during the COVID-19 crisis. Using the City of Austin, Texas as a case example, the authors demonstrate that effective local responses to supporting older adults requires coordination between local government and private and nonprofit organizations. They argue that services put into place as a result of COVID-19 should become permanent features of the local programmatic landscape because they meaningfully improve the quality of life of older adults, particularly seniors otherwise living without family and social support.

Hoffman, Webster & Bynum contend that COVID-19-related sheltering-in place risks deconditioning, reductions in formal and informal supports, and social isolation among older adults, potentially contributing to cascades of disability, injury, and psychological and cognitive decline that overwhelms the capacity of the nation's health and long-term care systems. To mitigate these risks, the authors recommend the provision of in-home acute and primary medical care, aggressive use of video telehealth and social interaction, and implementation of volunteer or paid intergenerational service. They conclude that local and national organization support for measures such as these could contribute to establishing resilient aging-friendly communities and structures and greater societal cohesion that bolster aging-in-place.

Finally, Xie and colleagues argue that community-based hybrid solutions involving both online and offline strategies that are tailored to diversity in language, literacy levels, and cultural norms are needed to deliver trustworthy information to older adults, family caregivers, and healthcare providers to enhance preparedness and prevention of COVID-19 and to manage daily lives. The authors propose that, together, high-tech and low-tech strategies help to ensure access to critical health information, as well as health care and other basic services (e.g., food, household supplies), and to promote the social interaction required to mitigate social isolation and loneliness resulting from social distancing.

Economic risks for older workers and retirees

Three articles examine economic risks for older workers and retirees, including with respect to worker protections, economic security, and pensions. Ghilarducci & Farmand point out that older workers disproportionately work in essential occupations in food distribution, trucking, janitorial, and home and personal care, and are thus particularly vulnerable to contracting COVID-19 from exposure at work due to inadequate PPE and a lack of paid sick leave. The authors argue that requiring paid sick leave, using the tax code for progressive stimulus, and providing additional health and safety protection are needed to further reduce the impact of COVID-19 on older workers in key support jobs.

Li and Mutchler report that the economic downturn resulting from the COVID-19 pandemic could have devasting consequences for older adults, given the high proportion of Americans aged 65 years or older living in counties where high infection rates co-occur with high economic insecurity risks. Policy makers need to consider that while Social Security serves as the foundation of economic security for older adults across the income continuum, it is often insufficient; a large segment of older people continue to rely on earnings well into later life, and cost of living varies greatly across geographic areas.

Tabor observes that retirees will need access to earned defined benefit pensions as a result of the COVID-19 pandemic, but many pension plan participants do not know where to go to claim their retirement benefits due to the lack of transparency associated with pension plan termination, an increasingly common occurrence. The author argues for the importance of ensuring that lost and unclaimed pension money is part of the economic recovery. This requires that the federal government mandate complete and timely disclosure of pension plan changes, create a national database for tracking the location of retirement plans, and ensure that pensioners can obtain information about their plans in the wake of regulatory changes broadening the use of e-mail in providing important disclosures.

Documenting and combating ageism

Three articles highlight the prevalence, adverse impacts, and strategies for mitigating the effects of ageism in the context of the COVID-19 pandemic. Reynolds provides a comprehensive biopsychosocial description of ageism and its effects on individuals and society. She argues that the pandemic exemplifies the extreme social consequences of ageism as illustrated by the case of the Lieutenant Governor of Texas who proposed that he and other grandparents would be willing to die to save the economy for the sake of their grandchildren. She identifies the relevance of the Elder Justice Act for addressing ageism in the wake of the pandemic, as well as various interventions to reduce ageism in society and the health and helping professions, specifically.

Previtali, Allen & Variamova also focus on the exacerbation of ageism during the pandemic, arguing that public policies meant to prevent the spread of COVID-19 purely on the basis of chronological age reinforces age stereotypes, violates older persons' rights to autonomy, treatment, work, and equality, overlooks differences within age groups, and fails to target beneficiaries on the basis of need. They urge policy makers to refrain from ageist practices and language that exacerbate society's ability to respond to COVID-19 and future emergencies while undermining intergenerational solidarity.

Ehni & Wahl observe that the correlation between age and the risk of severe and fatal COVID-19 infections have contributed to highly problematic policy suggestions exposing ageist attitudes and encouraging age discrimination based on negative stereotypes of the health and functioning of older adults. They highlight considerable heterogeneity within the older adult population and the hazards posed by mass deficit views of older age, as well as the unethical use of age limits for triage in medical care, inappropriate paternalistic treatment of older adults, and problematic assumptions that modern information and communication technologies are beyond the grasp of older individuals. It is critical, the authors conclude, that gerontology as a field inform policy guidance and understanding of the consequences of the crisis at large.

Recovery

The last article by Morrow-Howell, Galucia & Swinford looks forward to recovery from the COVID-19 pandemic. The authors identify challenges that need to be overcome, including economic setbacks (from barriers to reentering the workforce and lost retirement savings) and adverse health and well-being effects (from service disruptions, increased isolation and anxiety, and COVID-19 infection), exacerbated by the negative effects of persistent ageism, sexism, and racism on older adults. At the same time, the authors identify opportunities created in the midst of the crisis, including increased connectivity through technology and on-line platforms, stronger family and intergenerational connections, and increased quality life through greater recognition of the importance of self-care, time management, reduced isolation, and advanced directives and other legal documents. The authors also point to the opportunity to expand the workforce specializing in aging, addressing heretofore insufficient capacity in this area.

Conclusion

This issue came together very quickly, despite its length and the incredible professional and personal demands placed on the contributors as a result of the COVID-19 pandemic. Most contributors to the special issue are university-based scholars who needed to learn to teach remotely on the fly and to stay connected to dissertating students and other advisees and, in some cases, to figure out how to conduct master's thesis and dissertation defenses online. Contributors faced impediments conducting their own research, as research teams could no longer meet face-to-face, and primary data collection – for example, with respect to older adults and their family caregivers – became impossible under the prevailing circumstances. Contributors were inundated by Zoom meetings as universities, colleges, departments, and programs continued to operate from a distance, conducting routine business and determining how best to navigate this new alien environment in both the near and longer-term. While timely and important, requests for proposals from funders and contributions to special issues like this one, related to the effects and ramifications of COVID-19, further added to contributors' workloads during this time.

Like everyone else, contributors made significant adjustments to their personal lives in the context of work, K-12 school and child care closures, and sheltering in place orders in the midst of the pandemic. The interruption to everyday life is without precedence in most of our lifetimes. The threat to health and resulting stress and fatigue cannot be underestimated, exacerbated by a government response (federal and, in some cases, state) only designed, seemingly, to make matters worse. Many contributors have been forced to navigate new living arrangements as they and their partners now have to work at home (if they can work remotely) and their children are no longer able to attend child care or school. Many contributors have had to figure out how to school their children at home even though their professional responsibilities have barely let up, if at all, and may have even accelerated. Further adjustments are made to avoid virus spread because some households contain one or more essential workers. Direct, in-person visits with friends and family are discouraged. This is particularly challenging for contributors who previously relied on relatives and friends for child care. It is especially distressing for those contributors who have older parents living on their own who may face challenges getting their basic needs met, let alone face the adverse consequences of long-term social isolation, a concern intensified among contributors whose parents reside in a nursing home or assisted living facility due to the potential for contagion.

Yet, numerous scholars proposed contributions and virtually everyone approached to contribute said yes, producing relevant, high quality and insightful articles that expand the knowledge base and provide much needed guidance to individuals, policy makers, and practitioners during this critical time. Contributions were submitted on deadline, usually within two to three weeks of being asked; revisions were turned around even more quickly, often within two or three days and sometimes overnight. Double-blind peer review took place. Thus, none of this could have been accomplished without the help of the scholars who graciously agreed to review prospective contributions on the expedited timeframe requested. The editorial team owes a debt of gratitude for the selfless efforts of the individuals who agreed to perform this frequently unheralded but key function without which the promulgation of peer-reviewed scholarship would be impossible. Of course, the Journal's managing editor, Elizabeth Simpson, and the staff at Taylor and Francis, Inc., Jessica Ingle, Debraj Chattaraj, and Alyse Taggart, among others, proved instrumental in producing this timely issue as well.

Key points

- Older adults have been disproportionately impacted by the COVID-19 pandemic.
- Government and community actions have been taken to mitigate the spread of the virus and its adverse health and economic effects.
- Resulting policy actions can affect older adults negatively, including increased social isolation, economic risk and ageism.
- This special issue elucidates the pandemic's effects on older adults and their families, caregivers, and communities.
- This special issue proposes policies and strategies for protecting and improving the lives of older people, both during and after the pandemic.

Disclosure statement

No potential conflict of interest was reported by the author.

References

Center for Disease Control and Prevention. (2020a, May 28). *Provisions COVID-19 death counts by sex, age, and state*. Author. https://data.cdc.gov/NCHS/Provisional-COVID-19-Death-Counts-by-Sex-Age-and-S/9bhg-hcku

Center for Disease Control and Prevention. (2020b, May 29). *Coronavirus disease 2019 (COVID-19): Cases in the U.S.* Author. https://www.cdc.gov/coronavirus/2019-ncov/cases-updates/cases-in-us.html

Comas-Herrera, A., Zalakaín, J., Litwin, C., Hsu, A. T., Lane, N., & Fernández, J.-L. (2020, May 3). *Mortality associated with COVID-19 outbreaks in care homes: Early international evidence*. London School of Economics. https://ltccovid.org/wp-content/uploads/2020/05/Mortality-associated-with-COVID-3-May-final-6.pdf

Federal Interagency Forum on Aging-Related Statistics. (2016, August). *Older Americans 2016: Key indicators of well-being. Federal interagency forum on aging-related statistics*. U.S. Government Printing Office. https://agingstats.gov/docs/LatestReport/Older-Americans-2016-Key-Indicators-of-WellBeing.pdf

Girvan, G. (2020, May 7). Nursing homes & assisted living facilities account for 42% of COVID-19 deaths. *FREOPP*. https://freopp.org/the-covid-19-nursing-home-crisis-by-the-numbers-3a47433c3f70

Johns Hopkins University School of Medicine. (2020, May 29). *COVID-19 dashboard by the Center for Systems Science and Engineering (CSSE) at Johns Hopkins University (JHU)*. Author. https://coronavirus.jhu.edu/map.html

Kaiser Family Foundation. (2020, May 27). *KFF-health tracking—May 2020*. https://www.kff.org/report-section/kff-health-tracking-poll-may-2020-health-and-economic-impacts/

Raifman, M., & Raifman, J. (2020, April 27). Disparities in the population at risk of severe illness from COVID-19 by race/ethnicity and income. *American Journal of Preventive Medicine*. [Epub Ahead of Print]. https://doi.org/10.1016/j.amepre.2020.04.003

Reiniche, C. (2020, May 28). Total US unemployment shrinks for the first time since coronovirus layoffs began in March. *Business Insider*. https://www.businessinsider.com/total-us-unemployment-fell-first-time-coronavirus-layoffs-lockdown-march-2020-5

Rothwell, J. (2020, May 27). *The effects of COVID-19 on International labor markets: An update*. The Brookings Institution. https://www.brookings.edu/research/the-effects-of-covid-19-on-international-labor-markets-an-update/

Ryan, A., & Lazard, K. (2020, May 9). A new analysis: Coronavirus death rate surged in Massachusetts locations that already faced challenges. *The Boston Globe*. https://www.bostonglobe.com/2020/05/09/nation/disparities-push-coronavirus-death-rates-higher/

U.S. Census Bureau. (2020, May 29). *U.S. and world population clock*. Author. https://www.census.gov/popclock/

Wasser, M. (2020, May 28). State releases new data about coronavirus deaths and testing at Mass. Nursing homes. *CommonHealth*. https://www.wbur.org/commonhealth/2020/05/28/data-coronavirus-deaths-testing-nursing-homes

Webb Hopper, M., Nápoles, A. M., & Pérez-Stable, E. J. (2020, May 11). COVID-19 and racial/ethnic disparities. *Journal of the American Medical Association*. [Epub Ahead of Print]. https://doi.org/10.1001/jama.2020.8598. https://jamanetwork.com/journals/jama/fullarticle/2766098

Delivering Long-Term Services and Supports in the U.S.

The Coronavirus and the Risks to the Elderly in Long-Term Care

William Gardner ⓘ, David States, and Nicholas Bagley

ABSTRACT

The elderly in long-term care (LTC) and their caregiving staff are at elevated risk from COVID-19. Outbreaks in LTC facilities can threaten the health care system. COVID-19 suppression should focus on testing and infection control at LTC facilities. Policies should also be developed to ensure that LTC facilities remain adequately staffed and that infection control protocols are closely followed. Family will not be able to visit LTC facilities, increasing isolation and vulnerability to abuse and neglect. To protect residents and staff, supervision of LTC facilities should remain a priority during the pandemic.

Key Points:

- Elderly in long-term care (LTC) and their caregiving staff are at elevated risk from COVID-19.
- Outbreaks in LTC facilities can threaten the health care system.
- COVID-19 suppression should focus on testing and infection control at LTC facilities.
- Family will not be able to visit LTC facilities, increasing isolation of residents.
- Lack of family visits also increases residents' vulnerability to abuse and neglect.

The sick and elderly in long term care facilities are particularly vulnerable to COVID-19. Although the mortality rate of the disease is still uncertain, it is clear that it is far more lethal for adults aged 65 years and older than for children or younger adults (Wu & McGoogan, 2020). Worse, many aspects of long-term care facilities make them conducive to rapid spread of infectious disease. COVID-19 is thought to spread mainly through respiratory droplets produced when an infected person coughs or sneezes. This means that transmission risk is high between people who are in close contact (Centers for Disease Control, 2020). The risk of transmission is especially high in long-term care settings where older adults are particularly vulnerable to outbreaks of respiratory illness (Louie et al., 2007). In long-term care, large groups of patients cohabit in confined settings with communal meals and many group social activities. Moreover, many residents are incapable of practicing the levels of personal hygiene required to stop transmission. This perspective examines the heightened risk of long-term care recipients for COVID-19. It makes several policy recommendations for mitigating and addressing that risk.

A high-risk population in a high-risk setting

Long-term care recipients are a substantial population at risk for COVID-19. According to the National Center for Health Statistics (NCHS), "The 15,600 nursing homes in the country provided a total of 1,660,400 certified beds … The 28,900 residential care communities in the United States provided 996,100 licensed beds" (Harris-Kojetin et al., 2019). In 2016, there were an estimated 1,347,600 persons in nursing homes (95% CI: 1,334,333 to 1,360,867) and 811,500 persons in residential care communities (95% CI: 795,148 to 827,852), for a total of 2,159,100 persons in long-term care (95% CI: 2,129,480 to 2,188,720). There were an estimated 945,750 FTE (95% CI: 937,550 to 953,850) of staff working in nursing homes and 298,800 FTE (95% CI: 937,550 to 953,850) of staff working in residential care, for an estimated total of 1,244,500 FTEs of long-term care staff (95% CI: 1,228,571 to 1,260,249). Therefore, approximately 2.16 million adults live in long-term care facilities, cared for by 1.24 million staff. The majority of these facilities are private, for-profit, and owned by chains. There are also almost 300,000 adults who participate in day services centers and would be at elevated risk of infection if their center remains open (Harris-Kojetin et al., 2019). These numbers do not include the many elderly living in unlicensed and poorly regulated facilities (Lepore et al., 2019).

Clearly, infectious disease outbreaks are a danger to adults in long-term care even in ordinary times, *but these are not ordinary times*. A COVID-19 outbreak has already occurred in a nursing home in Kirkland, Washington:

> As of March 9, a total of 129 COVID-19 cases were confirmed among facility residents (81 of approximately 130), staff members, including health care person- nel (34), and visitors (14) … Overall, 56.8% of facility residents, 35.7% of visitors, and 5.9% of staff members with COVID-19 were hospitalized. Preliminary case fatality rates among residents and visitors as of March 9 were 27.2% and 7.1%, respectively; no deaths occurred among staff members. (McMichael et al., 2020)

We will see more of these stories in the coming days. The elderly and those with compromised health are the groups at the highest risk of dying from COVID-19. Most people in long-term care meet both criteria.

Long-term care facilities and the health care system

As outbreaks proliferate in long-term facilities, the health-care system will come under serious strain. To begin with, long-term care facilities are neither designed nor equipped to treat patients with serious COVID-19. They have limited abilities to isolate patients, and they do not have ventilators. Staff are not trained to care for serious respiratory illnesses. Moreover, they do not have the personal protective equipment to protect themselves from infection and doing their jobs in protective gear would be difficult.

This is by design, not negligence. Residential facilities care for elderly patients in a setting that is less expensive than a hospital. Once you start adding acute or intensive care beds to a long-term care facility, you will have just built another hospital (and a poorly functioning one at that). Long-term care facilities are meant to work in parallel with hospitals. When residents become acutely ill, they are transferred to hospitals that can provide more intensive levels of care.

About one-third of nursing homes house 100 or more patients (Harris-Kojetin et al., 2019). If COVID-19 sweeps through a single facility, this surge in case load could overwhelm local hospital capacity; or, the local hospital may already have every bed occupied, so that no new patient can be admitted. If patients cannot be moved to a hospital they will be in peril.

Maintaining adequate staffing in long-term care facilities will also pose challenges. The 1.5 million people who work in long-term care facilities will be at high risk when their facilities have COVID-19 outbreaks. Already, scores of employees were infected at Kirkland (Baker, 2020). When staff get infected, they will be quarantined. Who will take over those shifts? Even before the pandemic, it was hard to recruit qualified long-term care workers (Kacik, 2019). Further, absenteeism will be significant. Some staff members will not come to work because they are afraid of getting sick. Others are single parents. With school closures, they may need to stay home to care for their children. Staff who remain will end up working longer shifts. Care will deteriorate as staffing levels fall, raising the risk of COVID-19 outbreaks still further.

Long-term care facilities understand the risks. In response, they have begun adopting strict access and visitation restrictions. Indeed, on March 15, CMS announced that nursing homes should not allow any visitors unless it is for "an end-of-life situation" (Herman, 2020).

Elderly residents and their families

Locking down long-term care facilities – probably for several months (Anderson et al., 2020), and perhaps longer – raises its own concerns. Many long-term care residents are elderly and socially isolated; they depend on frequent visits from family and friends to socialize with them. Without these visits, residents may feel increasingly lonely, abandoned, and despondent. That's a medical problem in its own right, leading to depression, weight loss, and disruptive behavior.

As troubling, family visits are a crucial technique for monitoring quality of care. With visits curtailed and staff absenteeism rising, the quality of care – already low in many facilities – is likely to decline further. And we will have only limited visibility into the full scope of the problem.

How to protect the elderly in long-term care

In summary, we have 2.16 million sick and elderly patients in long-term care, served by 1.24 million staff, with both groups at high risk from COVID-19. Many of these facilities will be fragile in the face of the epidemic, and they will have limited medical backup from hospitals. There is a wave of COVID-19 cases coming, putting both residents and staff at acute risk.

So, what can we do? First, political leaders need to put the looming crisis in long-term care front and center. The danger of hospitals becoming overwhelmed is increasingly widely recognized. But we have heard little or no discussion of the long-term care population by the President or his team. Long-term care residences should be priority sites for COVID-19 testing and personal protective equipment.

Second, the staff at long-term care facilities must have paid sick leave. It is a setup for disaster if employees keep working despite being ill themselves. The deal that Congress has apparently cut with the White House will help, but it's patchy (New York Times Editorial Board, 2020), exempting business with more than 500 workers – which would include most nursing home chains – and allowing firms with fewer than 50 to apply for hardship exemptions.

Third, President Trump's emergency declaration unlocks the Center for Medicare and Medicaid Services' (CMS') authority to relax enrollment barriers for Medicaid beneficiaries (Centers for Medicare and Medicaid Services, 2020). The agency should exercise that authority immediately across the country. Many of the staff at long-term facilities are not well-compensated and will qualify for Medicaid, especially if they lose wages as a result of COVID-19. Bureaucratic roadblocks should not discourage them from enrolling in Medicaid.

Fourth, state officials must redouble inspections at long-term care facilities. They need to make sure that the facilities are adequately staffed, that the residents' needs are being met, and that infection control procedures are being followed. With family visits banned, we will otherwise have no visibility *at all* into nursing homes. States have extensive licensure and inspection data on existing facilities that could be used to target institutions with a history of poor compliance (June et al., 2020). If we do not watch closely, there is an acute risk that millions of elderly people might be effectively abandoned as the outbreak intensifies.

Fifth, when staff are ill, quarantined, or absent, we need to be ready to hire and quickly train replacements. CMS should consider relaxing certification and licensure requirements for health aides and nursing assistants. State policymakers should give the green light for trainees at nursing schools to start working (Nadell Farber, 2020). Attracting replacements may require raising compensation. So be it: that's how markets work. An emergency bill to increase the amount that Medicare and Medicaid pay for long-term care could save lives.

Conclusions

Vigilance about the health of the elderly in long-term care is essential not only for their health but also to protect the health care system from being overwhelmed by severe COVID-19 cases. For now, however, the most important thing we can do is minimize the transmission of the virus through disciplined hygiene and social distancing. The fewer people who get infected in the general population, the lower the risk of infection for long-term care residents. Likewise, the fewer of us in the general population who get hospitalized, the more hospital capacity will be available for long-term residents.

Disclosure statement

No potential conflict of interest was reported by the authors.

ORCID

William Gardner ⓘ http://orcid.org/0000-0003-1918-3540

References

Anderson, R. M., Heesterbeek, H., Klinkenberg, D., & Hollingsworth, T. D. (2020). How will country-based mitigation measures influence the course of the COVID-19 epidemic? *The Lancet*, 395(10228), 931–934. https://doi.org/10.1016/S0140-6736(20)30567-5

Baker, M. (2020, March 8). Nursing home hit by Coronavirus says 70 workers are sick. *The New York Times*, p. Section A, Page 16. https://www.nytimes.com/2020/03/07/us/corona virus-nursing-home.html

Centers for Disease Control. (2020). *How COVID-19 Spreads*. Atlanta, GA: Centers for Disease Control. https://www.cdc.gov/coronavirus/2019-ncov/prepare/transmission.html

Centers for Medicare and Medicaid Services. (2020). *CMS.gov: 1135 Waivers*. Washington, DC: Department of Health and Human Services. Retrieved March 22, 2020, from https://www.cms.gov/Medicare/Provider-Enrollment-and-Certification/SurveyCertEmergPrep/1135-Waivers

Harris-Kojetin, L., Sengupta, M., Lendon, J. P., Rome, V., Valverde, R., & Caffrey, C. (2019). *Long-term care providers and services users in the United States, 2015–2016*. Vital Health Statistics

Herman, B. (2020, March 15). *Feds tell nursing homes to ban all visitors*. Axios. https://www.axios.com/nursing-homes-visitors-ban-coronavirus-adf1f996-2d06-4de9-b836-a493221ea77b.html

June, J. W., Meng, H., Dobbs, D., & Hyer, K. (2020). Using deficiency data to measure quality in assisted living communities: A Florida statewide study. *Journal of Aging & Social Policy*, *32*(2), 125–140. https://doi.org/10.1080/08959420.2018.1563471

Kacik, A. (2019). *Nursing home staffing levels often fall below CMS expectations*. Modern Healthcare. https://www.modernhealthcare.com/providers/nursing-home-staffing-levels-often-fall-below-cms-expectations

Lepore, M., Greene, A. M., Porter, K., Lux, L., Vreeland, E., & Hawes, C. (2019). Unlicensed care homes in the United States: A clandestine sector of long-term care. *Journal of Aging & Social Policy*, *31*(1), 49–65. https://doi.org/10.1080/08959420.2018.1485397

Louie, J. K., Schnurr, D. P., Pan, C.-Y., & Kiang, D., Carter, C.,Tougaw, S., … Trochet, G. (2007). A Summer outbreak of Human Metapneumovirus Infection in a Long-Term-Care Facility. *The Journal of Infectious Diseases*, *196*(5), 705–708. https://doi.org/10.1086/519846

McMichael, T., Sargis, S., Pogosjans, C., Kay, M., Lewis, M. A., & Baer, A.; Investigation, C. C.-19. (2020, March 18). *COVID-19 in a long-term care facility — King County, Washington, February 27–March 9, 2020*. MMWR Morbidity and Mortality Weekly Report. https://doi.org/org/http://dx.doi.10.15585/mmwr.mm6912e1

Nadell Farber, O. (2020, March 14). *Medical students can help combat Covid-19. Don't send them home*. STAT. https://www.statnews.com/2020/03/14/medical-students-can-help-combat-covid-19/

New York Times editorial Board. (2020, March 18). The giant hole in Pelosi's coronavirus bill. *The New York Times*, p. Section A, page 26. https://www.nytimes.com/2020/03/14/opinion/coronavirus-pelosi-sick-leave.html

Wu, Z., & McGoogan, J. M. (2020). Characteristics of and Important lessons from the Coronavirus Disease 2019 (COVID-19) Outbreak in China: Summary of a Report of 72 314 cases from the Chinese center for disease control and prevention. *JAMA*. https://doi.org/10.1001/jama.2020.2648

"We are Alone in This Battle": A Framework for a Coordinated Response to COVID-19 in Nursing Homes

Liza L. Behrens ⓘ and Mary D. Naylor ⓘ

ABSTRACT

As of May 2020, nursing home residents account for a staggering one-third of the more than 80,000 deaths due to COVID-19 in the U.S. This pandemic has resulted in unprecedented threats to achieving and sustaining care quality even in the best nursing homes, requiring active engagement of nursing home leaders in developing solutions responsive to the unprecedented threats to quality standards of care delivery during the pandemic. This perspective offers a framework, designed with the input of nursing home leaders, to facilitate internal and external decision-making and collective action to address these threats. Policy options focus on assuring a shared understanding among nursing home leaders and government agencies of changes in the operational status of nursing homes throughout the crisis, improving access to additional essential resources needed to mitigate the crisis' impact, and promoting shared accountability for consistently achieving accepted standards in core quality domains.

As of May 2020, nursing home residents account for a staggering one-third of the more than 80,000 deaths due to COVID-19 in the U.S. This pandemic has resulted in unprecedented threats to achieving and sustaining the quality of care even in the best nursing homes. Nursing homes are required to implement effective, data-driven quality assurance and performance improvement (QAPI) programs that are systematically focused on improving the care and lives of their residents (Center for Medicare and Medicaid Services [CMS], 2016a). During this crisis, QAPI requirements have been narrowed to center on two quality domains, adverse events, and infection control (Center for Medicare and Medicaid Services, 2020b). Under normal circumstances, nursing homes rely on established standards and guidelines to operationalize QAPI programs (Zale & Selvan, 2010). However, a key response to the devastating impact of COVID-19 on residents has been the massive amount of new guidance nursing homes continually receive from multiple federal, state, and local (e.g., public health department) governmental agencies related to these core domains. This top-down, poorly coordinated communication strategy is highly ineffective, often confusing, and enormously stressful to nursing home leaders who, in the best of times, have limited capacity to process and act on information from numerous sources (D'Adamo et al., 2020).

Under normal circumstances, most nursing homes are stretched to provide essential care to residents coping with complex physical, functional, and cognitive needs (White et al., 2019). This pandemic has created a crisis situation due to the challenging needs of residents with COVID-19 and the unparalleled growth in demands for quality data from multiple agencies. Even more troubling is the fact that these homes lack the essential resources required to protect their residents and staff. One nursing home leader stated, "we are alone in this battle," reflecting the sense of abandonment that is shared by many in the industry as they work tirelessly, but not collectively, to respond to unparalleled threats (J. Duffey, personal communication, April 20, 2020).

Immediate solutions are critically needed to position nursing home leaders to maximize available resources, rapidly communicate major gaps in these resources, and be assured of timely assistance from governmental agencies to prevent major interruptions in the delivery of established standards of care quality that all residents deserve. A framework, designed by the authors and critically reviewed by nursing home leaders, provides a path forward to better position nursing home leaders and their teams to achieve these goals. This perspective describes this framework and offers ideas for its use by decision-makers, both internal to nursing homes (e.g., nursing home administrators, directors of nursing), and external to nursing homes (e.g., county health departments, policymakers at all levels). It also suggests policy opportunities to advance widespread use of this roadmap to assure acceptable levels of care quality throughout and beyond COVID-19.

Framework to guide quality assurance

A framework to guide operational decision-making during this crisis, "Nursing Home Capacity to Provide Quality Care During COVID-19 Pandemic" was designed, independently reviewed by six leaders from four Philadelphia nursing homes and refined based on their input. The "Ethical Framework for Health Care Institutions Responding to Novel Coronavirus SARS-CoV-2" (Berlinger et al., 2020) was developed to assist health systems and community centers associated with hospitals to discuss, review, and update institutional policies concerning the care of patients during times of diminishing resources such as the COVID-19 pandemic. While its full adoption in these settings is unclear, health system leaders have acknowledged its utility in addressing ethical issues raised by the COVID-19 pandemic (Meagher et al., 2020). In recognition of the complexities associated with balancing person-centered care with public health demands in the nursing home settings, this source framework (Berlinger et al., 2020) was adapted to characterize four stages of operations: Standard, Contingency, Crisis, and Catastrophic. "Standard Operations" reflects a capacity to deliver care to residents that meets accepted quality standards. "Contingency Operations" represents a moderate decrease in this capacity, leading to interference with the consistent delivery of established levels of quality. "Crisis Operations" suggests a significant decline in capacity that results in substantial and ongoing interference with achieving quality standards. "Catastrophic Operations" represents a sentinel failure, where delivery of care consistent with established standards is not possible.

Consistent with federal and state guidelines, categories of resources essential to mitigate COVID-19 represented in this framework include: Testing, Personal Protective Equipment (PPE), Bed Availability, Staff, Leadership, Registered Nurse Infection Preventionist, Culture of Care, and Physical Environment (Center for Medicare and Medicaid Services, 2020b, 2020c; Commonwealth of Pennsylvania Department of Health, 2020a, 2020b; Wright, 2020). Figure 1 depicts the dynamic and interdependent relationships between these categories and stages of operations. For example, limited access to testing and PPE in one nursing home contributes to increased infections among staff which, in turn, reduces the availability of requisite staff to deliver care consistent with accepted standards. The net effect is a facility in "Crisis Operations." If reductions in staff are protracted and a high proportion of residents are subsequently diagnosed with COVID-19, the situation in this nursing home converts to "Catastrophic Operations." Alternatively, adequate access to testing and PPE enables another nursing home to maintain accepted levels of quality and, thus, this facility remains in the "Standard Operations" stage.

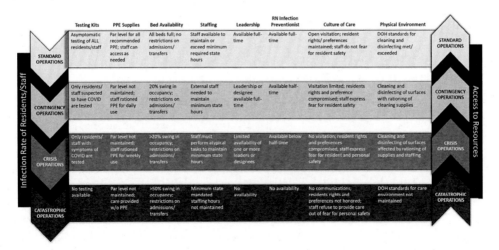

Figure 1. Operational framework to guide decision-making during the COVID-19 pandemic*. Par Level = pre-determined quantity of a resource item that a nursing home should always have, PPE = personal protective equipment, RN = registered nurse, DOH = department of health, COVID = COVID-19 or coronavirus.*Adapted from the "Ethical Framework for Health Care Institutions Responding to Novel Coronavirus SARS-CoV-2" (Berlinger et al., 2020).

Use of framework for internal decision-making

The proposed framework provides a path for nursing home leaders to anticipate and continuously monitor critical resource categories during the COVID-
19 pandemic and to use findings to both plan for operational changes or
initiate interventions in response to new operational threats. Using data on
variables identified under each resource category (see Figure 1), QAPI team
members could develop plans responsive to threats likely to contribute to
adverse events and infection control. For example, in a preparedness exercise
a nursing home might assume that 50% of residents and staff are infected and
PPE is in short supply. With these data, they would then conclude that they are
in "Crisis Operations." Their goal, in turn, would be to improve operations to
the "Contingency" level. Guided by the resource categories defined in the
framework, they might decide to halt all new admissions (Bed Availability)
until all residents and staff suspected to have COVID-19 are tested (Testing
Kits), resources are secured for all staff to receive a ration of PPE for daily use
(PPE), external staff support is enlisted from external agencies or pools to meet
minimum state hours (Staffing), and leadership reaches out to external experts
for leadership support (Leadership). A communication strategy could be
designed to continually update family members and staff on progress in
mitigating risks (Culture of Care). Additionally, the plan might include offering staff assigned to COVID-19 residents alternative housing, emotional support, and additional remuneration (Culture of Care). Finally, the plan might
include cleaning and disinfecting all surfaces prior to clustering infected
residents in one area (Physical Environment). Any set of circumstances that
moves a nursing home from "Standard Operations" to another level should
trigger the implementation of plans to return to a higher level of operations.

Use of framework for external support

While leaders may be able to implement some dimensions of proposed contingency plans, most will not be able to do so without external support. Support
from county, state, and federal leaders is critical to enable nursing homes to
acquire and maintain the additional resources needed to mitigate COVID-19
risks (D'Adamo, Yoshikawa, Ouslander, 2020). The proposed framework can be
used to facilitate effective collaboration and coordination among nursing home
leaders, governmental agencies and other key stakeholders, with attention to the
communication of timely and accurate data (McClelland et al., 2017). Nursing
home leaders who provided input in the design of this framework (Figure 1)
suggested that a streamlined set of core data relevant to each of the resource
categories be reported daily to local, state and federal agencies. The use of
a standardized format is essential to assure that consistent and reliable information is shared with these agencies and burden on an overwhelmed nursing home

staff is minimized. In turn, this data could trigger targeted and more immediate responses. For example, if one or more nursing homes in a community are determined to be in "Crisis Operations," an external team of quality experts might be enlisted to focus on the needs of specific facilities. Through collaborations with local academia and state government, Missouri has implemented such a state-wide program to support local QAPI teams (Rantz et al., 2009). Nursing homes that have successfully mitigated the impact of COVID-19 can be identified from these data; then, strategies employed by them to maintain or return to "Standard Operations" can be shared with others. Overall, the operations' trajectories and lessons learned can inform the development of policies that will better position nursing homes for future crises.

To assure nursing homes are positioned to deliver accepted standards of care quality to residents in the core quality domains of adverse events and infection control, immediate action on the following federal and state policies is needed:

- Implement a single, standardized mechanism for routine communication by nursing homes of changes in operational status during COVID-19 to local, state, and federal agencies;
- Fill immediate gaps in essential resources (e.g., testing, PPE, additional staffing, RN infection control nurse) to nursing homes in "Contingency" or "Crisis" stages of operations;
- Provide emergency support (e.g., interim management team, staff from local staffing core or national guard) to nursing homes in "Catastrophic" stage of operation;
- Enact legislation modeled on the state of Missouri to provide external support to nursing homes in "Contingency" or "Crisis" stages of operations; and
- Assure public reporting of responses by local, state, and federal agencies to nursing homes in "Crisis" or "Catastrophic" stages of operations.

Conclusion

Active engagement of nursing home leaders in developing solutions responsive to the unprecedented threats to care quality posed by COVID-19 is imperative. This perspective offers a framework designed with the input of nursing home leaders to facilitate internal and external decision-making and collective action to address these threats. Policy options focused on assuring a shared understanding of changes in the operational status of nursing homes throughout this crisis, improving access to additional essential resources needed to mitigate the impact of this crisis, and promoting shared accountability for consistently achieving accepted standards in core quality domains are identified. Nursing home residents are arguably the most vulnerable population to the human devastation wrought by this pandemic. Nursing home leaders cannot be left " … alone in this battle" in providing residents with the quality of care they need and deserve.

Key points

- The needs of nursing home residents during the COVID-19 pandemic demand a coordinated response among nursing home leaders and government agencies.
- Consistent use of an operational framework during a coordinated response can inform decisions related to quality.
- A standardized strategy to communicate resource needs to governmental agencies is essential.
- Accountability for care quality needs to be shared among internal and external nursing home stakeholders.

Disclosure statement

No potential conflict of interest was reported by the authors.

Funding

This work was supported by the National Institute of Nursing Research, Ruth L. Kirschstein National Research Service Award [T32NR009356].

ORCID

Liza L. Behrens PhD, RN ⓘ http://orcid.org/0000-0002-6143-2654
Mary D. Naylor PhD, RN, FAAN ⓘ http://orcid.org/0000-0001-9287-153X

References

Berlinger, N., Wynia, M., Powell, T., Hester, D. M., Milliken, A., Fabi, R., … Jenks, N. P. (2020). *Ethical framework for health care institutions responding to Novel Coronavirus SARS-CoV-2 (COVID-19): Guidelines for institutional ethics services responding to COVID-19.* The Hastings Center. https://www.thehastingscenter.org/ethicalframeworkcovid19/

Center for Medicare and Medicaid Services. (2020b, May 11). *COVID-19 emergency declaration blanket waivers for health care providers.* Centers for Medicare and Medicaid Services. https://www.cms.gov/files/document/summary-covid-19-emergency-declaration-waivers.pdf

Center for Medicare and Medicaid Services. (2020c, April 30). *Coronavirus commission for safety and quality in nursing homes.* Author. https://www.cms.gov/files/document/coronavirus-commission-safety-and-quality-nursing-homes.pdf

Center for Medicare and Medicaid Services (CMS). (2016a). Medicare and Medicaid programs; Reform of requirements for long-term care facilities. https://www.federalregister.gov/documents/2016/10/04/2016-23503/medicare-and-medicaidprograms-reform-of-requirements-for-long-term-care-facilities

Commonwealth of Pennsylvania Department of Health. (2020a, April 19). *Staffing resources for nursing care facilities during COVID-19 pandemic: Frequently asked questions.* Pennsylvania

Department of Health. https://www.health.pa.gov/topics/Documents/Diseases%20and%20Conditions/COVID-19%20LTC%20Staffing%20Resources.pdf

Commonwealth of Pennsylvania Department of Health. (2020b, May 5). *Health.pa.gov; COVID-19 information for nursing homes*. Pennsylvania Department of Health. Retrieved May 14, 2020, from https://www.health.pa.gov/topics/disease/coronavirus/Pages/Nursing-Homes.aspx

D'Adamo, H., Yoshikawa, T., & Ouslander, J. G. (2020). Coronavirus disease 2019 in geriatrics and long-term care: The ABCDs of COVID-19. *The Journal of the American Geriatrics Society, 68*(5), 912–917. Advanced online publication. https://doi.org/10.1111/jgs.16445

McClelland, E., Amlot, R., Rogers, M. B., Rubin, J., Tesh, J., & Pearce, J. M. (2017). Psychological and physical impacts of extreme adverse events on older adults: Implications for communications. *Disaster Medicine and Public Health Preparedness, 11* (1), 127–134. https://doi.org/10.1017/dmp.2016.118

Meagher, K. M., Cummins, N. W., Bharucha, A. E., Badley, A. D., Chlan, L. L., & Wright, R. S. (2020). COVID-19 ethics and research. *Mayo Clinic Proceedings, 95*(6), 1119–1123. https://doi.org/10.1016/j.mayocp.2020.01.019

Ouslander, J. G. (2020). Coronavirus disease19 in geriatrics and long-term care: An update. *The Journal of the American Geriatrics Society, 68*(5), 918–921. Advanced online publication. https://doi.org/10.111/jgs.16464

Rantz, M. J., Cheshire, D., Flesner, M., Petroski, G. F., Hicks, L., Alexander, G., Aud, M. A., Siem, C., Nguyen, K., Boland, C., & Thomas, S. (2009). Helping nursing homes "at risk" for quality problems: A statewide evaluation. *Geriatric Nursing, 30*(4), 238–249. https://doi.org/10.1016/j.gerinurse.2008.09.003

White, E. M., Aiken, L. H., & McHugh, M. D. (2019). Registered nurse burnout, job dissatisfaction, and missed care in nursing homes. *Journal of the American Geriatrics Society, 67*(10), 2065–2071. https://doi.org/10.1111/jgs.16051

Wright, D. R. (2020, March 13). *Guidance for infection control and prevention of Coronavirus disease 2019 (COVID-19) in nursing homes (REVISED)* (Ref: QSO-20-14-NH). Centers for Medicare and Medicaid Services. https://www.cms.gov/files/document/qso-20-14-nh-revised.pdf

Zale, J. M., & Selvan, M. S. (2010). Interfaces between quality improvement, law, and medical ethics. In P. Varkey (Ed.), *Medical quality management* (pp. 197–222). Jones and Bartlett Publishers.

COVID-19 Pandemic: Exacerbating Racial/Ethnic Disparities in Long-Term Services and Supports

Tetyana P. Shippee ⓘ, Odichinma Akosionu, Weiwen Ng, Mark Woodhouse, Yinfei Duan, Mai See Thao, and John R. Bowblis

ABSTRACT

What services are available and where racial and ethnic minorities receive long-term services and supports (LTSS) have resulted in a lower quality of care and life for racial/ethnic minority users. These disparities are only likely to worsen during the COVID-19 pandemic, as the pandemic has disproportionately affected racial and ethnic minority communities both in the rate of infection and virus-related mortality. By examining these disparities in the context of the pandemic, we bring to light the challenges and issues faced in LTSS by minority communities with regard to this virus as well as the disparities in LTSS that have always existed.

Introduction

Many older adults in the United States are in need of long-term services and supports (LTSS) provided in nursing homes, assisted living, at home, and other settings. Traditionally, LTSS focused on institutional care in the nursing home, but the last two decades saw an expansion of the use of home and community-based services. These home and community-based services include visits by a nurse or nurse aide, transportation, meal delivery, in-home therapy, and homemaker services provided at an older adult's home or delivered in other residential care settings such as an assisted living (Centers for Medicare and Medicaid Services, 2019). While individuals utilizing LTSS have always been considered a vulnerable population, the COVID-19 pandemic has brought unique challenges to this population, as these older LTSS utilizers are at a high risk of COVID-19 infection and premature mortality.

LTSS utilizers are reliant on caregivers, increasing their exposure to COVID-19 due to their inability to socially distance. Moreover, their age and high prevalence of chronic health conditions, including heart disease, diabetes, dementia, and respiratory illnesses, increase mortality risks once exposed to virus.

In this perspective, we focus on the role of racial and ethnic disparities in LTSS in the United States in the context of the COVID-19 pandemic. The LTSS setting is characterized by racial and ethnic disparities in financing, access, quality, and service delivery (Gorges et al., 2019; Rivera-Hernandez et al., 2019). These disparities are likely to increase during the COVID-19 pandemic, with emerging data that show people of color and indigenous people have a higher burden of illness and death from COVID-19 than their white peers (Hedgpeth et al., 2020; Scott, 2020). Furthermore, the pandemic is bringing to light the gaps in care due to already existing racial and ethnic disparities in LTSS and provides an opportunity to advance equity in LTSS during the pandemic and beyond.

Existing barriers that lead to racial/ethnic disparities in the context of COVID-19

There are many existing barriers to the provision of quality LTSS for users from minority racial and ethnic groups that are likely exacerbated during the COVID-19 pandemic. In this section, we describe these barriers, their resulting effects on racial and ethnic disparities, as well as how responses to COVID-19 need to address these barriers. We highlight (1) cumulative health disparities for minority populations over the life course, (2) unequal clinical care and quality of life for nursing home users from communities of color, (3) impediments to quality experienced by low-English proficiency nursing home users, (4) inordinate impact on care quality due to challenges faced by an LTSS workforce that is disproportionately composed of immigrants and racial/ethnic minorities, and (5) disparities in home and community-based services.

Cumulative health disparities put minority populations at greater risk

Cumulative health disparities for older adults from racial/ethnic minority groups place them at a higher risk during COVID-19. Older adults from communities of color and indigenous people are more likely to experience cumulative adversity in their lifetime, the outcomes of which are magnified by the lack of health insurance and adequate access to health care over the life course. (Buchmueller et al., 2016; Chen et al., 2016). These barriers lead to undiagnosed medical issues and worse health outcomes when health conditions are identified and treated. Hence, these already existing disparities are likely to disproportionately affect older adults from racial/ethnic minority communities who thus become sicker and more likely to die from virus-related complications. This disproportionate risk for adverse outcomes should make testing and adequate access to hospital care a priority in minority communities.

Disparities in the quality of nursing home services are a barrier to pandemic response

Even before the pandemic, segregation in the provision of institutional LTSS resulted in worse outcomes for older adults from communities of color and indigenous people (Mack et al., 2020; Smith et al., 2008). Racial and ethnic disparities in the community are amplified in the LTSS setting, as minorities that use LTSS are often younger, have greater physical impairments, and more likely to use nursing homes (Fabius et al., 2018; Rahman & Foster, 2015). Moreover, long-term care has been identified as one of the most racially segregated sectors of health care (Rahman & Foster, 2015). System-level disparities that affect what services are available and where minorities receive LTSS manifest themselves in both institutional and community-based LTSS options that result in segregation and lower quality of services for minority users (Buchmueller et al., 2016; Mack et al., 2020; Rahman & Foster, 2015).

A wealth of data shows that racial/ethnic minorities receive care in lower performing nursing homes than their white peers (Konetzka & Werner, 2009). Black nursing home residents receive a lower clinical quality of care than their white peers, with outcomes including a higher risk of physical restraints, in-dwelling catheters, feeding tubes, and antipsychotic medication than their white peers (Grabowski & McGuire, 2009). Black residents are also less likely to receive the flu or other vaccines (Cai et al., 2011; Luo et al., 2014), and more likely to have un- or under-treated pain (Hunnicutt et al., 2017). Evidence suggests that Hispanic residents receive a lower quality of care and are less likely to recover from incontinence than white residents (Bliss et al., 2014). The concentration of residents of color within lower quality nursing homes suggests that they may be at a higher risk of COVID-19 infection and mortality.

Minority racial/ethnic groups are also likely to report lower quality of life. Quality of life measures non-clinical aspects of resident's lives in nursing homes and includes satisfaction with activities offered, meals, and relation-ships with staff and other residents. Significant disparities exist across most domains of quality of life, and these differences remained after controlling for health status and facility characteristics (Shippee et al., in press). In addition, facilities with high proportions of racial/ethnic minority residents report lower average quality of life than facilities that provide care to mainly white residents. Consistently, activities and social work staffing are asso-ciated with a better quality of life (Shippee et al., 2015, 2016, in press), yet many of these have been furloughed during the COVID-19 pandemic. Their work is essential for maintaining the resident quality of life and facilities need to identify creative strategies in how residents can continue to engage with activity staff.

The systemic disparities in quality of care and life in nursing homes for racial/ethnic minority groups need immediate attention during the COVID-19 pandemic. Furthermore, nursing homes with a high proportion of residents of color and indigenous residents are more likely to be in urban settings and are more reliant on Medicaid (Shippee et al., in press). Urban settings currently have a greater number of cases of COVID-19 and spreading the virus is more likely. Medicaid, because of its historically low reimbursement, causes additional challenges as high-Medicaid facilities may have fewer financial resources to hire staff when existing staff get sick. Additionally, in the early stages of the pandemic and even today, states prioritized COVID-19 testing to first responders and health-care workers in hospitals, leaving nursing homes to find private laboratories to conduct COVID-19 testing. As a result, nursing homes that service a disproportionate share of minority residents are likely to be at greater risk of infection and more likely to have fewer financial resources to test for and combat the virus if it becomes present in the facility.

Challenges faced by low English proficiency nursing home residents

Language barriers impact health-care access and quality of care (Eichler et al., 2009). Those with limited English proficiency report worse quality of care compared to racial and ethnic minorities (Yeo, 2004), lower access to qualified medical interpreters (Flores, 2005), and lower odds of receiving consultation with a health-care provider and getting a flu shot compared to English-speaking patients (Lebrun, 2012). Language barriers are a pressing issue that needs to be addressed, as supported by our case-study with Hmong nursing home residents (Thao et al., 2019). We found those who did not speak English relied on English-speaking Hmong residents and their family members to communicate their needs. These residents often received their care last because of the lack of interpreters and self-reported worse quality of care compared to non-Hmong residents. Hmong residents with limited English proficiency also reported more experiences of social isolation in nursing homes.

Compared to native English speakers, residents with limited English proficiency may face substantial barriers during the pandemic. Such challenges can be the lack of access to readily translated information resulting in misinformation, possibility of lower virus testing, and exacerbated mental health issues stemming from social isolation. At a time where social distancing is encouraged, social distancing for already linguistically isolated older adults in nursing homes can be more threatening. Hence, more attention is needed to communicate strategies and responses to users of LTSS with limited English proficiency.

Protecting LTSS users starts with protecting the LTSS workforce

LTSS in all settings requires direct care workers to deliver services – such as bathing, grooming, feeding, and transferring – which involves physical contact between individuals and workers (Harris-Kojetin et al., 2013; Walton & Rogers, 2017). This implies that workers and those receiving care have an increased chance of virus transmission. Yet, direct care is often considered low-skilled work and is associated with low compensation. Typical salaries for these workers were under 30,000 USD per year in 2018, and immigrants and racial/ethnic minorities disproportionally fill these positions (Hurtado et al., 2012; Travers et al., 2020; True et al., 2020). Studies show that black direct care staff are more likely to report work-related strain and burnout compared to their white counterparts (Hurtado et al., 2012; Travers et al., 2020). This is compounded by the fact that nursing home staff from communities of color are more likely to work in under-resourced, for-profit nursing homes, with a high proportion of residents funded through Medicaid prior to the pandemic (Hurtado et al., 2012). While all LTSS workers face risks, preexisting disparities for workers of color and immigrant LTSS direct care workers place them at even higher risk associated with COVID-19 (Bates et al., 2018; True et al., 2020).

Another challenge for the LTSS workforce is that nursing homes located in communities with a higher prevalence of COVID-19 infections are more likely to have a higher number of resident COVID-19 cases (Choi et al., 2020; Rahman & Foster, 2015; True et al., 2020). Staff that work in these facilities, especially staff of color, are more likely to rely on public transportation to get to work, placing them and the residents at a higher risk of COVID-19 infection and mortality. They are also more likely to live in underserved neighborhoods that are disproportionately affected by the virus. All these existing barriers increase the risk of these staff inadvertently infecting residents in the facilities in which they work (Choi et al., 2020; True et al., 2020). In the current pandemic, increased exposure to these stressful events may increase the negative impact on staff members' mental and physical health, and in turn have consequences for resident care quality and health. It is likely that with COVID-19, direct care workers will be asked to do more work and provide even more care than before. With restrictions on who can visit facilities, direct care workers may not be getting extra assistance from volunteers and family members who would have visited. Potential workforce shortages, the extra strain from increased duties, and potentially higher exposure to COVID-19 will disproportionately affect staff and the quality of care they provide.

Disparities in home and community-based LTSS

Disparities among users of home and community-based LTSS can create a greater need in minority communities during the pandemic. Among those who utilize home and community-based services, the quality of care for racial/ethnic minority users has been lower than for white users. For example, home health-care providers who serve a higher proportion of indigenous persons had lower quality scores than providers who serve a lower proportion of indigenous persons (Towne et al., 2015). Another study found that black home and community-based service recipients had higher rates of avoidable hospitalizations than white recipients while receiving those services (Gorges et al., 2019). Overall, some studies suggest that even if disparities in access to home and community-based care are removed, the quality of the care received by racial/ethnic minority users may still be of lower quality than that received by their white peers.

While the quality of home and community-based services may be lower in minority communities, they still provide a valuable resource for those who have access to these services. COVID-19 has closed many community-based providers. Without access to these services, the needs of those from minority communities who may have preexisting physical, emotional, and social needs, and the ability to have those needs met through aging network services and the health-care system, are only likely to be amplified. For example, adult day centers in most states have closed for the duration of stay home orders (WCCO, 2020) and they are increasingly used by people of color (Centers for Disease Control and Prevention [CDC], 2020), hence creating an unmet need for an already vulnerable population. Also, home care agencies are struggling to retain clients and staff because of fears by both groups of contracting the virus (Morrow-Howell et al., 2020). While COVID-19 affects all groups, those from communities of color and indigenous groups that may be more heavily reliant on home and community-based services for food, transportation, and medical assistance (in part due to systemic disparities over the life course) may be made more vulnerable to having unmet needs, placing them at greater risk of adverse health outcomes unrelated to COVID-19.

Recommendations for today and into the future

Report COVID data in LTSS by race/ethnicity

Actions taken today to identify and remediate issues caused by the pandemic require good underlying data. Solid information regarding how COVID-19 is affecting the LTSS population, and racial/ethnic minority users, in particular, is unknown. Individual states vary in reporting of virus cases, and most do not break down the data by race/ethnicity or by use of LTSS. Among the few that do release more demographic data that information is incomplete (e.g.,

Virginia was missing race/ethnicity for two-thirds of confirmed cases at the time of this brief) (Farmer, 2020). This lack of information is a barrier that needs to be immediately addressed; without understanding the scope of the pandemic's impact on racial/ethnic minority communities, it is not possible to develop adequate strategies to address it.

Establish priority testing, personal protective equipment, and other supports for high-proportion minority facilities

With the stress that the pandemic is placing on all frontline workers, particularly in nursing homes and assisted living facilities, immediate attention is needed to ensure that these institutions have adequate resources to stop the virus from gaining a foothold and spreading within these facilities. While all facilities need help, the documented systemic disparities in quality for racial/ethnic minority groups indicate a need to focus on providing resources (e.g., relief staff, virus testing) to facilities with a high proportion of minority residents. These facilities are often in urban areas and have a payer-mix of residents that provide them with fewer financial resources to combat the COVID-19 pandemic. Yet, government assistance and priority testing for these groups are not happening (Farmer, 2020).

Take action to address existing racial/ethnic disparities

Once the pandemic has passed, these underlying disparities for racial and ethnic minorities, both in access and quality of LTSS services, will not improve without additional action. For example, future efforts need to address persistent racial/ethnic segregation of LTSS and that residents of color and indigenous residents disproportionally receive lower quality services. While the Centers for Medicare and Medicaid Services (CMS) has made attempts to improve overall nursing home quality via public reporting of quality measures and made improvements and adjustments to survey and certification process of LTSS providers, most of these changes have benefited higher performing facilities that primarily serve white residents and racial/ethnic disparities continue to exist (Konetzka et al., 2015). We need to examine how existing policies may be perpetuating or increasing the disparities and take action to address them.

Include quality of life as a key metric of LTSS quality

Furthermore, CMS has focused on reporting clinical measures of quality rather than the quality of life. The pandemic has increased attention to the importance of social engagement and the risks of social isolation. Numerous news and resource sites focus on the risks and consequences of social disconnection and present strategies for combatting isolation. The corona-virus has shown why the quality of LTSS should not only be measured by clinical measures but needs to include comprehensive measures of well-being such as quality of life. The inclusion of quality of life is particularly salient for LTSS racial/ethnic minority users who already reported lower quality of life (Shippee et al., in press) and higher risk for isolation in LTSS prior to the pandemic (Li & Cai, 2014).

Improve pay and work conditions for LTSS direct care staff

Another area that the pandemic has highlighted is the role of frontline workers. Because the services provided as part of LTSS require human interaction, staff play a vital role in the quality of the services. Many of the disparities in LTSS are likely sensitive to staffing quality. Yet, LTSS staff make low wages and there is a long-standing problem of recruiting and retaining direct care staff (True et al., 2020). This crisis is an opportunity for policy solutions that focus on better pay and better conditions for LTSS direct care workers, many of whom are immigrants and come from com-munities of color. Indeed, some nursing homes have temporarily increased wages and provided other incentives to staff during the pandemic. LTSS providers may find that increasing pay results in more efficient and produc-tive workers.

Conclusion

The COVID-19 pandemic has exacerbated prevailing racial/ethnic dispari-ties. It is important to communicate the evidence regarding disparities as policymakers and popular media grapple with racial/ethnic disparities in COVID-19 deaths, often neglecting to put it in context of existing system-level disparities that have led to these outcomes. The racial/ethnic disparities across LTSS are not due to race, but inherent inequalities built into the health-care sector and other areas that lead to minority communities having worse health outcomes. The current pandemic has highlighted an ongoing, often hidden problem that without improved policies and actions today will continue into the future. Given the spotlight that the pandemic has placed on inequality in the long-term care system, now is the time for policymakers to share data and to learn about the sources of system-level issues that drive racial/ethnic segregation in LTSS and gaps in quality for racial/ethnic min-ority LTSS users. The hope is that the attention given to these disparities now is not short-lived and can help illuminate inequalities experienced by racial/ethnic minority groups to build momentum toward health equity in LTSS.

Key points

- Racial/ethnic minority users of LTSS have increased risk during the COVID-19 pandemic due to individual and system-level factors.
- The barriers that increase risk will remain after the pandemic passes without improved policies today.
- The pandemic highlights the role of social support and isolation, important factors in racial and ethnic disparity in quality of life.
- This crisis spotlights challenges faced by LTSS staff, particularly those who are immigrants and from communities of color.

Disclosure statement

John R. Bowblis provides consulting services to the health-care industry, which sometimes include long-term care providers. All other authors report no known conflicts of interest.

Funding

This project was funded by the National Institute on Minority Health and Health Disparities (R01-MD010729, PI: Shippee). Tetyana Shippee also acknowledges funding from the MN Department of Human Services.

ORCID

Tetyana P. Shippee PhD   (iD)   http://orcid.org/0000-0003-1804-2527

References

Bates, T., Amah, G., & Coffman, J. (2018). *Racial/ethnic diversity in the long-term care workforce.* UCSF Health Workforce Research Center on Long-Term Care UCSF Health Workforce Research Center on Long-Term Care. https://healthworkforce.ucsf.edu/sites/healthworkforce.ucsf.edu/files/REPORT-2018.HWRC_diversity_.4-18.pdf

Bliss, D. Z., Gurvich, O., Savik, K., Eberly, L. E., Harms, S., & Wyman, J. F. (2014). Racial and ethnic disparities in time to cure of incontinence present at nursing home admission. *Journal of Health Disparities Research and Practice, 7*(3), 96–113. https://www.ncbi.nlm.nih.gov/pmc/articles/PMC4540235/

Buchmueller, T. C., Levinson, Z. M., Levy, H. G., & Wolfe, B. L. (2016). Effect of the affordable care act on racial and ethnic disparities in health insurance coverage. *American Journal of Public Health, 106*(8), 1416–1421. https://doi.org/10.2105/AJPH.2016.303155

Cai, S., Feng, Z., Fennell, M. L., & Mor, V. (2011). Despite small improvement, black nursing home residents remain less likely than whites to receive flu vaccine. *Health Affairs, 30*(10), 1939–1946. https://doi.org/10.1377/hlthaff.2011.0029

Centers for Disease Control and Prevention [CDC]. (2020). *Adult day services centers.* https://www.cdc.gov/nchs/fastats/adsc.htm

Centers for Medicare and Medicaid Services. (2019). *Home- and community-based services.* https://www.cms.gov/Outreach-and-Education/American-Indian-Alaska-Native/AIAN/LTSS-TA-Center/info/hcbs

Chen, J., Vargas-Bustamante, A., Mortensen, K., & Ortega, A. N. (2016). Racial and Ethnic Disparities in Health Care Access and Utilization Under the Affordable Care Act. *Medical Care, 54*(2), 140–146. https://doi.org/10.1097/MLR.0000000000000467

Choi, K. H., Denice, P., Haan, M., & Zajacova, A. (2020, May 13). Studying the social determinants of COVID-19 in a data vacuum. *SocArXiv.* https://doi.org/10.31235/osf.io/yq8vu

Eichler, K., Wieser, S., & Brügger, U. (2009). The costs of limited health literacy: A systematic review. *International Journal of Public Health, 54*(5), 313–324. https://doi.org/10.1007/s00038-009-0058-2

Fabius, C. D., Thomas, K. S., Zhang, T., Ogarek, J., & Shireman, T. I. (2018). Racial disparities in Medicaid home and community-based service utilization and expenditures among persons with multiple sclerosis. *BMC Health Services Research, 18*(1), 773. https://doi.org/10.1186/s12913-018-3584-x

Farmer, B. (2020). Long-standing racial and income disparities seen creeping into COVID-19 care. *Kaiser Health News.* https://khn.org/news/covid-19-treatment-racial-income-health-disparities/

Flores, G. (2005). The impact of medical interpreter services on the quality of health care: A systematic review. *Medical Care Research and Review, 62*(3), 255–299. https://doi.org/10.1177/1077558705275416

Gorges, R. J., Sanghavi, P., & Konetzka, R. T. (2019). A national examination of long-term care setting, outcomes, and disparities among elderly dual eligibles. *Health Affairs, 38*(7), 1110–1118. https://doi.org/10.1377/hlthaff.2018.05409

Grabowski, D. C., & McGuire, T. G. (2009). Black-White disparities in care in nursing homes. *Atlantic Economic Journal: AEJ, 37*(3), 299–314. https://doi.org/10.1007/s11293-009-9185-7

Harris-Kojetin, L., Sengupta, M., Park-Lee, E., & Valverde, R. H. (2013). *Long-term care services in the United States: 2013 overview.* Hyattsville, MD: National Center for Health Statistics. https://stacks.cdc.gov/view/cdc/22285

Hedgpeth, D., Fears, D., & Scruggs, G. (2020, April 4). Indian Country, where residents suffer disproportionately from disease, is bracing for coronavirus. *Washington Post.* https://www.washingtonpost.com/climate-environment/2020/04/04/native-american-coronavirus/

Hunnicutt, J. N., Ulbricht, C. M., Tjia, J., & Lapane, K. L. (2017). Pain and pharmacologic pain management in long-stay nursing home residents. *Pain, 158*(6), 1091–1099. https://doi.org/10.1097/j.pain.0000000000000887

Hurtado, D. A., Sabbath, E. L., Ertel, K. A., Buxton, O. M., & Berkman, L. F. (2012). Racial disparities in job strain among American and immigrant long-term care workers. *International Nursing Review, 59*(2), 237–244. https://doi.org/10.1111/j.1466-7657.2011.00948.x

Konetzka, R. T., Grabowski, D. C., Perraillon, M. C., & Werner, R. M. (2015). Nursing home 5-star rating system exacerbates disparities in quality, by payer source. *Health Affairs, 34*(5), 819–827. https://doi.org/10.1377/hlthaff.2014.1084

Konetzka, R. T., & Werner, R. M. (2009). Review: Disparities in long-term care building equity into market-based reforms. *Medical Care Research and Review, 66*(5), 491–521. https://doi.org/10.1177/1077558709331813

Lebrun, L. A. (2012). Effects of length of stay and language proficiency on health care experiences among Immigrants in Canada and the United States. *Social Science & Medicine, 74*(7), 1062–1072. https://doi.org/10.1016/j.socscimed.2011.11.031

Li, Y., & Cai, X. (2014). Racial and ethnic disparities in social engagement among US nursing home residents. *Medical Care, 52*(4), 314–321. https://doi.org/10.1097/MLR.0000000000000088

Luo, H., Zhang, X., Cook, B., Wu, B., & Wilson, M. R. (2014). Racial/ethnic disparities in preventive care practice among U.S. nursing home residents. *Journal of Aging and Health, 26*(4), 519–539. https://doi.org/10.1177/0898264314524436

Mack, R. S., Jesdale, B. M., Ulbricht, C. M., Forrester, S. N., Michener, P. S., & Lapane, K. L. (2020). Racial segregation across U.S. nursing homes: A systematic review of measures and outcomes. *The Gerontologist, 60*(3), e218–e231. https://doi.org/10.1093/geront/gnz056

Morrow-Howell, N., Galucia, N., & Swinford, E. (2020). Recovering from the COVID-19 pandemic: A focus on older adults. *Journal of Aging & Social Policy*, 1–9. https://doi.org/10.1080/08959420.2020.1759758

Rahman, M., & Foster, A. D. (2015). Racial segregation and quality of care disparity in US. *Journal of Health Economics, 39*, 1–16. https://doi.org/10.1016/j.jhealeco.2014.09.003

Rivera-Hernandez, M., Kumar, A., Epstein-Lubow, G., & Thomas, K. S. (2019). Disparities in nursing home use and quality among African American, Hispanic, and White medicare residents with Alzheimer's disease and related dementias. *Journal of Aging and Health, 31*(7), 1259–1277. https://doi.org/10.1177/0898264318767778

Scott, D. (2020). *Covid-19's devastating toll on black and Latino Americans, in one chart.* https://www.vox.com/2020/4/17/21225610/us-coronavirus-death-rates-blacks-latinos-whites

Shippee, T. P., Henning-Smith, C., Rhee, G., Held, R., & Kane, R. A. (2016). Racial differences in minnesota nursing home residents' quality of life: The importance of looking beyond individual predictors. *Journal of Aging and Health, 28*(2), 199–224. https://doi.org/10.1177/0898264315589576

Shippee, T. P., Henning-Smith, C. L., Kane, R., & Lewis, T. (2015). Resident- and facility-level predictors of quality of life in long-term care. *The Gerontologist, 55*(4), 643–655. https://doi.org/10.1093/geront/gnt148

Shippee, T. P., Ng, W., & Bowblis, J. R. (in press). Does living in a higher proportion minority facility improve quality of life for racial/ethnic minority residents in nursing homes? *Innovation in Aging.*

Smith, D. B., Feng, Z., Fennell, M. L., Zinn, J., & Mor, V. (2008). Racial disparities in access to long-term care: The illusive pursuit of equity. *Journal of Health Politics, Policy and Law, 33* (5), 861–881. https://doi.org/10.1215/03616878-2008-022

Thao, M.-S., Akosionu, O., Davila, H., & Shippee, T. P. (2019). *The invisible labor of Culturally Sensitive Care (CSC): A hmong nursing home case study* [Paper presentation]. Gerontological Society of America Annual Scientific Meeting, Austin, TX.

Towne, S. D., Probst, J. C., Mitchell, J., & Chen, Z. (2015). Poorer quality outcomes of medicare-certified home health care in areas with high levels of native American/Alaska native residents. *Journal of Aging and Health, 27*(8), 1339–1357. https://doi.org/10.1177/0898264315583051

Travers, J. L., Teitelman, A. M., Jenkins, K. A., & Castle, N. G. (2020). Exploring social-based discrimination among nursing home certified nursing assistants. *Nursing Inquiry, 27*(1), e12315. https://doi.org/10.1111/nin.12315

True, S., Cubanski, J., Garfield, R., Rae, M., Claxton, G., & Chidambaram, P. (2020). *COVID-19 and workers at risk: Examining the long-term care workforce.* https://www.kff.org/medicaid/issue-brief/covid-19-and-workers-at-risk-examining-the-long-term-care-workforce/?utm_campaign=KFF-2020-Medicaid&utm_source=hs_email&utm_medium=email&utm_content=86855544&_hsenc=p2ANqtz-_lP7AwFxEYqlHmG5FM3pOFDsyr4pEhfDoldSbNFOF5tsTktGkIWQ2uExwLMu5pRSa12BxQyThwTWs5ieylTb7fYzFWnA&_hsmi=86855544

Walton, A. L., & Rogers, B. (2017). Workplace hazards faced by nursing assistants in the United States: A focused literature review. *International Journal of Environmental Research and Public Health, 14*(5), 544. https://doi.org/10.3390/ijerph14050544

WCCO. (2020). Coronavirus updates: Minnesota orders adult day care centers to close. *CBS Minnesota.* https://minnesota.cbslocal.com/2020/04/01/coronavirus-updates-minnesota-orders-adult-day-care-centers-to-close/

Yeo, S. (2004). Language barriers and access to care. *Annual Review of Nursing Research, 22* (0739–6686 (Print)), 59–73. https://doi.org/10.1891/0739-6686.22.1.59

The Unique Challenges Faced by Assisted Living Communities to Meet Federal Guidelines for COVID-19

Debra Dobbs⃝, Lindsay Peterson, and Kathryn Hyer

ABSTRACT

This perspective addresses the challenges that assisted living (AL) providers face concerning federal guidelines to prevent increased spread of COVID-19. These challenges include restriction of family visitation, use of third-party providers as essential workers, staffing guidelines, transfer policies, and rural AL hospitalizations. To meet these challenges we recommend that AL providers incorporate digital technology to maintain family-resident communication. We also recommend that states adopt protocols that limit the number of AL communities visited by home health care workers in a 14-day period, appeal to the federal government for hazard pay for direct care workers, and to extend the personal care attendant program to AL. It is further recommended that states work with AL communities to implement COVID-19 comprehensive emergency management plans that are well-coordinated with local emergency operation centers to assist with transfers to COVID-19 specific locations and to assist in rural areas with hospital transfers. Together, these recommendations to AL providers and state and federal agencies address the unique structure and needs of AL and would enable AL communities to be better prepared to care for and reduce those infected with COVID-19.

Introduction

Since one of the first COVID-19 cases in the United States was confirmed January 21, 2020, in a Washington state nursing home, there have been at least 1.15 million confirmed cases and close to 70,000 deaths as of May 3, 2020 (Centers for Disease Control, 2020). Approximately 83% of the deaths from COVID-19 in the U.S. have occurred in the 65 and older population (National Center for Health Statistics, 2020). The approximately 2.16 million adults who live in long-term care facilities (including nursing homes and assisted living (AL) communities) and cared for by 1.24 million staff (Gardner et al., 2020) are most at risk for infection from COVID-19.

Nationally, it is reported that about one-fifth of all deaths have been in nursing homes, and in some states as many as half of the deaths are in long-term care facilities (Stockman et al., 2020).

Since the outbreak occurred in the United States a number of articles have been published about how COVID-19 has affected residents and staff in long-term care settings (Dosa et al., 2020; Gardner et al., 2020). Media reports have focused more on the challenges in nursing homes than in AL communities, particularly at the larger outlets. For example, the Washington Post reported that 40% of 650 nursing homes with COVID-19 cases identified by State health departments had been cited more than once for infection-control deficiencies in the last four years (Cenziper et al., 2020). The New York Times has reported widely on the numbers of deaths in nursing homes (e.g. Harris et al., 2020).

This perspective argues that more attention needs to be paid to AL, which has been a dominant sector of long-term care for more than 20 years. It highlights the unique characteristics of AL communities relative to nursing homes in the U.S. It then outlines federal guidelines for long-term care facilities for COVID-19. The challenges those guidelines pose for AL with respect to visitation, third-party providers, staffing, transfers, and rural settings are then highlighted together with recommendations in light of those challenges.

The assisted living sector: a primer

There are an estimated 30,200 licensed AL communities across the United States, providing care to more than 835,000 residents (Sengupta et al., 2016). AL has a philosophy to enable a person to age-in-place for as long as possible by providing 24-hour supervision for unscheduled needs for activities of daily living but not nursing care (Chapin & Dobbs-Kepper, 2001). AL also provides programming for socialization and at least 2 meals a day. Unlike federally regulated nursing homes, AL communities are regulated at the state level and therefore vary widely in the services they provide and types of residents they may accept based on licensure type. For example, some states have separate licensure for AL communities that serve persons with psychiatric illnesses or provide memory care, while other states license AL communities to serve only less-impaired individuals.

There are wide state variations in staffing, with fewer than one-third of states requiring any specific numbers or types of licensed staff in their regulations (Roberts et al., 2020). Compared to nursing homes, where infection control programs are federally mandated, AL has varying degrees of regulation for infection control based on the state; only one-fourth of all states have an actual infection control program (Zimmerman et al., 2020) which has consequences for COVID-19. Bucy and colleagues (2020) reported that 31 states required infection control policies in AL, but the requirements varied in level of detail. Only six states directly referenced isolation practices for residents with communicable diseases.

Federal guidelines in long-term care facilities for COVID-19

The Centers for Disease Control Long Term Care Team and Infection Control Team have published webinars on how to prepare nursing homes and assisted living communities for COVID-19 (Centers for Disease Control, 2020). The Centers for Medicare and Medicaid (CMS) also recently released guidelines for long-term care facilities to reduce the spread of COVID-19 (CMS, 2020). The federal recommendations and guidelines apply equally to AL as to nursing homes. However, while similar in some of the services provided and population cared for, nursing homes and AL communities are different in philosophy, regulation and design. The National Center for Assisted Living recently offered clarifications to AL providers in response to federal guidance about state requirements for reporting COVID positive resident and staff cases and the need for personal protective equipment (PPE) (National Center for Assisted Living, 2020).

Relative to nursing homes, AL communities face several challenges in following federal guidelines for COVID-19. These challenges relate to: 1) restrictions on family visitation; 2) use of third-party providers as essential workers; 3) lower levels of direct care staffing; 4) limitations in facilitating transfers; and 5) additional challenges for rural AL communities. These challenges are discussed next along with recommendations for addressing them.

Challenge to restricting family visits to resident care

Federal guidelines have been established to restrict visitation from family and other nonrelatives. This is particularly challenging for AL communities that do not have the amount of activity, social work and direct care staff as nursing homes do, to fill the void created by these limitations. Family plays a vital role in providing additional care and socialization for AL residents (Port et al., 2005). Family members are the ones who make sure their loved ones get out into the community on a regular basis. The visitation limits are an even a greater challenge for AL residents with dementia, who may not understand why the one person whom they may remember, their spouse, daughter, or son, is no longer coming to see them.

Recommendation

Technology can be one solution to maintaining socialization and well-being within AL. AL administrators have reported using Google hangouts,

Skype and Zoom video to facilitate family and resident daily communication. More staff time needs to be devoted to assisting with technology needs, especially for residents with dementia, as they do not have the cognitive capability to use this technology without assistance. Access to wifi can be spotty in residents' rooms and is reported to be costly to upgrade (Zimmerman et al., 2020). In contrast to AL, nursing homes have a program through CMS to pay for service upgrades to wifi whereby Civil Money Penalty (CMP) Reinvestment funds are set aside to provide residents with adaptive communicative technologies (Indiana Health Care Association, 2020). The CMP funds can also be used for upgrades to wifi connections for any type of communication including telehealth visits. Finally, AL communities should take advantage of apartment style privacy that include individual rooms with patios and large windows that can enable families to communicate in person through windows or social distancing on patios when the weather permits and family members wear protective masks.

Challenge of third-party providers as essential workers and the risk of infection

Another difference between nursing homes and AL communities is the increased risk of infection in AL communities because of third-party providers and home health care visits. Home health care workers are deemed essential during the pandemic. All states allow the use of third-party providers in AL as this policy allows residents to receive services that states do not permit residential care providers to perform, such as skilled nursing services or assistance with activities of daily living that typically are provided only twice a week by AL staff (Carder et al., 2015). Home health care workers are at greater risk of spreading infection if they work in more than one AL community.

Recommendation

States need to adopt protocols that limit the number of AL communities visited by home health care workers in a 14-day period during this pandemic to help reduce the spread of infection from one AL community to another. An adequate supply of personal protective equipment (PPE) needs to be available for home health care workers, including masks, gloves and gowns for each new resident they care for. Some AL communities across the country are housing direct care workers on-site and paying them bonuses so they can contain the spread of infection (Belanger, 2020). This may not be feasible for all ALs, but for those who can afford it, is worth considering.

Challenge for AL to meet federal staffing guidelines

CMS has recommended the use of separate staffing teams for COVID-19 positive residents and consistent assignment of staff to the same set of residents. The AL industry faces challenges to meet these guidelines because of low levels of direct care staff, a lack of nursing staff and lack of infection control programs for airborne illness such as COVID-19. Staffing shortages will continue to rise with increased care demands due to COVID-19 and low wages. Personal care aides in AL on average make even less than certified nursing assistants in nursing homes, approximately two dollars less per hour (Payscale, 2020). There is a real fear among some AL administrators that direct care staff will weigh the benefits and rewards of their jobs caring for a highly vulnerable population and decide it is not worth the risk. What is making that decision more likely is the fact they could earn more money with the CARES Act stimulus funding ($1,200.00 plus 500.00 USD dollars per child for workers who have adjusted gross income less than 75,000 USD in addition to unemployment benefits) (Department of Treasury, 2020).

Recommendation

The implementation in AL of infection control programs for COVID-19 and educating staff about the importance of social distancing, handwashing and wearing PPE during each resident encounter is essential. Also important is increasing what workers are paid, given they are expected to care for highly vulnerable residents, in many cases without the PPE necessary because AL is not given priority. Any state requests for federally funded hazard pay for essential workers (e.g., police, firefighters, hospital nurses) should include long-term care nursing and direct care staff. In the face of staff shortages, some states have enacted COVID-19 Personal Care Attendant Programs to provide nursing homes with additional staff to care for residents during a State of Emergency and to train new workers to obtain skills necessary to become a certified nursing assistant (Florida Health Care Administration, 2020). States should extend this to AL communities.

Challenge For AL in transfer policies

Transfer policies have also been developed by CMS for COVID-19 (CMS, 2020) that recommend collaboration with state and local leaders to designate distinct facilities or units within a facility to separate COVID-19 negative residents from COVID-19 positive residents and individuals with unknown COVID-19 status. These transfer policies are more likely to be successfully implemented in large chain, corporate-owned AL communities that already have existing relationships with other AL communities from the same owners. Smaller, independently-owned AL communities will struggle to find alternate locations or space within their existing communities for COVID-19 wings or units.

Recommendation

States agencies should develop a template for AL communities as well as nursing homes for a COVID-19 comprehensive emergency management plans (CEMPs) similar to those required for disaster planning (Peterson et al., 2020). CEMPs are helpful planning tools and provide a framework that addresses emergency prevention, preparedness, response, recovery and mitigation. Because CEMPs are already in existence in states for disasters, it would not take long to modify for COVID-19. Local emergency operation centers would need to assist in the coordination of shared shelter agreements for AL communities that do not have alternate locations or spaces for COVID-19 positive residents. Shared shelter agreements could be with another AL or nursing home designated specifically for COVID-19 positive patients.

Additional challenges for rural AL communities

COVID-19 also has affected long-term care facilities in rural areas where a lack of available hospital beds has increased the likelihood of spread of the infection. Circumstances are dire in some places. One rural Florida community reported that "the local hospital is scheduled to close at the end of the month and the next closest hospital is 30 minutes away" (Klas, 2020). Another study reported a case in Idaho where a patient had to travel for nine hours to reach the hospital (Henning-Smith et al., 2017). Nursing homes, by comparison, may be part of existing networks of healthcare providers that can coordinate hospital transfers (McSweeney-Feld et al., 2017).

Recommendation

State agencies should assist AL providers in rural areas to make sure hospital arrangements are in writing in a COVID-19 CEMP. AL providers should coordinate with nursing homes in their areas to develop relationships to facilitate emergency transfers due to COVID-19 infections. Emergency operation officials should be tasked with a role in facilitating these arrangements.

Conclusion

This perspective has outlined some challenges AL communities face in their attempt to adhere to COVID-19 federal guidelines developed for long-term care facilities. Among these challenges are meeting the needs of residents who have traditionally relied on family members for socialization and care. This is especially critical for residents with dementia. The use of technology, with the assistance of staff, to coordinate family communication is essential to maintain resident well-being. Furthermore, AL communities need to work closely with home health care agencies to reduce the spread of COVID-19 infection as they travel from community to community. Challenged by low staffing potentially worsened by the COVID-19 threat, AL communities need to train staff on how to protect residents and themselves from infection. Higher pay is also needed, considering the risk to the direct care staff. Federal hazard pay may be a viable temporary solution. Another answer may be to extend the personal care attendant program that is available to nursing homes to the assisted living sector. Concerning preparation, emergency operations centers in local counties need to coordinate with AL communities in the transfer of residents who need to be isolated during a pandemic emergency. Rural AL providers should be given special assistance, working with local nursing homes, health departments and hospitals in other counties to provide care for those in need of treatment for COVID-19. The implementation of COVID-19-specific CEMPs could facilitate preparation for both transfers and rural hospitalizations due to COVID-19. Together, these recommendations to AL providers, state and federal agencies address the unique structure and needs of AL and would enable AL communities to be better prepared to care for those infected with COVID-19.

Key Points

- Federal guidelines for COVID-19 need to take AL policies and structure into account.
- Digital technology with staff assistance is key to resident-family communication.
- AL providers should appeal to the federal government for hazard pay for direct care workers.
- The Personal Care Attendant Program in nursing homes should be extended to AL.
- COVID-19 comprehensive emergency management plans are needed for COVID-19 related transfers.

Disclosure statement

No potential conflict of interest was reported by the authors.

Funding

This work was supported by RO1 AG060581-01 (Hyer, K. PI) Strategic Approaches to Facilitating Evacuation by Health Assessment of Vulnerable Elderly in Nursing Homes II.

ORCID

Debra Dobbs ⓘ http://orcid.org/0000-0002-9282-7624

References

Belanger, T. (2020). *The coronavirus is killing too many nursing home residents: Here's one idea for protecting them.* New York Times. Retrieved May 4, 2020, from https://www.nytimes.com/2020/05/03/opinion/coronavirus-nursing-homes.html

Bucy, T., Smith, L., Carder, P., Winfree, J., & Thomas, K. (2020). Variability in state regulations pertaining to infection control and pandemic reponse in US assisted living communities. *Journal of the American Medical Directors Association, 21*(5), 701–705. https://doi.org/10.1016/j.jamda.2020.03.021

Carder, P., O'Keeffe, J., & O'Keeffe, C. (2015). *Compendium of residential care and assisted living reguation and policy: 2015 edition.* Research Triangle Park, NC: RTI Press.

Centers for Disease Control. (2020). *Preparing nursing homes and assisted living facilities for COVID-19.* Washington, DC. Retrieved April 20, 2020, from CDC.gov/COVID-19

Centers for Disease Control and Prevention. (2020). *Coronavirus 19 U.S. Cases.* Washington, DC: Centers for Medicare and Medicaid Services. Retrieved May 4, 2020, from https://www.cdc.gov/coronavirus/2019-ncov/cases-updates/cases-in-us.html

Centers for Medicare and Medicaid Services. (2020). *COVID-19 long-term care facility guidance.* CDC. Retrieved April 18, 2020, from https://www.cms.gov/files/document/4220-covid-19-long-term-care-facility-guidance.pdf

Cenziper, D., Jacobs, J., & Mulcahy, S. (2020). Hundreds of nursing homes with cases of coronavirus have violated federal infection-control rules in recent years. *Washington Post.* Washington, DC: Retrieved April 22, 2020, from https://www.washingtonpost.com/business/2020/04/17/nursing-home-coronavirus-deaths

Chapin, R., & Dobbs-Kepper, D. (2001). Aging in place in assisted living: Philosophy versus policy. *The Gerontologist, 41*(1), 43–50. https://doi.org/10.1093/geront/41.1.43

Dosa, D., Jump, R. L. P., LaPlante, K., & Gravenstein, S. (2020, March 13). Long-term care facilities and the coronavirus epidemic: Practical guidelines for a population at highest risk. *Journal of the American Medical Directors Association, 21*(5), 569–571. https://doi.org/10.1016/j.jamda.2020.03.004

Florida Health Care Association. (2020). *Temporary COVID-19 personal care attendant program.* Tallahassee, FL: Florida Health Care Association. Retrieved April 23, 2020, from https://www.fhca.org/facility_operations/pcaprogram

Gardner, W., States, D., & Bagley, N. (2020). The coronavirus and the risks to the elderly in long-term care. *Journal of Aging & Social Policy,* 1–6. https://doi.org/10.1080/08959420.2020.1750543

Harris, A. J., Leland, J., & Tully, T. (2020). Nearly 2,000 dead as coronavirus ravages nursing homes in N.Y. Region. *New York Times.* Retrieved April 26, 2020, from https://www.nytimes.com/2020/04/11/nyregion/nursing-homes-deaths-coronavirus.html

Henning-Smith, C., Casey, M., Prasad, S., & Kozhimmanil, K. (2017). *Medical barriers to nursing home care for rural residents*. University of Minnesota Rural Health Research Center.

Indiana Health Care Association. (2020) *Civil money penalty reinvestment application coronavirus disease 2019 (COVID-19) communicative technology request*. Indianapolis, IN: Indiana Health Care Association. Retrieved May 4, 2020, from https://www.ihca.org/wp-content/uploads/2020/04/496260d9-e5bf-4760-8191-b1d166e5c8eb.pdf

Klas, M. (2020). 'There was an outbreak': Rural Florida nursing home overwhelmed by COVID-19. *Tampa Bay Times*. https://www.tampabay.com/news/health/2020/04/10/there-was-an-outbreak-rural-florida-nursing-home-overwhelmed-by-covid-19/

McSweeney-Feld, M. H., Molinari, C., & Oetjen, R. (Eds.). (2017). *Dimensions of long-term care management* (2nd ed.). Health Administration Press.

National Center for Health Statistics. (2020). *Provisional death counts for coronavirus disease*. Washington, DC: National Center for Health Statistics. https://www.cdc.gov/nchs/nvss/vsrr/covid19/index.htm

American Health Care Association/National Center for Assisted Living. (2020). *NCAL issues guidance on reporting COVID-19 cases in skilled nursing facilities and assisted living communities*. Washington, DC: AHCA. Retrieved April 25, 2020, from https://www.ahcancal.org/News/news_releases/Pages/AHCANCAL-Issues-Guidance-on-Reporting-COVID-19-Cases-in-Skilled-Nursing-Facilities-and-Assisted-Living-Communities.aspx

Payscale. (2020). *Hourly rate of certified nursing assistants*. Payscale, Inc. Retrieved April 22, 2020, from https://www.payscale.com/research/US/Job=Certified_Nurse_Assistant_(CNA)/Hourly_Rate

Peterson, L. J., June, J., Sakib, N., Dobbs, D., Dosa, D., Thomas, K., Jester, D. J., & Hyer, K. (2020). Assisted living communities during Hurricane Irma: The decision to evacuate or shelter in place and resident acuity. *Journal of the American Medical Directors Association*. https://doi.org/10.1016/j.jamda.2020.01.104.

Port, C. L., Zimmerman, S., Williams, C. S., Dobbs, D., Preisser, J. S., & Williams, S. (2005). Families filling the gap: Comparing family involvement for assisted living and nursing home residents with dementia. *The Gerontologist*, *45*(Suppl. 1), 87–95. https://doi.org/10.1093/geront/45.suppl_1.87

Roberts, M., Peterson, L. J., & Hyer, K. (2020). State of the states' assisted living websites: Information available to consumers. *The Gerontologist*, 1–7. https://doi.org/10.1093/geront/gnz174

Sengupta, M., Valverde, R., Lendon, J. P., Rome, V., Caffrey, C., & Harris-Kojetin, L. D. (2016). *Long-term care providers and services users in the Untied States - State estimates supplement: National study of long-term care providers, 2013-2014*. Washington, DC: National Center for Health Statistics.

Stockman, F., Richtel, M., Ivory, D., & Smith, M. (2020, April 17). They're death pits': Virus claims at least 7,000 lives in U.S. nursing homes. *New York Times*. https://www.nytimes.com/2020/04/17/us/coronavirus-nursing-homes.html

United States Department of Treasury. (2020). *The CARES act works for all Americans*. Washington, DC. Retrieved April 24, 2020, from https://home.treasury.gov/policy-issues/cares

Zimmerman, S., Katz, P., Kunze, M., O'Neil, K., & Resnick, B. (2020). The need to include assisted living in responding to the COVID-19 pandemic. *Journal of American Medical Directors' Association*, *21*(5), 572–573. https://doi.org/10.1016/j.jamda.2020.03.024

Financing Long-Term Services and Supports in the U.S.

Emergency Flexibility for States to Increase and Maintain Medicaid Eligibility for LTSS under COVID-19

Lynn A. Blewett (iD) and Robert Hest

ABSTRACT

Medicaid provides essential coverage for health care and long-term services and supports (LTSS) to low-income older adults and disabled individuals but eligibility is complicated and restrictive. In light of the current public health emergency, states have been given new authority to streamline and increase the flexibility of Medicaid LTSS eligibility, helping them enroll eligible individuals and ensure that current beneficiaries are not inadvertently disenrolled. Though state budgets are under increased pressure during the economic crisis created by the coronavirus, we caution states against cutting Medicaid LTSS eligibility or services to balance their budgets. These services are critical to an especially vulnerable population during a global pandemic.

Introduction

Medicaid provides essential health care coverage to low-income older adults and disabled individuals who are at particular risk during the COVID-19 pandemic. More than one-third of all U.S. COVID-19 deaths have occurred in nursing facilities (Yourish et al., 2020), and the conditions – including staffing difficulties and infection control – are all under scrutiny. Medicaid covers more than 60% of all nursing home residents receiving long-term care services (Harris-Kojetin et al., 2019) and is a fundamental resource for low-income older adults and disabled individuals who, without access to the program, would be destitute. Medicaid financial eligibility for older adults is among the most restrictive of all Medicaid eligibility categories. Even still, states may be tempted to control state spending by restricting eligibility. In this essay, we discuss the implications of Medicaid financial eligibility and recent emergency waivers that provide states with more flexibility to react swiftly to the devastation that COVID-19 is inflicting upon older adults, particularly those in nursing homes. We conclude with a caution not to look to eligibility restrictions for LTSS as a means to manage strained state budgets during a time of great need for the most vulnerable among us.

Medicaid financial eligibility for older adults

States provide Medicaid to eligible individuals using state criteria and federal minimum standards. There are two key aspects of eligibility rules that can be adjusted by states: financial rules (household income and asset limitations) and rules surrounding the need for LTSS based on a functional needs assessment. In general, individuals aged 65 years or older who receive Supplemental Security Income (SSI) benefits and need an institutional level of care are eligible for Medicaid LTSS services. SSI is an income support program for aged, blind, or disabled individuals with incomes at or below 74% of federal poverty guidelines. Forty-two states and the District of Columbia provide automatic Medicaid enrollment for SSI recipients without a separate application (Medicaid and CHIP Payment and Access Commission [MACPAC], n.d.). Many states use the "special income rule" to extend eligibility to older adults with incomes up to 300% of the SSI benefit level, approximately 2,250 USD per month in 2018 for an individual (Musumeci et al., 2019). Older adults are also required to pass an asset test to qualify for Medicaid, most commonly 2,000 USD for an individual and 3,000 USD for a couple.

In addition, in order to qualify for Medicaid LTSS, individuals must demonstrate the need for help with self-care or household activities, the existence of particular medical conditions, or a certain level of cognitive impairment (Kaiser Family Foundation (KFF), 2016). In addition to basic eligibility determinations, as of 2019, 34 states offered eligibility for those defined as "Medically Needy," i.e., individuals with incomes too high to meet Medicaid income eligibility requirements but who have high levels of health care spending (Musumeci et al., 2019). These individuals are allowed to deduct their health care expenses from their income to qualify for Medicaid.

Finally, approximately 10 million Medicaid beneficiaries are also eligible for Medicare coverage, so-called "dual eligibles." Dual-eligible beneficiaries have some of the greatest health care needs and lowest incomes of all individuals covered by Medicare or Medicaid and represent a disproportionate percent of Medicaid and Medicare spending (Medicaid and CHIP Payment and Access Commission (MACPAC), 2016). Dual eligibles whose incomes or assets are too high to qualify for full Medicaid services ("full duals") can qualify for a partial benefit in which Medicaid pays their Medicare premiums and, in some cases, some or all of their Medicare cost sharing ("partial duals").

COVID-19 response, focused on eligibility

During the COVID-19 pandemic, it is essential for states to leverage existing and new Medicaid administrative waiver authority to provide needed services to a known vulnerable, at-risk population. Leveraging this authority to promote enrollment is especially salient given the evidence suggesting that Medicaid is not reaching a sizable portion of the eligible population, potentially due to the burdens created by its complex eligibility determination process. Evidence suggests that policy changes like automatic Medicaid enrollment for disabled SSI participants (Rupp & Riley, 2016), increased generosity of home and community-based service benefits (Pezzin & Kasper, 2002), and relative restrictiveness of income and asset counting (Ungaro & Federman, 2009) all have a significant influence on take-up of Medicaid among eligible individuals.

Then, once individuals are enrolled, states must be proactive in adjusting their policies to prevent inadvertent disenrollment. Because of the complexities of enrollment and renewal, many beneficiaries lose coverage throughout the year. One recent study found that over a five-year study period, 18.2% of dual eligibles lost Medicaid coverage for reasons other than death, including18.5% of full Medicaid recipients, and 29.9% of partial Medicaid recipients (Roberts et al., 2019).

States have new authority under the COVID-19 public health emergency to expand eligibility and offer additional services. The Centers for Medicare and Medicaid Services (CMS) has issued guidance including a toolkit that outlines state options under existing and new waiver authority. Existing authority includes the use of Medicaid state plan amendments (SPAs) and section 1115 research and demonstration waivers. Washington state, for example, has received approval of a 1115 waiver that allows for self-attestation of individual income and assets and level of care to qualify for LTSS and for the state to modify eligibility criteria for LTSS (Centers for Medicare & Medicaid Services (CMS), 2020b). This allows for ease of enrollment by not requiring documentation of income upon enrollment but instead relying on an individual's statement of income. An additional 1115 waiver authority includes the ability for states to waive the 30-day institutional stay requirement and asset transfer rules, further expanding eligibility for Medicaid LTSS (Musumeci & Chidambaram, 2020).

States can also use authority provided under a new section 1135 waiver and section 1915(c) Appendix K, which provide for temporary flexibility to state Medicaid programs during a public health emergency (Centers for Medicare & Medicaid Services (CMS), 2020a). Section 1135 waivers, activated in certain public health emergencies, give states a range of additional flexibilities with the goal of ensuring Medicaid enrollees have sufficient access to needed services and health care items. For example, 44 states have used 1135 waiver authority to suspend for 30 days Level 1 and Level 2 pre-admission screenings and annual resident reviews (KFF, 2020). Under 1915(c) Appendix K, more than 30 states have approved waivers to allow them to conduct virtual or remote eligibility assessments and evaluations, and nearly as many have approved waivers extending deadlines to conduct reevaluations or assessments of eligibility (KFF, 2020). Connecticut has used authority under 1915(c) Appendix K to allow eligibility redeterminations to be conducted virtually and to extend the time for redeterminations to up to 12 months (Allen, 2020). Other provisions afforded under Appendix K allow states to waive level-of-care renewals for up to 12 months, temporarily suspend prior authorization requirements and extend medical necessity authorizations (Musumeci & Chidambaram, 2020). As of April 16, 2020, 27 states have approved 1915(c) Appendix K waivers (KFF, 2020).

This new flexibility provided for under emergency authority granted by the federal government gives states the ability to reduce the administrative burdens of applications and streamline eligibility redeterminations and relax eligibility requirements, allowing them to better provide needed coverage during a time of a global pandemic.

The need for Medicaid during a time of state budget constraints

Expenditures on Medicaid LTSS continue to be a large and growing part of Medicaid spending and state budgets. In FY 2018, it was the largest single component of state spending, accounting for 29% of all state expenditures (National Association of State Budget Officers, 2019). Medicaid pays for 51% of all expenditures on LTSS (Office of Disability, Aging and Long-Term Care Policy, 2018), and becomes a target as states look for ways to constrain spending. In addition, while users of LTSS represented just 5.9% of enrollees in 2013, they made up more than 40% ($168 billion) of all spending (Office of Disability, Aging and Long-Term Care Policy, 2018). The pressure from Medicaid on state budgets will only continue to grow throughout this crisis as Medicaid expenditures grow and state tax revenues fall.

The recently passed Families First Coronavirus Response Act (FFCRA) provided some financial relief to states by increasing the state federal medical assistance percentage (FMAP) by 6.2 percentage points for the duration of the COVID-19 public health emergency (Manatt Health, 2020). The FMAP rate determines the federal share of state Medicaid spending for most health care services and varies by state, determined by a formula based on states' per-capita incomes, providing higher FMAP rates to lower-income states. States in receipt of the enhanced match are not allowed to reduce their eligibility standards for existing programs and must cover COVID-19 testing and treatment without additional cost sharing. The National Governors Association (NGA) and others are calling for an additional increase of 5.8 percentage points to bring this emergency FMAP increase in line with that provided in the 2009 Recovery Act (National Governors Association, 2020). Most recently, the U.S. House of Representatives passed the Health and Economic Recovery Omnibus

Emergency Solutions Act (HEROES) which included an addition of 7.8 percentage points (added to the CARES Act 6.2 percentage point enhancement) for a total one-year increase of 14 percentage points starting July 1, 2020 (Flinn, 2020)

State budgets are now under extraordinary pressure as safety net spending is critical at a time when tax revenue is falling. In past times of constrained state budgets, state lawmakers have often looked to cutting Medicaid eligibility and services for savings. This continues to be the case in the current economic crisis. New York, which recently passed a budget with 1.6 USD billion in Medicaid cuts, nearly half of which came from cuts to LTSS (Lewis, 2020); Ohio announced 210 USD million in cuts to its Medicaid program (Roubein & Goldberg, 2020); and California's proposed budget includes a reduction of Medi-Cal eligibility for low-income seniors from 138% to 123% FPL (Wright, 2020).

Conclusion

Eligibility for Medicaid LTSS for older adults is already at the minimum required income levels in most states, requiring moderate- and low-income seniors to become impoverished before they can access needed care and services. At the same time, the care provided under Medicaid LTSS is essential, especially in a pandemic, considering that low-income, older adults are at the greatest risk of severe illness and death from COVID-19. It is critical that eligibility and flexibility be maintained, as the current crisis poses new challenges to states' enrollment and eligibility processes and creates new demands for services. Perhaps this crisis can forge policies that streamline eligibility determinations and reduce complexity across states. The steps taken by states and CMS to increase this flexibility are encouraging, but more should be done to ensure that older adults get the services they need, that existing beneficiaries are not disenrolled due to administrative complexity, and that states not cut Medicaid eligibility for LTSS during this time of great need.

Key Points

- Medicaid provides essential health care and long-term services and supports (LTSS) to low-income older adults who are at particular risk from COVID-19;
- States have been given emergency authority to add flexibility to a complicated Medicaid eligibility process to ensure that eligible individuals get coverage;
- Policymakers who must balance state budgets during this economic crisis should not cut essential eligibility for needed services during a time of great need.

Disclosure statement

No potential conflict of interest was reported by the authors.

ORCID

Lynn A. Blewett MA, PhD http://orcid.org/0000-0003-0409-8394

References

Allen, K. (2020, April 2). *HMA review of state appendix K waivers in response to COVID-19.* Health Management Associates. https://www.healthmanagement.com/blog/hma-review-of-state-appendix-k-waivers-in-response-to-covid-19/

Centers for Medicare & Medicaid Services. (2020a, April 2). *COVID-19 frequently asked questions (FAQs) for state medicaid and children's health insurance program (CHIP) agencies.* https://www.medicaid.gov/state-resource-center/downloads/covid-19-faqs.pdf

Centers for Medicare & Medicaid Services. (2020b, April 21). *Washington COVID-19 public health emergency demonstration.* https://www.medicaid.gov/medicaid/section-1115-demonstrations/downloads/wa-covid19-phe-ca.pdf

Flinn, B. (2020, May 15). *HEROES act highlights for medicaid and home and community-based services.* Leading Age. https://leadingage.org/legislation/heroes-act-highlights-medicaid-and-home-and-community-based-services

Harris-Kojetin, L., Sengupta, M., Lendon, J. P., Rome, V., Valverde, R., & Caffrey, C. (2019). *Long-term care providers and services users in the United States, 2015–2016.* DHHS Publication No. 2019–1427, National center for health statistics. https://www.cdc.gov/nchs/data/series/sr_03/sr03_43-508.pdf

Kaiser Family Foundation. (2016, August 2). *Medicaid's role in meeting seniors' long-term services and supports needs.* https://www.kff.org/medicaid/fact-sheet/medicaids-role-in-meeting-seniors-long-term-services-and-supports-needs/

Kaiser Family Foundation. (2020, April 29). *Medicaid emergency authority tracker: Approved state actions to address COVID-19.* https://www.kff.org/medicaid/issue-brief/medicaid-emergency-authority-tracker-approved-state-actions-to-address-covid-19/

Lewis, R. C. (2020, April 3). Medicaid cuts make the state budget, with some tweaks. New York, NY. https://www.cityandstateny.com/articles/policy/budget/medicaid-cuts-make-state-budget-some-tweaks.html

Manatt Health. (2020, March 27). *Summary of healthcare provisions of COVID-19 Stimulus Package #3 (CARES Act).* https://www.manatt.com/Manatt/media/Documents/Articles/Manatt-Insights_Summary-of-Healthcare-Provisions-of-COVID-19-Stimulus-Package-_3-(CARES-A(205712565-2).pdf

Medicaid and CHIP Payment and Access Commission. (2016, October). *Medicaid and medicare plan enrollment for dually eligible beneficiaries.* https://www.macpac.gov/wp-content/uploads/2016/10/Medicaid-and-Medicare-Plan-Enrollment-for-Dually-Eligible-Beneficiaries.pdf

Medicaid and CHIP Payment and Access Commission. (n.d.). *Eligibility for long-term services and supports.* Retrieved April 4, 2020, from https://www.macpac.gov/subtopic/eligibility-for-long-term-services-and-supports/

Musumeci, M., & Chidambaram, P. (2020, April 16). *COVID-19 issues and medicaid policy options for people who need long-term services and supports.* Kaiser Family Foundation. https://www.kff.org/medicaid/issue-brief/covid-19-issues-and-medicaid-policy-options-for-people-who-need-long-term-services-and-supports/

Musumeci, M., Chidambaram, P., & Watts, M. O. (2019, June 14). *Medicaid financial eligibility for seniors and people with disabilities: Findings from a 50-state survey.* Kaiser Family

Foundation. https://www.kff.org/report-section/medicaid-financial-eligibility-for-seniors-and-people-with-disabilities-findings-from-a-50-state-survey-issue-brief/

National Association of State Budget Officers. (2019). *State expenditure report: Fiscal Years 2017–2019.* https://www.nasbo.org/reports-data/state-expenditure-report

National Governors Association. (2020, April 21). *Governors' letter regarding COVID-19 aid request.* https://www.nga.org/policy-communications/letters-nga/governors-letter-regarding-covid-19-aid-request/

Office of Disability, Aging and Long-Term Care Policy. (2018, May). *An overview of long-term services and supports and medicaid: Final report.* U.S. Department of Health and Human Services Assistant Secretary for Planning and Evaluation. https://aspe.hhs.gov/system/files/pdf/259521/LTSSMedicaid.pdf

Pezzin, L. E., & Kasper, J. D. (2002). Medicaid enrollment among elderly medicare beneficiaries: Individual determinants, effects of state policy, and impact on service use. *Health Services Research, 37*(4), 827–847. https://doi.org/10.1034/j.1600-0560.2002.55.x

Roberts, E. T., Hayley Welsh, J., Donohue, J. M., & Sabik, L. M. (2019). Association of state policies with medicaid disenrollment among low-income medicare beneficiaries. *Health Affairs, 38*(7), 1153–1162. https://doi.org/10.1377/hlthaff.2018.05165

Roubien, R., & Goldberg, D., (2020, May 5). States cut medicaid as millions of jobless workers look to safety net. *POLITICO Magazine.* https://www.politico.com/news/2020/05/05/states-cut-medicaid-programs-239208

Rupp, K., & Riley, G. F. (2016). State medicaid eligibility and enrollment policies and rates of medicaid participation among disabled supplemental social security income recipients. *Social Security Bulletin, 76*(3), 17. https://www.ssa.gov/policy/docs/ssb/v76n3/v76n3p17.html

Ungaro, R., & Federman, A. D. (2009). Restrictiveness of eligibility determination and medicaid enrollment by low-income seniors. *Journal of Aging & Social Policy, 21*(4), 338–351. https://doi.org/10.1080/08959420903166993

Wright, A., (2020, May 14) *New California budget proposes major cuts to health and other needed services, even worse without federal assistance.* Health Access California. https://health-access.org/2020/05/new-ca-budget-proposes-major-cuts-to-health-and-other-needed-services-even-worse-without-federal-assistance/

Yourish, K. K., Lai, R., Ivory, D., & Smith, M. (2020, May 11). One-third of all U.S. Coronavirus deaths are nursing home residents or workers. *New York Times.* https://www.nytimes.com/interactive/2020/05/09/us/coronavirus-cases-nursing-homes-us.html

COVID-19 and the Future of Long-Term Care: The Urgency of Enhanced Federal Financing

Judy Feder

ABSTRACT

The economic threat posed by responses to COVID 19 endangers financing for long-term care across the states that is already inadequate and inequitable. Increasing the federal share of Medicaid spending as unemployment rises would mitigate fiscal pressure on states and preserve public services. But unlike the demand for Medicaid's health care protections, which rises when economic activity declines, the demand for long-term care protections will grow even in a healthy economy as the population ages. Enhanced federal support is urgent not only to cope with the virus today but also to meet the long-term care needs of the nation's aging population in the years to come. Long-term care financing policy should be modified to either adjust federal matching funds by the age of each state's population, or fully federalize the funding of LTC expenses of Medicaid beneficiaries who are also eligible for Medicare.

That deaths in nursing homes account for over a quarter of COVID-19 fatalities in the U.S. (Chidambaram, 2020) dramatically links the virus to long-term care (LTC). Less visible but equally powerful is the link between the economic shutdown aimed at stemming the virus and long-term care financing. Although deficiencies in LTC quality (Drucker & Silver-Greenberg, 2020) and financing (Feder & Komisar, 2012) predate COVID-19, the horror of the virus has the potential to generate effective policy action to address these deficiencies: specifically, enhanced federal funding for Medicaid's long-term care benefits. Medicaid's adequacy has always varied with states' ability and willingness to invest in services, whether at home or in nursing homes, in return for federal matching grants. But the virus and the shutdown are overwhelming the fiscal capacity of even states willing to support Medicaid services. This perspective argues that enhanced federal support is urgent not only to cope with the virus today but also to meet the LTC needs of the nation's aging population in the years to come.

Medicaid and long-term care

Medicaid is the nation's safety net for long-term care – help with the basic tasks of daily life, like dressing, bathing, and eating, for people who cannot manage on their own. In 2018, Medicaid spent 197 USD billion to finance 52% of the nation's long-term care spending (Watts et al., 2020). But Medicaid LTC benefits vary considerably across states (Kaiser Family Foundation, 2016). A 2012 report found that half the states reached about a third or less of their low-income population with long-term care needs, and the least generous states achieved only about a third of the reach of the most generous states (Feder & Komisar, 2012). Another metric showed even greater variation: long-term care spending per low income person in the state, which reflects not only who gets served but how much service they get. The most generous states spent six times as much as the least generous states for all long-term care services, and eight times as much for services at home or in the community.

Although the Great Recession slowed states' investment in home and community-based services, the availability of those services has increased over the last decade (Snyder & Rudowitz, 2016). But variation and inadequacies in home care persist (Hauser et al., 2018). Policies that limit access to care take many forms – arbitrary limits on the number of visits a beneficiary receives, requirements for financial contribution or "spend-down," and, most important, caps on enrollment, which are allowable under "waivers" from Medicaid's statutory guarantee of benefits to persons assessed as eligible for covered care (Watts et al., 2020). Limited Medicaid services mean that family caregivers face the primary responsibility for caregiving, at enormous health and economic cost (National Academy of Medicine, 2016; Reinhard et al., 2019), and that people in need suffer harm from insufficient care (Freedman & Spillman, 2014).

Enhanced federal financing over the short-term

Despite the design of Medicaid's federal match to provide greater support to lower than to higher income states, federal support has never been sufficient to overcome variation in state commitments. Deterioration in states' fiscal capacity, however, poses an immediate threat to all states' support for long-term care (as well as other Medicaid services), no matter how willing states are to pay. The magnitude and duration of states' revenue losses associated with the COVID-induced shutdown is of historic proportions. Drawing on other experts' estimates as well as its own, the Center on Budget and Policy Priorities projects that after a substantial revenue drop-off in the current fiscal year (ending June 30 in most states), the fiscal 2021 shortfall will be greater than that in the worst year of the Great Recession – equivalent to a quarter of state revenues – and that significant losses will continue well into fiscal 2022 (McNichol et al., 2020). Fiscal pressure will be compounded, of course, by heightened pressure to provide social and health assistance, as incomes plummet, local economies struggle, and disease persists. Given balanced budget requirements and past experience, cutbacks in even limited benefits seem more likely than not. After all, cuts made During the Great Recession continue to leave education, unemployment benefits, infrastructure, and other services underfunded after almost a decade of recovery.

In previous recessions, an enhanced match – or increase in the rate at which the federal government matches state Medicaid spending – has been adopted to provide immediate relief to states and reduce state burdens in meeting greater demands (McNichol et al., 2020). The Families First Coronavirus Response Act included a modest 6.2 percentage point bump in the Medicaid match tied to the public health emergency, conditional on states' retention of current eligibility levels or "maintenance of effort" (Broaddus, 2020). The case has been made that circumstances call for an even larger increase in the match and a permanent mechanism for increasing the match rate in response to increases in states' unemployment levels (Fiedler & Powell, 2020; Holahan et al., 2020). An enhanced match could help sustain LTC along with other Medicaid services under the virus' immediate threat.

Looking for a longer term fix in federal financing

Unlike the demand for Medicaid's health care protections, which rises when economic activity declines, the demand for long-term care protections will grow even in a healthy economy. That is not just because some states' benefits already fall far short of need. It is also because the need for long-term care is growing with the aging of the population. Beginning in just over ten years (2031), as the oldest baby boomers start turning 85, the number and the share of the population aged 85 and older will start to increase. The number of people aged 85 years or older will double to 18 million from 2030 to 2050; and the share of the older population in that age group will grow from 12% to 21% (Ortman et al., 2014). As the population ages, the need for long-term care will increase. In 2018, just over four in ten people age 85 or older needed long-term care, more than twice the rate among people aged 75–84 (Hado & Komisar, 2019).

The population is aging in every state. But the effects – and the fiscal burden – of an aging population will be larger in some states than others. Key to the adequacy of public resources to support the needs of older people will be the availability of working people to generate resources and tax revenues – measured as the ratio of one age group to the other. In 2010, the number of people aged 65+ per 100 people aged 18–64 ranged from 12 in the "youngest" state to 28 in the oldest state. By 2030, this ratio is projected to grow in all states and the range to expand from 21 in the youngest states to 51 in the oldest. In 2030, more than half of the states will have a ratio greater than the highest state has today. On the whole, the "oldest" states today will continue to be among the "oldest" in 2030 (Feder & Komisar, 2012). It is questionable whether any state has the capacity to meet the growing demand for long-term care.

Regardless, the greater the imbalance between the older population and the working age population, the greater the challenge states will face in sustaining, let alone improving, the adequacy of long-term care services. Under current law, then, the inadequacy and inequity that already characterizes Medicaid long-term care services across the states is likely to grow substantially worse in the years to come. Only an expansion of federal financing is likely to prevent or reverse growing inadequacy and inequity in the availability of Medicaid support for long term care.

Enhanced federal match for long-term care

To prevent deterioration and promote improvement in LTC protections, Congress should permanently increase federal fiscal responsibility for LTC financing alongside a countercyclical boost tied to unemployment rates. Paralleling the match enhancements that are tied to unemployment, the long-term care enhancement could be tied to an age-based index (Feder & Komisar, 2012). Matching rate enhancements could vary with the "age" of the state; for example, the enhancements could initially range from perhaps an addition of 5 percentage points to the current federal share for states that are now the "youngest" to an addition of 10 or 15 percentage points for states that are now the "oldest." "Maintenance of effort" requirements, a floor in terms of benefits and eligibility, along with enforcement of quality standards, would be required to assure improvements in coverage. Federal matching rates could be further increased for improvements in access.

A state's "age" would be measured based on the ratio of its population age 75 or over with incomes below 300% of the federal poverty level (the population most likely to need Medicaid long-term care services) to its working aged population (the population providing the bulk of the financial resources in the state). The goal would be to have the federal government assume much of the burden associated with responding to each state's actual aging. To that end, each state's "age" would be periodically recalculated and the federal enhancement would increase with the increase in a state's "age" (that is, ratio of people age 75 or older with income below 300% of poverty to the working age population). The relationship between the ratio and the enhancement would be fixed, so as states age, the maximum enhancement would also rise (as ratios increase in all states). The total federal share in each state could be limited to a maximum enhancement of 20 or 25% or capped at, say, 90%.

Full federal financing for dual eligibles

Full federal financing for Medicaid long-term care, especially for low income Medicare beneficiaries (dual eligibles) is also a possibility, whether in the short- or long-term. A shift from federal-state to full federal financing of dual eligibles' Medicaid long-term care would resemble the establishment of the Supplemental Security Income (SSI) program for low-income older adults and people with disabilities in 1972. SSI then replaced federal matching grants to states with a federally-financed, federal-state administered "floor" of income protection. Similarly, federal assumption of long-term care responsibilities for dual eligibles would likely include establishment of a nationally-uniform benefit standard, perhaps set somewhere in the middle of today's range of state long-term care programs.

Federal assumption of long-term care responsibilities for Medicare beneficiaries who also qualify for Medicaid has historically been favored by state governors (Bruen & Holahan, 2003) who might be particularly responsive to the shift at this time. A new federally-financed long-term care program for dual eligibles would entail national rules – on eligibility, benefits, quality assurance, and payment rates – even if, as in SSI, states continued to manage the benefit. Establishing and sustaining a nationally-uniform benefit floor across all states by fully federalizing Medicaid LTC benefits for Medicare beneficiaries would likely accomplish more than a capped enhanced match to achieve a higher level of service across all states – enhancing both adequacy and equity into the future.

Conclusion

COVID-19 clearly elevates attention to the importance of federal relief to sustaining states' capacity to protect low income Americans from health and economic catastrophe, regardless of where they live. Although social insurance for long-term care could likely even further promote adequacy and quality (Cohen et al., 2018), political concern about states' fiscal burdens may "open a window" (Kingdon, 1984) for targeted federal fiscal relief through the Medicaid program as a specific path to overcoming longstanding barriers to improving long-term care financing.

It is difficult at this moment to predict the long-term impact of COVID-19 on long-term care financing or any other social policy. As of May 1, 2020, we have seen agreement across party lines on a mammoth investment of federal funds to address the dire economic as well as health conditions facing the American public. But we've also seen conflict between the parties over the bolstering of the federal government's role in social welfare – specifically, though not solely, when the issue is relief for the states. Action to date may reflect what one expert has described as only a "temporary truce in the small government versus big government battle … " – unlikely to galvanize the support needed to enhance federal long-term-care financing proposed here (Jason Furman as cited in Balz, 2020). To quote another, however, it might be that in " … a country deep in crisis … once inconceivable political interventions suddenly appear possible" (Goldberg, 2020). If the latter is correct, this proposal to enhance federal financing for long-term care to provide both immediate relief to states and long-term benefits to people who need others' help to survive may be "an idea whose time has come" (Kingdon, 1984).

Key Points

- Medicaid is the nation's safety net for long-term care (LTC), but Medicaid LTC benefits vary significantly across states, overburdening family-caregivers and harming people who receive insufficient care.
- The shutdowns aimed at stemming COVID-19 are overwhelming states' abilities to support long-term care along with other Medicaid services.
- A short-run increase in federal support to states can mitigate the COVID-19 threat; but a permanent increase is essential to meet the needs of an aging population.

Disclosure statement

No potential conflict of interest was reported by the author.

References

Balz, D. (2020, April 19). Government is everywhere now. Where does it go? *The Washington Post*. https://www.washingtonpost.com/graphics/2020/politics/pandemic-government-role/

Broaddus, M. (2020, April 21). *Families first's medicaid funding boost a useful first step, but far from enough*. Center on Budget and Policy Priorities. https://www.cbpp.org/blog/families-firsts-medicaid-funding-boost-a-useful-first-step-but-far-from-enough

Bruen, B., & Holahan, J. (2003, November). *Shifting the cost of dual eligibles: Implications for states and the Federal government*. The Henry J. Kaiser Commission on Medicaid and the Uninsured. https://www.kff.org/wp-content/uploads/2013/01/shifting-the-cost-of-dual-eligibles-implications-for-states-and-the-federal-government-issue-paper.pdf

Chidambaram, P. (2020, April 23). *State reporting of cases and deaths due to Covid-19 in long-term care facilities*. The Henry J. Kaiser Family Foundation. https://www.kff.org/medicaid/issue-brief/state-reporting-of-cases-and-deaths-due-to-covid-19-in-long-term-care-facilities/

Cohen, M., Feder, J., & Favreault, M. (2018, January). *A new public-private partnership: Catastrophic public and front-end private LTC insurance*. The Urban Institute. https://www.umb.edu/mccormack.umb.edu/uploads/gerontology/Public_Catastrophic_Insurance_Paper_for_Bipartisan_Policy_Center_1-25-2018.pdf

Drucker, J., & Silver-Greenberg, J. (2020, March 14). Trump administration is relaxing oversight of nursing homes. *The New York Times*. https://www.nytimes.com/2020/03/14/business/trump-administration-nursing-homes.html

Feder, J., & Komisar, H. (2012). *The importance of federal financing for long-term care*. Georgetown University. https://www.thescanfoundation.org/sites/default/files/georgetown_importance_federal_financing_ltc_2.pdf

Fiedler, M., & Powell, W. (2020, April 2). *States will need more Fiscal relief. Policymakers should make that happen automatically*. The Brookings Institution. https://www.brookings.edu/blog/usc-brookings-schaeffer-on-health-policy/2020/04/02/states-will-need-more-fiscal-relief-policymakers-should-make-that-happen-automatically/

Freedman, V., & Spillman, B. (2014, April 11). *Disability and care needs of older Americans*. Office of the Assistant Secretary for Planning and Evaluation. Department of Health and Human Services. https://aspe.hhs.gov/report/disability-and-care-needs-older-americans-analysis-2011-national-health-and-aging-trends-study

Goldberg, M. (2020, April 20). A Biden presidency could be better than progressives think. *The New York Times*. https://www.nytimes.com/2020/04/20/opinion/joe-biden-progressive.html

Hado, E., & Komisar, H. (2019, August). *Fact sheet: Long-term services and supports*. AARP Public Policy Institute. https://www.aarp.org/content/dam/aarp/ppi/2019/08/long-term-services-and-supports.doi.10.26419-2Fppi.00079.001.pdf

Hauser, A., Fox-Grage, W., & Ujvari, K. (2018). *Across the states: Profiles of long-term services and support*. AARP Public Policy Institute. https://www.aarp.org/content/dam/aarp/ppi/2018/08/across-the-states-profiles-of-long-term-services-and-supports-full-report.pdf

Holahan, J., Haley, J. M., Buettgens, M., Elmendorf, C., & Wang, R. (2020, April). *Increasing federal medicaid matching rates to the states during the Covid-19 epidemic*. The Urban Institute. https://www.urban.org/sites/default/files/publication/102098/increasing-federal-medicaid-matching-rates-to-provide-fiscal-relief-to-states-during-the-covid-19-pandem_0_0.pdf

Kaiser Family Foundation. (2016, August). *Medicaid's role in meeting seniors' long-term services and supports needs*. http://files.kff.org/attachment/Fact-Sheet-Medicaids-Role-in-Meeting-Seniors-Long-Term-Services-and-Supports-Needs#http://files.kff.org/attachment/Fact-Sheet-Medicaids-Role-in-Meeting-Seniors-Long-Term-Services-and-Supports-Needs%20%20

Kingdon, J. (1984). *Agendas, alternatives, and public policies*. Longman.

McNichol, E., Leachman, M., & Marshall, J. (2020, April 14). *States need significantly more Fiscal relief to slow the emerging deep recession*. Center on Budget and Policy Priorities. https://www.cbpp.org/research/state-budget-and-tax/states-need-significantly-more-fiscal-relief-to-slow-the-emerging-deep

Musemeci, M., Watts, M., & Chidambaram, P. (2020, February 4). *Key state policy choices about medicaid home and community-based services*. The Henry J. Kaiser Family Foundation. https://www.kff.org/report-section/key-state-policy-choices-about-medicaid-home-and-community-based-services-issue-brief/

National Academy of Medicine. (2016). *Family caregiving for an aging America*. National Academies Press. https://www.kff.org/report-section/key-state-policy-choices-about-medicaid-home-and-community-based-services-issue-brief/

Ortman, J., Velkoff, V., & Hogan, H. (2014). *An aging nation: The older population in the United States*. U.S. Census Bureau. https://www.census.gov/library/publications/2014/demo/p25-1140.html#https://www.census.gov/library/publications/2014/demo/p25-1140.html

Reinhard, S., Feinberg, L. F., Choula, R., & Evans, M. (2019, November 14). *Valuing the invaluable 2019 update: Charting a path forward.* AARP Public Policy Institute. https://www.aarp.org/ppi/info-2015/valuing-the-invaluable-2015-update.html

Snyder, L., & Rudowitz, R. (2016, June 21). *Trends in state Medicaid programs: Looking back and looking forward.* Kaiser Family Foundation. https://www.kff.org/medicaid/issue-brief/trends-in-state-medicaid-programs-looking-back-and-looking-ahead/

Watts, M., Musumeci, M., & Chidambaram, P. (2020, February 4). *Medicaid home and community-based services enrollment and spending.* The Henry J. Kaiser Family Foundation. https://www.kff.org/medicaid/issue-brief/medicaid-home-and-community-based-services-enrollment-and-spending/

Long-Term Services and Supports in Other Contexts

COVID-19 and Long-Term Care Policy for Older People in Canada

Daniel Béland ⓘ and Patrik Marier

ABSTRACT
Older people are especially vulnerable to COVID-19, including and especially people living in long-term care facilities. In this Perspective, we discuss the impact of the COVID-19 pandemic on long-term care policy in Canada. More specifically, we use the example of recent developments in Quebec, where a tragedy in a specific facility is acting as a dramatic "focusing event". It draws attention to the problems facing long-term care facilities, considering existing policy legacies and the opening of a "policy window" that may facilitate comprehensive reforms in the wake of the COVID-19 pandemic.

Introduction

Older people are especially vulnerable to COVID-19, including and especially people living in long-term care facilities (Gardner et al., 2020), most notably in nursing homes. For instance, in Canada, as of mid-April 2020, nearly half of known COVID-19 deaths are tied to nursing homes, a situation that has received ample media coverage while generating fresh policy discussions about the state of long-term care policies for older people in the country (Aiello, 2020). Comparatively high mortality rates are not only the case for public long-term care facilities but also for privately-owned yet publicly regulated facilities. In this article, we discuss the policy status of both public and private facilities in the aftermath of the COVID-19 pandemic using the example of a widely debated case in the province of Quebec, which we understand as a "focusing event" (Kingdon, 2010). This current "focusing event" draws attention to the fate of these facilities, in light of existing policy legacies (Pierson, 1993), and the

---

This article has been republished with minor changes. These changes do not impact the academic content of the article.

possible opening of a "policy window" (Kingdon, 2010) for reform in the wake of COVID-19.

Federalism, the public-private dichotomy and long-term care in Canada

Like many other countries, Canada faced a rapid increase in the number of COVID-19 cases in mid-late March and early-April 2020: as of April 12, "there are 23,318 cases of COVID-19 cases and, sadly, 653 deaths. We have completed tests for more than 404,000 people, and 5.6% of those tests were confirmed as positive." (Public Health Agency of Canada, 2020). Early on, it became clear that, like in other countries, older people living in long-term care facilities proved especially vulnerable to COVID-19. As of April 25, 64.8% of all reported COVID-19 deaths occurred in these facilities in Quebec, referred to as CHSLD (*Centres d'hébergement de soins de longue durée*) (Institut national de santé publique (INSPQ), 2020). As media stories about the high death tolls in a number of long-term care facilities in provinces such as British Columbia, Ontario, and Quebec emerged, the federal government issued new guidelines to help these facilities protect their residents against COVID-19 (Osman, 2020).

In the Canadian context, however, it is the provinces, and not the federal government, who have the constitutional jurisdiction over the operation of public facilities and the regulation of private facilities in the field of long-term care for older people. This fact stresses two key aspect of existing policy legacies in Canada: federalism (Banting, 2005) and the public-private dichotomy, with respect to the level of regulation in a given jurisdiction (Béland & Gran, 2008). These two issues created significant policy challenges before the COVID-19 outbreak, which has simply exacerbated them. First, regarding federalism, Ottawa has much more fiscal capacity than the provinces and it allocates money to them for health and social programs through three major federal transfers: the Canada Health Transfer, the Canada Social Transfer, and equalization, which only targets poorer provinces. Yet, most of the funding for health care, including for long-term care public facilities, come from the provinces, which are increasingly struggling to finance health care costs in a context of accelerated population aging and, more decently, declining tax revenues caused by the sudden, pandemic-related economic downturn (on fiscal federalism in Canada see (Béland et al., 2017).

Second, the central role of long-term care facilities in the provinces generates crucial regulatory issues. In the following discussion about Quebec, we focus on this issue related to the public-private dichotomy in social policy (in terms of the level of government intervention in the market), which remains fuzzy and leads to calls for government intervention in case of perceived market failure (Béland & Gran, 2008). This is especially the case in the context of the unprecedented COVID-19 crisis, which has generated enhanced public legitimacy for bolder government action (Mérand, 2020). Yet as John W. Kingdon (2010) suggests, bold government action is typically much more likely in the context of relatively short "policy windows," during which policymakers and the public are more receptive to new policy alternatives that break away from existing policy legacies, which tend to be self-reinforcing, under most conditions (Pierson, 1993). As Kingdon (2010) also shows, dramatic "focusing events" can shape the policy agenda and direct public attention toward particular policy problems. This dynamic is apparent in the current Canadian context, as far as multiple COVID-19 deaths in nursing homes is pushing their reform to the forefront of the agenda during a period of crisis capable of opening a "policy window" during which change becomes more likely. It is at this point that "policy entrepreneurs" – actors capable of promoting particular policy solutions within the political area to address a problem on the policy agenda – can seize the moment and promote new policy alternatives.

The next section explores existing long-term care policy legacies in Quebec and a recent "focusing event" – a sudden occurrence that captures public attention – that is shaping the policy agenda toward a possible reform of both public and private long-term care in the province. The article concludes by discussing whether the nature of the current COVID-19 "policy window" and the issue of how the federal government could step in and provide more funding to help provinces like Quebec could lead to reform of long-term care for older people in a post-COVID-19 world.

Long-term care in Quebec: existing policy legacies

As elsewhere in Canada, long term care in Quebec operates at the margins of the health care system. It is an "extended service" within the federal Canada Health Act, meaning that the federal government does not provide standards (it is left to the provinces to fund public facilities and to regulate both public and private facilities) and this sector has even been ignored in high profile health care commissions and strategic consultations (Canadian Healthcare Association (CHA), 2009). This lack of attention to long-term care contributes to an insidious policy feedback that accentuates the curative bias of the health care system and divert policy attention *away* from long-term care (Marier, Forthcoming).

In Quebec, as in the other nine provinces, nursing homes receive most of the media and policy attention when it comes to both long term care policy discussions and residential settings for seniors, although only 3.4% of older adults (65+) reside in them (Séguin et al., 2018). In the aftermath of the 2008 financial crisis, Quebec slightly decreased the number of beds available resulting in the number of beds per older adults above the age of 75 dropping by 17% between 2010 and 2017 period (Commissaire à la santé et au bien-être, 2017). This could have been part of a renewed focused on home care, in the context of aging at home strategies. However, despite two decades of advocating a shift toward home care, nursing home expenditures have constantly represented 80-82% of the long-term care budget in Canadian provinces (Grignon & Spencer, 2018), meaning that there has not been a noticeable shift in resources. Hence, as a result, this reduction in the number of beds in Quebec has led to more stringent admission criteria, rising waiting lists to access nursing homes, and a stronger reliance on unpaid family caregivers.

In Quebecand in other provinces, the marginal status combined with budgetrestraints have fostered deficiencies within long-term care systems, including, as noted, lengthy waiting lists, as well as lack of available rooms, poor working conditions, and the increasing role of the private sector in nursing homes. These deficiencies have been well known for quite some time, but the entire COVID-19 episode represents a clear focusing event that draws attention on key policyissues. For instance, the expansion and increasing use of private providers in the delivery of care has been a preoccupation of various governmental watchdogs across Canada, such as ombudsperson offices and seniors' advocates. Accessibility to a private provider, can take two forms in Quebec. First, individuals can opt to pay out of pocket and reside in a private nursing home (*privé non-conventionné*). In this case, the operator must satisfy basic norms and the Ministry of Health and Social Services (MHSS) provides a permit, but these private nursing homes have a lot of autonomy, as they can, for example, establish their own admission requirements. Second, the MHSS can temporary lease rooms inprivate facilities to alleviate pressures on public facilities where individuals pay the same rate as in the public sector. In some cases, these are part of long-standing agreements with the ministry, which operate under the same guidelines as public nursing homes (*privé conventionné*).

In recent years in Quebec, the ministry has been increasingly purchasing temporary rooms in private nursing homes operating without an agreement (i.e. *privé non-conventionné*). In the 2017–18 annual report of the Ombudsperson, it states that this "type of arrangement, in certain cases, does not provide the appropriate degree of monitoring for the health status of individuals" (Protecteur du citoyen, 2018: 74, authors' translation). One of these private establishments, CHSLD Herron, is currently under criminal investigation after 31 out of 150 residents died in less than a month following reports of gross negligence; so far, five of these deaths have been attributed to COVID 19, but this number is expected to rise since authorities just received access to residents' files. In response, the Quebec government deployed inspections for all similar private facilities (Ocampo, 2020).

It is important to note that in Quebec, the ongoing difficulties experienced by CHSLDs go well beyond private facilities. The entire system is under stress with 142 facilities reporting COVID cases (CBC News, 2020), which prompted modifications of earlier guidelines related to nursing homes and even an emergency call to recruit additional staff beyond the health care workers to caregivers, former employees and even university professors in related fields.

Conclusion

The tragic and widely debated situation in the CHSLD Herron and other facilities is creating a dramatic "focusing event" that draws the attention on the flawed policy legacies of long-term care policy in Quebec and in Canada more generally. Consequently, the issue of improving both public and private long-term care for older people has moved to the top of the social policy agenda. In this context of acute media and political attention toward this policy issue, the CODIV-19 crisis is opening a genuine "policy window" during which comprehensive reform of the sector is likely to be debated. Yet, only time will tell whether policymakers in Quebec and elsewhere across the country will seize the moment and try to make sure the public health crisis we are witnessing never occurs again.

Additional funding from the federal government, which could also integrate fully long-term care within the Canada Health Act, would seem, at first, to be a course of action worthy of consideration. In fact, this is something Prime Minister Justin Trudeau alluded to in his April 24 briefing, which immediately led to complaints from provinces, especially Quebec and Ontario, of potential federal intrusion in provincial jurisdictions. A retraction quickly followed on the part of the federal government (Marquis, 2020). In the past 40 years, the provinces have developed different models of long-term care, which results in specific organizational structures regulating relationships among provincial administrations, regional health authorities, the private sector, and community organizations (Marier, Forthcoming). These two elements result in policy and political complexities when seeking a pan-Canadian solution. Nonetheless, this situation does not prevent the federal government to negotiate a new form of fiscal transfer to the provinces dealing directly with long-term care for older people.

In the provinces, there will also be stark pressures on governments to bolster the budget dedicated to long-term care and alter current practices on the ground. Each province faces a specific institutional environment. For instance, Quebec is currently studying the possibility of taking control of private CHSLDs and make them public (Gerbert, 2020). However, this kind of solution is possible in Quebec because the private sector only plays a marginal role within the long-term care system, but this is definitely not the case in other provinces such as British Columbia and Ontario. In these two provinces, more than 50% of nursing homes are privately owned and nonprofit organization also operate a substantial number of them as well (Marier, Forthcoming). This specific situation creates different constraints and opportunities for reform compared to the ones present in Quebec and in other provinces.

Key Points

- COVID 19 has laid bare multiple ongoing issues with nursing homes;
- COVID 19 represents a focusing event opening a policy window to address long-standing issues with nursing homes, and long-term care in general;
- The case of Quebec, Canada, provides an illustration of these ongoing dynamics.

Disclosure statement

No potential conflict of interest was reported by the author.

ORCID

Daniel Béland ⓘ http://orcid.org/0000-0003-2756-5629

References

Aiello, R. (2020, April 13). Nearly half of known COVID-19 deaths in Canada linked to long-term care homes: Tam. *CTV News*. https://www.ctvnews.ca/canada/nearly-half-of-known-covid-19-deaths-in-canada-linked-to-long-term-care-homes-tam-1.4893419

Banting, K. G. (2005). Canada: Nation-building in a federal welfare state. In F. G. Castles, S. Leibfried, & H. Obinger (Eds.), *Federalism and the welfare state: New world and European experiences* (pp. 89–137). Cambridge University Press.

Béland, D., & Gran, B. (Eds.). (2008). *Public and private social policy: Health and pensions policies in a new era*. Palgrave Macmillan.

Béland, D., Lecours, A., Marchildon, G. P., Mou, H., & Olfert, M. R. (2017). *Fiscal federalism and equalization policy in Canada: Political and economic dimensions*. University of Toronto Press.

Canadian Healthcare Association. (2009). *New directions for facility-based long term care*.

CBC News. (2020, April 14). *Here's a list of Quebec's long-term care homes with confirmed COVID-19 cases*. https://www.cbc.ca/amp/1.5532549

Commissaire à la santé et au bien-être. (2017). Les personnes de 75 ans et plus en attente d'une place d'hébergement en CHSLD. *Info-performance, 16*, 10.

Gardner, W., States, D., & Bagley, N. (2020). The coronavirus and the risks to the elderly in long-term care. *Journal of Aging & Social Policy*, 1–6. https://doi.org/10.1080/08959420.2020.1750543

Gerbert, T. (2020, April 24). François Legault songe à rendre tous les CHSLD publics. *Radio-Canada*. https://ici.radio-canada.ca/nouvelle/1696784/quebec-chsld-prives-salaires-preposes-conventionne-gouvernement

Grignon, M., & Spencer, B. G. (2018). The funding of long-term care in Canada: What do we know, what should we know? *Canadian Journal on Aging/La Revue canadienne du vieillissement, 37*(2), 110–120. https://doi.org/10.1017/S0714980818000028

Institut national de santé publique (INSPQ). (2020, April 25). *Données détaillées COVID-19 au Québec*. Quebec City: Institut national de santé publique (INSPQ). https://www.inspq. qc.ca/covid-19/donnees/details

Kingdon, J. W. (2010). *Agendas, alternatives, and public policies* (2nd ed.). Longman.

Marier, P. (Forthcoming). *The four lenses of population aging: Planning for the future in Canadian Provinces*. University of Toronto Press.

Marquis, M. (2020, April 25). CHSLD et fédéral: Justin Trudeau clarifie ses propos. *La Presse*. https://www.lapresse.ca/covid-19/202004/25/01-5270868-chsld-et-federal-justin-trudeau-clarifie-ses-propos.php

Mérand, F. (2020, March 14). Le grand retour de l'État. *Le Devoir*. https://www.ledevoir.com/ opinion/idees/574948/le-grand-retour-de-l-etat

Ocampo, R. (2020, April 11). Legault annonce que les CHSLD privés non-conventionnés seront tous inspectés. *Le Devoir*. https://www.ledevoir.com/societe/sante/576894/legault-annonce-que-les-chsld-prives-non-conventionnes-seront-tous-inspectes

Osman, L. (2020, April 13). *Long-term care deaths expected to rise as growth of total cases slows: Tam. The National Post*. https://nationalpost.com/pmn/news-pmn/canada-news-pmn/long-term-care-home-deaths-expected-to-rise-tam

Pierson, P. (1993). When effect becomes cause: Policy feedback and political change. *World Politics, 45*(4), 595–628. https://doi.org/10.2307/2950710

Protecteur du citoyen. (2018). *Rapport annuel d'activités 2017-18*. Le Protecteur du citoyen.

Public Health Agency of Canada. (2020, April 12). *Statement from the Chief Public Health Officer of Canada on COVID-19*. Ottawa: Public Health Agency of Canada. https://www. canada.ca/en/public-health/news/2020/04/statement-from-the-chief-public-health-officer-of-canada-on-covid-19.html

Séguin, A.-M., Van Pevenage, I., & Dauphinais, C. (2018). La plupart des personnes très âgées vivent-elles en CHSLD? In V. Billette, P. Marier, & A.-M. Séguin (Eds.), *Les vieillissements sous la loupe: Entre mythes et réalités* (pp. 65–74). Presses de l'Université Laval.

COVID-19: Implications for the Support of People with Social Care Needs in England

Adelina Comas-Herrera ⓘ, Jose-Luis Fernandez, Ruth Hancock, Chris Hatton ⓘ, Martin Knapp, David McDaid ⓘ, Juliette Malley, Gerald Wistow, and Raphael Wittenberg

ABSTRACT
This perspective examines the challenge posed by COVID-19 for social care services in England and describes responses to this challenge. People with social care needs experience increased risks of death and deteriorating physical and mental health with COVID-19. Social isolation introduced to reduce COVID-19 transmission may adversely affect well-being. While the need for social care rises, the ability of families and social care staff to provide support is reduced by illness and quarantine, implying reductions in staffing levels. Consequently, COVID-19 could seriously threaten care availability and quality. The government has sought volunteers to work in health and social care to help address the threat posed by staff shortages at a time of rising need, and the call has achieved an excellent response. The government has also removed some barriers to effective coordination between health and social care, while introducing measures to promote the financial viability of care providers. The pandemic presents unprecedented challenges that require well-co-coordinated responses across central and local government, health services, and non-government sectors.

Care and support with personal and practical tasks are needed by many older adults and people with disabilities across the United Kingdom (UK). In England alone, the social care system received 1.9 million requests for support in 2018/19 (NHS Digital, n.d.). Social care helps people become

Contributorship statement

and remain independent, retain their dignity, achieve better wellbeing, and be safe from abuse and neglect. It includes all forms of personal and practical support for children, young people, and adults who need extra assistance, including supported housing or residential care, as well as helping unpaid family carers. While health care provided through the National Health Service (NHS) is mainly free of charge and is dominated by public providers, social care – which is the responsibility of local authorities ('councils') – is means-tested and provided mainly by for-profit ('private') and non-profit ('voluntary') organizations as well as by millions of unpaid family and other carers. For example, in England in 2015, nearly 200,000 community-dwelling people with dementia relied exclusively on unpaid care (Wittenberg et al., 2019).

People with social care needs experience increased risks of death and deteriorating physical and mental health with COVID-19. For many, the consequences of infections can be serious, and people with dementia and learning disabilities have a higher prevalence of risk-related conditions such as respiratory and cardiovascular disease, diabetes, and dysphagia. In this perspective we examine challenges posed by COVID-19 for social services in England (which accounts for 84% of the UK population). We also describe the social care sector's response to COVID-19 in light of these challenges. Since administrative structures and national policies are set independently by the four countries of the UK, we focus here on England, but the challenges currently faced in the other countries of the UK are not dissimilar.

The challenge posed by COVID-19 for social services

The UK faces an unprecedented challenge in responding to COVID-19. The four UK governments – England, Scotland, Wales, and Northern Ireland – are implementing stringent measures to slow the spread of the virus and avoid overwhelming the National Health Service (NHS) and social care services. Nationally, the Coronavirus Act 2020 emergency legislation (UK Government, n.d.) suspends the statutory obligations of local authorities[1] to conduct detailed assessments of care and support needs and to meet these needs. However, many individuals still require help with care tasks involving frequent face-to-face contact with care workers and local authorities are still expected to take all reasonable steps to continue to meet needs.

Moreover, the ability of both families and the social care workforce to provide care is itself seriously hampered by illness and self-isolation. Shortages of personal protective equipment (PPE) increase both risk of disease transmission and anxiety in staff, volunteers, carers, and people with care needs. Precarity of employment for much of the social care workforce is an enduring issue, with most paid at or close to minimum wage. There are already serious concerns about the financial situation of care providers, as austerity policies in recent years have resulted in reductions in the fees local authorities pay to providers. COVID-19 may further threaten their financial viability if staff absences reduce their capacity, if more vacancies arise from higher than normal numbers of residents' deaths or if there are fewer admissions.

In the context of already significant pressures on the sector, COVID-19 could seriously threaten care availability and quality. Countries that are ahead in terms of infection rates, such as Spain and the United States, provide stark warnings (Barnett & Grabowski, 2020; Davey, 2020): some care homes are already overwhelmed by large numbers of deaths and substantial levels of sickness absence. Early international evidence suggests that nearly half of all COVID-19 deaths in five European countries were among care home residents (Comas-Herrera & Zalakain, 2020). COVID-19 could similarly pose a risk to the quality of care in care homes and other congregate settings in England.

The lockdown increases other risks, including domestic abuse and social isolation, with health consequences (Courtin & Knapp, 2017). Pressure on online delivery services means that interrupted access to food and other essentials may turn into urgent social care issues. Unpaid carers also face an invidious dilemma as they are sources of both support and risk. While nonresident carers are wondering whether they should still visit, co-resident carers, often with their own support needs, may face even greater responsibilities if no-one else can now visit.

The immediate response of the social services sector

There needs to be the best possible coordination between health and social care bodies, food-distribution systems, civil contingency, and military services to mobilize community resources to provide support to older adults and others in need of social care. Without such coordination some of those needing care may not get the full range of support they require, and services may prove less effective and efficient due, for example, to duplication of processes.

The response to the call for NHS volunteers (Royal Voluntary Service, n. d.) has far exceeded its target, but registration for additional support (UK Government, 2020) is based on a restricted set of medical conditions rather than *circumstances* requiring such support, thereby excluding many in need of assistance. Volunteers potentially play vital roles in supporting social care, for instance, through, for example, delivering food and medicine to vulnerable people during a lockdown, and providing telephone support to help reduce social isolation and loneliness.[2] For this to work well, co-ordination between local authorities responsible for social care and NHS bodies responsible for health care is essential. A rapid training program would also help ensure volunteers can support people safely and effectively.

As noted above, the NHS and local authority social care services operate within separate and distinct administrative structures. Integration of their activities has long been advocated but with very limited results (Smith et al., 2019). Baggage from past relationships could obstruct integrated approaches that the current emergency demands. The reported face-off between NHS hospitals and residential care service providers funded through social care in North West England is a worrying development: it emerged over the apparent reluctance of residential and nursing homes to accept discharged hospital inpatients without testing for COVID-19, particularly as staff lacked PPE (Health Service Journal, n.d.).

Other recent developments are potentially more positive, not least policymakers' attempts to remove barriers long considered 'too difficult to handle', especially barriers to effective coordination between health, social care, and other public services. One example is the remarkably comprehensive (given timescales) guidance published on 19 March 2020 about the discharge of patients from hospital to their own homes or care homes, aiming to streamline in-patient pathways and processes through more clearly specified responsibilities and accountabilities (NHS England, 2020). Charges/co-payments for social care services after hospital discharge have been temporarily removed, and restrictions on information-sharing between health and social services relaxed. There remain many risks arising from these regulatory changes, however, including relaxation of councils' statutory duty to assess and meet needs, already fragile social care services being swamped by unmanageable levels of demand on hospital and community services, and unsustainable staffing pressures.

Timely data on suspected infection rates and deaths amongst people using social care services and support staff availability are key to monitoring and targeting of support to at-risk populations, and there are some encouraging international developments (Comas-Herrera & Fernandez-Plotka, 2020). As receipt of publicly-funded social care in England is subject to an assessment of care needs and an assessment of incomes and savings, many people with social care needs do not seek services and remain unknown to local authorities or voluntary organizations best-placed to respond to their circumstances. These people include those who pay for their own care and adults supported solely by their families. Engaging non-government providers is crucial to identifying those individuals. Many adults with dementia or learning disabilities are not eligible for long-term social care support, and councils may be unaware of what is happening to them or to recent care leavers and other younger people at high risk.

Preventing and controlling infection in both care homes and among vulnerable groups in the community will continue to be hampered unless there is both a more rapid distribution of PPE and much better access to testing for care home residents, social care staff, family members providing significant personal care and volunteers in front-line roles, as is happening in South Korea (Comas-Herrera & Fernandez-Plotka, 2020). The central government Department of Health and Social Care (DHSC) has published a plan for PPE which provides guidance on who needs it, what type and in what circumstances. It also explains the arrangements for PPE delivery to those who need it, and actions being taken to buy more PPE from abroad and make more in the UK. Public Health England has updated guidance on PPE in the light of COVID-19. To date, however, policy has focused on challenges facing the NHS to a greater extent than those facing social care.

Technology could be used more extensively to ensure access to up-to-date safety guidance. The UK government launched an app for the public that provides updates. Specialist initiatives are needed for social care staff on minimizing the risk of spreading infection. Similar technology might match people with urgent needs to available staff and volunteers, for example, to obtain shopping or medical supplies. Social care staff who find themselves having to perform palliative care tasks for which they are not trained could be supported by medical personnel through telehealth.

Measures are needed to expand the workforce. Some countries are already widening the potential pool by, for example, recruiting students, allowing staff with restricted visas to work more hours and offering pay supplements. Other measures include planning for rapid-response teams to support care homes or other services that become overwhelmed, or isolating staff and care home residents together, which has been successful in containing outbreaks in South Korea (together with PPE and testing) and is starting to happen in New Zealand, Spain, and the UK. People who have recently left the NHS have been invited to return, and 20,000 retired health care professionals are re-joining the NHS. In social care, councils and (some) service providers are urgently seeking former carers to contribute as volunteers to expand capacity (The Independent, n.d.). Even if there was no variation in volunteer response across England, there remains the challenge of how these volunteers are co-ordinated and deployed.

Measures to ensure the financial viability of social care providers announced by the government are welcome. They include a COVID-19 response fund that is providing support for local authorities to manage social care pressures, as well as direct financial support for charities to help them provide key services and support for vulnerable people. Other measures include government funding of 80% of the previous income of self-employed workers unable to work as normal in the sector. Support is also needed for families and other carers (e.g., extending eligibility for Carers Allowance, a small weekly payment to carers (mainly below state pension age) providing at least 35 hours of support per week).

At the same time, the social care sector needs to be careful that reductions in obligations during the crisis, such as the right to assessment of care needs, do not become permanent, as this could reduce longer-term access to services.

Moving forward

These extraordinary challenges to social care require immediate, well-co-coordinated responses across different tiers of government and the non-government sectors, and with the general public. It is critical that information about best practices is shared as it emerges; the National Institute for Health and Care Excellence (NICE), which is producing rapid guidelines and evidence summaries on COVID-19, the Local Government Association representing all local authorities, and central government departments all have responsibilities here. We can learn from international experience, which offers an advance warning of difficulties ahead, but also good examples of how best to respond. Previous patterns of unconstructive, sometimes self-destructive, fighting between the NHS and councils must be avoided. Innovation is always easier said than done, but has never been more urgently needed.

Notes

1. Local government authorities in England are responsible for a wide range of services, including social care. Elected councilors are responsible for the overall direction of policy in each local authority. There are 152 local authorities in England with responsibilities for social care.
2. NHS Volunteer Responders has been set up to support the NHS and the care sector during the COVID-19 outbreak. The program enables volunteers to provide care or to help a vulnerable person. It includes Community Response Volunteers who deliver shopping, medication, or other essential supplies to the homes of people who are self-isolating and Check and Chat Volunteers providing short-term telephone support to individuals who are at risk of loneliness as a consequence of self-isolation. See https://www.goodsamapp.org/NHS.

Key Points

- COVID-19 poses risks to the health and wellbeing of people with social care needs.
- It reduces the ability of families, friends, and social care staff to provide support.
- The availability and quality of care are at risk due to the pandemic.
- The UK government has introduced measures to assist social care providers.

- The challenges posed by COVID-19 require well-coordinated intera-gency responses.

Disclosure statement

No potential conflict of interest was reported by the authors.

ORCID

Adelina Comas-Herrera ⓘ http://orcid.org/0000-0002-9860-9062
Chris Hatton ⓘ http://orcid.org/0000-0001-8781-8486
David McDaid ⓘ http://orcid.org/0000-0003-0744-2664

References

Barnett, M. L., & Grabowski, D. C. (2020). Nursing homes are ground zero for COVID-19 pandemic. *JAMA Health Forum*, 1(3), e200369–e200369. https://doi.org/10.1001/JAMAHEALTHFORUM.2020.0369

Comas-Herrera, A., & Fernandez-Plotka, J.-L. (2020). *Summary of international policy measures to limit impact of COVID19 on people who rely on the long-term care sector.* LTCcovid.org, International Long-Term Care PolicyNetwork, CPEC-LSE. Retrieved from https://ltccovid.org/2020/03/29/summary-of-international-policy-measures-to-limit-impact-of-covid19-on-people-who-rely-on-the-long-term-care-sector/

Comas-Herrera, A., & Zalakain, J. (2020). *Mortality associated with COVID-19 outbreaks in care homes: Early international evidence.* LTCcovid.org, International Long-Term Care PolicyNetwork, CPEC-LSE. Retrieved from https://ltccovid.org/2020/04/12/mortality-associated-with-covid-19-outbreaks-in-care-homes-early-international-evidence/

Coronavirus: 20,000 retired NHS staff have returned to fight Covid-19, Johnson says | The Independent. (n.d.). Retrieved April 3, 2020, from https://www.independent.co.uk/news/uk/politics/coronavirus-latest-retired-nhs-workers-staff-return-boris-johnson-a9433001.html

Courtin, E., & Knapp, M. (2017). Social isolation, loneliness and health in old age: A scoping review. *Health & Social Care in the Community*, 25(3), 799–812. https://doi.org/10.1111/hsc.12311

Davey, V. (2020). *Report: The COVID-19 crisis in care homes in Spain, recipe for a perfect storm (LTCcovid).* LTCcovid.org, International Long-Term Care PolicyNetwork, CPEC-LSE. Retrieved from https://ltccovid.org/2020/03/30/report-the-covid19-crisis-in-care-homes-in-spain-recipe-for-a-perfect-storm/

NHS Digital. (n.d.). *Adult social care activity and finance report, England - 2018-19 [PAS] - NHS digital.* NHS England. Retrieved April 3, 2020, from https://digital.nhs.uk/data-and-information/publications/statistical/adult-social-care-activity-and-finance-report/2018-19

NHS England. (2020). *COVID-19 hospital discharge service requirements contents.* NHS England. Retrieved from https://www.england.nhs.uk/coronavirus/wp-content/uploads/sites/52/2020/03/covid-19-discharge-guidance-hmg-format-v4-18.pdf

NHS told to 'up its game' in helping social care respond to crisis | News | Health Service Journal. (n.d.). Wilmington Healthcare. Retrieved April 3, 2020, from https://www.hsj.co.uk/news/nhs-told-to-up-its-game-in-helping-social-care-respond-to-crisis/7027193.article

Royal Voluntary Service. (n.d.). *GoodSAM.* Retrieved April 3, 2020, from https://www.goodsamapp.org/nhs

Smith, J., Wistow, G., Holder, H., & Gaskins, M. (2019). Evaluating the design and implementation of the whole systems integrated care programme in North West London: Why
   commissioning proved (again) to be the weakest link. *BMC Health Services Research*, *19*(1),
   228. https://doi.org/10.1186/s12913-019-4013-5

UK Government. (2020). *Get coronavirus support as a clinically extremely vulnerable person -
   GOV.UK*. UK Government. Retrieved April 3, 2020, from https://www.gov.uk/coronavirus-
   extremely-vulnerable

UK Government. (n.d.). *Coronavirus Act 2020 — UK Parliament*. UK Government. Retrieved
   April 3, 2020, from https://services.parliament.uk/bills/2019-21/coronavirus.html

Wittenberg, R., Knapp, M., Hu, B., Comas-Herrera, A., King, D., Rehill, A., ... Kingston, A.
   (2019). The costs of dementia in England. *International Journal of Geriatric Psychiatry*, *34*
   (7), 1095-1103. https://doi.org/10.1002/gps.5113

COVID-19 and Long-Term Care Policy for Older People in Hong Kong

Terry Lum (iD), Cheng Shi, Gloria Wong (iD), and Kayla Wong

ABSTRACT

Hong Kong is a major international travel hub and a densely populated city geographically adjacent to Mainland China. Despite these risk factors, it has managed to contain the COVID-19 epidemic without a total lockdown of the city. Three months on since the outbreak, the city reported slightly more than 1,000 infected people, only four deaths and no infection in residential care homes or adult day care centers. Public health intervention and population behavioral change were credited as reasons for this success. Hong Kong's public health intervention was developed from the lessons learned during the SARS epidemic in 2003 that killed 299 people, including 57 residential care residents. This perspective summarizes Hong Kong's responses to the COVID-19 virus, with a specific focus on how the long-term care system contained the spread of COVID-19 into residential care homes and home and community-based services.

Hong Kong is an international travel hub closely connected to all major cities in Mainland China and internationally. It has ranked consistently as the most traveled city in the world (Euromonitor International, 2019). With about 7.5 million residents, it received more than 65 million visitors in 2018, a great majority of whom, 43.7 million, were from mainland China (Census & Statistics Department, 2020). When the news of COVID-19 emerged in Wuhan in January, Hong Kong was expected to be hit hard by the epidemic because of its immense population density, geographic proximity to Mainland China, fluid boundaries with neighboring areas, and a large number of mainland and international visitors. Instead of being severely impacted, however, Hong Kong's responses to contain the infection and death rates have been recognized as highly effective (Gibney, 2020).

Based on the lessons the city learned from fighting the severe acute respiratory syndrome (SARS) epidemic in 2003, Hong Kong residents responded swiftly by wearing surgical masks in public areas, following strict hand hygiene practices, and maintaining social distance. The Government also implemented a range of public health measures to contain a potential community outbreak and to prevent any transmission of the virus from hospitals to nursing homes (Lee, 2003). The results are very encouraging: since early February, the transmission rate has been cut to below one (Cowling et al., 2020). As of May 17, 2020, more than three months into the epidemic, Hong Kong recorded 1,053 infections and four deaths (0.4% of confirmed cases). No infections have been reported in residential care homes or other long-term care facilities.

A recent article published in *Lancet Public Health* concluded that the reduced transmission of COVID-19 in Hong Kong was associated with the public health interventions implemented by the Government and population behavior changes (Cowling et al., 2020). Hong Kong seems to provide a good example to the world in how to effectively curb COVID-19 without a total lockdown, a strategy adopted by many other countries. This perspective summarizes the experience of Hong Kong in combating COVID-19, with a specific focus on the long-term care system.

Long-term care in Hong Kong

Long-term care services in Hong Kong are part of the social welfare system, while the health-care system plays only a supportive role. The Hong Kong Government funds a great majority of long-term care services through its social welfare budget but it does not directly provide services itself. Almost all home and community-based services (HCBS) are provided by nonprofit non-governmental organizations (NGOs) while about 60% of residential care services are provided by private-for-profit companies and the other 40% by NGOs. There are two types of residential care homes in Hong Kong, namely Care and Attention Homes for frail elders and Nursing Homes for very frail elders. There is no means test to determine eligibility for government-funded long-term care services and services are provided at a nominal fee for all residents. For example, service recipients pay only 4% copayment for home-based services, 10% for adult day center services, and 10–20% for residential care services (Working Group on Elderly Services Programme Plan, Elderly Commission of Government of Hong Kong SAR, 2017). The average copayment for residential care is currently about 264 USD per month and that can be waived for low income older adults. All residential care homes are licensed by the Social Welfare Department of the Hong Kong Government and operate according to the code of practice set by the Government. As of March 31, 2020, there were 76,343 residential care beds in Hong Kong, 63% (or 47,988 beds) were non-government-funded and 37% (or 28,355 beds) were government-funded (Social Welfare Department, 2020). Almost 80% of non-government-funded residential care beds were also funded by the Social Welfare Department through its means-tested welfare program for older people living in poverty (Working Group on Elderly Services Programme Plan, Elderly Commission of Government of Hong Kong SAR, 2017).

The Hong Kong Government is not only the funder and regulator of long-term care services; it is also a gatekeeper for service eligibility via a centralized care needs assessment. Since 2000, the Social Welfare Department has used the Minimum Data Set for Home Care Assessment Instrument (MDS-HC) to assess eligibility for government-funded long-term care services. All assessments are undertaken by assessors accredited by the Social Welfare Department. Most of these are medical social workers working for the Government or social workers in community elderly centers. Social workers employed by care providers are not allowed to become accredited assessors in order to avoid a potential conflict of interest. Older adults assessed as having no impairment or mild impairment only are not eligible for any government-funded long-term care services. Those assessed as having a moderate to severe level of impairment are eligible for government-funded HCBS, such as chore services, meal delivery, or adult day care centers. Only those assessed as having severe impairment are eligible for residential care services. There is no needs assessment for privately funded residential care services.

Because of rapid population aging, the Hong Kong Government has significantly expanded its long-term care services in recent years. In particular, the "money follows the older person" funding scheme has been introduced as a pilot project, which means the money goes directly to the older persons who are eligible for government-funded care services by means of a voucher. Using the voucher, participants in the pilot project directly contract with care providers of their choice for services.

Lessons from SARS in 2003

While older people, particularly those who are frail and living in residential care homes, are particularly vulnerable to COVID-19 in many countries (Comas-Herrera et al., 2020), as of May 17, Hong Kong recorded zero infections in residential care homes and adult day care centers. This achievement is the combined effect of evidence-based public health interventions, such as social distancing and rigorous hygiene practice of care home staff and residents, and behavioral changes of Hong Kong residents, all of which were learned during the SARS epidemic.

In 2003, SARS infected 8,098 individuals worldwide and killed 774 people. Hong Kong, because of its geographic proximity to Mainland China and high population density, bore the heaviest disease burden in this epidemic, with 1,775 people infected (22% of the total infected worldwide) and 299 deaths

(39% of total deaths worldwide) (Leung et al., 2009). Among those who were infected in Hong Kong, 324 were older adults aged 65 years or over (18% of the total number infected) and 72 were care home residents (22% of the total number of older adults infected), of whom 57 died (79% of care home residents infected) (Kong, 2006). SARS also infected 11 care home staff and killed two of them (Anonymous, 2003). A local study found that care home residents were 5 times more likely to be infected than the general public during the SARS epidemic and 81% of infected care home residents acquired SARS in hospitals (Kong, 2006). Furthermore, care home residents had a much higher mortality rate (78.1%) than community-dwelling older adults (44%) and non-older adults (6.3%) (Kong, 2006). After the SARS epidemic, the Government published the first "Guidelines on Prevention of Communicable Diseases in Residential Care Homes for the Elderly" in 2004 and required all care home operators to designate an Infection Control Officer to coordinate and implement infection control measures within the home according to the Guidelines.

The lessons learned from Hong Kong's experience with the SARS epidemic include: (1) older adults are more vulnerable to SARS as they have both a high infection rate and a high mortality rate once infected; (2) care home residents are particularly vulnerable as their risk of contracting SARS was 5 times that of the general population; (3) most infections of care home residents are acquired during hospital visits, therefore cutting the transmission between hospitals and care homes should be an important defense to protect care home residents; (4) a higher proportion of elderly SARS patients require intensive care and mechanical ventilation and have longer hospital stays, thereby increasing the burden on the health-care system. Since both SARS and COVID-19 are caused by the novel coronavirus, these lessons have been put into practice from the beginning of the COVID-19 epidemic.

Response to COVID-19

To prevent and control the spread of COVID-19, the Hong Kong Government adopted a bundle of containment measures, including intense surveillance for infection in incoming travelers and in local communities, isolation of infected patients in hospitals for treatment and their close contacts in special quarantine facilities for observation, travel restrictions and bans, school closures, flexible working arrangements, and prohibition of gatherings of more than four people in public. Hong Kong residents also changed their behavior immediately after the outbreak, such as wearing a face mask in public areas by almost everyone to prevent silent transmission by asymptomatic-infected individuals, enhanced hand hygiene by frequent use of hand sanitizers and handwashing, and voluntarily maintaining social distance. Immediately after the COVID-19 outbreak in Mainland China in late January, 74.5% of adults in Hong Kong used face masks to protect themselves (Cowling et al., 2020). That number rapidly increased to 97.5% by mid-February. Also, 90.2% of adults reported that they avoided going to crowded places and 92.5% reported washing or sanitizing their hands more often in mid-February (Cowling et al., 2020). Even without a total lockdown, a strategy adopted in many other regions, Hong Kong was able to contain the spread of COVID-19 by public health interventions and behavioral changes of the population.

To prevent the spread of COVID-19 into long-term care facilities, Hong Kong's Social Welfare Department issued the first operation guideline to NGO care providers as early as January 28, 2020, announcing three measures that would remain in place between January 29 and February 17. First, all residential care services for older adults would continue as normal but visiting doctors to these care homes would be reduced. Second, all day care centers for older people would suspend their services to reduce the risk of infection arising from the gathering of people, but centers would remain open at limited capacity to serve those who do not have anyone at home to care for them during the day time. Three, HCBS would be limited to providing only home-delivered meals, escort to medical appointments, nursing care, and administration of medicine. Subsequently, the Social Welfare Department extended this special service delivery arrangement several times and as of May 17, 2020, these special arrangements remain in place.

To cope with the additional resources needed in long-term care facilities during the COVID-19 outbreak, the Social Welfare Department provided financial support for NGO service providers to procure sanitary and personal protective equipment and to hire additional temporary staff for extra cleaning and hygiene practice (Wong et al., 2020). To reduce the risk of infection among older people during clinic visits, the Hospital Authority that runs all public hospitals and specialist outpatient clinics suspended all non-essential medical services, including regular doctor visits for chronic diseases. Instead, older people with chronic diseases can now refill their medicines without physically seeing a doctor.

Although residential care services are provided as usual, service providers imposed stringent visitation rules and hygiene practices immediately above and beyond the requirements of the infectious control Guidelines. All face-to-face visits by outsiders including family members and volunteers were terminated. Instead, remote meetings via information technology channels (e.g., Zoom and Face Time) have been organized in some care homes to maintain residents' social connections. The body temperature of all staff who work in care homes is checked before work and anyone with a fever or other signs of respiratory infection will not be allowed to work. All staff are required to wear a face mask all day while working. All residents are required to wear a face mask in public areas inside the care homes. They are asked to eat and to stay in their rooms most of the time. Strict hand hygiene practice is observed. These practices have effectively stopped the virus from entering care homes, leading to zero infections among care home residents.

As noted, Hong Kong has implemented "money follows the older person" as a pilot project for long-term care. COVID-19 hit care providers under this new funding mode the hardest. In the traditional funding mode, the Government agrees to a service quota with service providers and provides funding based on the agreed quota, rather than the actual services used. Providers, therefore, are not at risk of having reduced or no income regardless of whether their services are used or not. However, under the "money follows the older person" mode, the Government does not have a direct funding relationship with these providers. Instead, resources go to older adults in the form of service vouchers. Older adults can exchange the vouchers for services with any government-designated care provider. However, due to COVID-19, many older adults have stayed at home and the volume of HSBS used has plunged. These providers have seen a very significant drop in their income. In the context of COVID-19, however, voucher-based care arrangements expose service providers to extra financial risk of not having regular income to support their staff when voucher clients cease to show up to use their services.

Conclusion

COVID-19 will likely be a long-lasting challenge for most countries. Total lockdown is not a longer-term option to stop the spread of the virus as it is economically very costly and disruptive to daily life. The approaches developed and tested in Hong Kong may shed new light on how to prevent and control the spread of an epidemic and to protect vulnerable older people in long-term care facilities including residential care homes.

Key points

(1) Densely population and internationally connected, Hong Kong managed to contain the spread of COVID-19 without imposing a total lockdown of the city.
(2) Lessons from the SARS epidemic in 2003 have been applied to contain COVID-19.
(3) Early on, the Government directed residential care homes to continue as normal but provided resources for preventive and hygiene practices.
(4) A visiting doctor service to residential care homes continued to provide non-urgent medical care to residents.
(5) These measures, together with population behavior changes, have successfully contained the spread of the COVID-19 in long-term care facilities.

Disclosure statement

No potential conflict of interest was reported by the authors.

ORCID

Terry Lum PhD, MSW ⓘ http://orcid.org/0000-0003-1196-5345
Gloria Wong PhD ⓘ http://orcid.org/0000-0002-1331-942X

References

Anonymous. (2003, June 9). The death of a nursing home staff. *Ming Pao Daily.*

Census & Statistics Department. (2020). *Table E511: Visitors arrivals by country/region of residents.* Author. https://www.censtatd.gov.hk/hkstat/sub/sp130.jsp?productCode=D5600551

Comas-Herrera, A., Zalakaín, J., Litwin, C., Hsu, A. T., Lane, N., & Fernández, J.-L. (2020, May 3). *Mortality associated with COVID19 outbreaks in care homes: Early international evidence.* International Long-Term Care Policy Network. https://ltccovid.org/2020/04/12/mortality-associated-with-covid-19-outbreaks-in-care-homes-early-international-evidence/

Cowling, B. J., Ali, S. T., Ng, T. W. Y., Tsang, T. K., Li, J. C. M., Fong, M. W., Liao, Q., Kwan, M. Y., Lee, S. L., Chiu, S. S., Wu, J. T., Wu, P., & Leung, G. M. (2020, April 17). Impact assessment of non-pharmaceutical interventions against Coronavirus disease 2019 and influenza in Hong Kong: An observational study. *The Lancet Public Health, 5*(5), e279–e288. https://doi.org/10.1016/S2468-2667(20)30090-6

Euromonitor International. (2019). *Top 100 city destinations: 2019 edition.* Author. http://go.euromonitor.com/rs/805-KOK-719/images/wpTop100Cities19.pdf

Gibney, E. (2020, April 27). Whose Coronavirus strategy worked best? Scientists hunt most effective policies. *Nature, 581*(7806), 15–16. https://doi.org/10.1038/d41586-020-01248-1

Kong, T. K. (2006). SARS: Geriatric considerations. In J. C. K. Chan & V. C. W. Taam Wong (Eds.), *Challenges of severe acute respiratory syndrome* (pp. 451–476). Elsevier (Singapore) Pte Ltd.

Lee, S. H. (2003). The SARS epidemic in Hong Kong: What lessons have we learned? *Journal of the Royal Society of Medicine, 96*(8), 374–378. https://doi.org/10.1177/014107680309600803

Leung, G., Ho, L., Lam, T., & Hedley, A. (2009). Epidemiology of SARS in the 2003 Hong Kong epidemic. *Hong Kong Medical Journal, 15*(Supp 9), S12–16. https://www.hkmj.org/system/files/hkm0912sp9p12.pdf

Social Welfare Department. (2020). *Provision of residential care services for the elderly (subsidised versus non-subsidised places)* (as at 31. 3.2020). Author. https://www.swd.gov.hk/storage/asset/section/632/en/3.Provision_of_RCHEs_(Subsidised_versus_Non-subsidised_Places) (31.3.20).pdf

Wong, K., Lum, T., & Wong, G. (2020, April 27). *The COVID-19 long-term care situation in Hong Kong: Impact and measures.* International Long-Term Care Policy. https://ltccovid.org/wp-content/uploads/2020/04/Hong-Kong-COVID-19-Long-term-Care-situation-27-April-2020-1.pdf

Working Group on Elderly Services Programme Plan, Elderly Commission of Government of Hong Kong SAR. (2017). *Elderly services programme plan.* Author. https://www.elderlycommission.gov.hk/en/download/library/ESPP_Final_Report_Eng.pdf

High Risk Older Adults in Communities

Who are the Most At-Risk Older Adults in the COVID-19 Era? It's Not Just Those in Nursing Homes

Marc A. Cohen and Jane Tavares

ABSTRACT

COVID-19 has taken a terrible toll on the nursing home population. Yet, there are **five times** the number of seniors living in the community who are also extremely vulnerable because they suffer from respiratory illnesses. Using the 2018 wave of the Health and Retirement Study we analyze this group of roughly 7 million seniors living in the community and find that they have multiple risk factors that make them particularly exposed. We also show how current strategies for protecting this population may be exacerbating risks and suggest concrete steps for better protecting this group.

Much has been written about the terrible toll – current and projected – of the COVID-19 pandemic on the older adult population, and in particular, those living in nursing homes. Currently, there are roughly 1.3 million nursing facility residents (Kaiser Family Foundation, 2019), most of whom are older adults. This group is at very great risk for contracting the disease and is already paying a heavy price in the pandemic (Mosk et al., 2020). For many reasons, mortality rates are highest in homes where one or more residents have become infected. Some have estimated that upwards of 20% of nursing home residents will die from the illness (Syre, 2020). Moreover, more than three million older adults are living in close communal contact in independent living, assisted living, and senior housing facilities, thus placing them at high risk as well (Weisman, 2020).

The focus on this extremely vulnerable population is certainly warranted. However, even as nursing homes have been identified as a top priority for COVID-19 testing, it is important to note that there are **five times** the number of elders living in the community who would also be classified as extremely vulnerable, in large part because they currently suffer from respiratory illnesses (Condon & Herschaft, 2020). These include diseases such as asthma, Chronic Obstructive Pulmonary Disease (COPD), emphysema, and other conditions. In fact, our analysis of the 2018 wave of the Health and Retirement Study indicates that 12.6% of the roughly 55 million adults age 65 and over, or about 6.9 million elders, suffer from such respiratory ailments (AARP, n.d.; Institute for Social Research, 2020). This high prevalence among seniors explains, in part, why COVID-19 is particularly lethal among this age group (Begley, 2020). For instance, an estimated 13.4% of patients 80 and older have an infection fatality ratio, compared to 1.25% of those in their 50s, and 0.3% of those in their 40s (Verity et al., 2020).

In this perspective we characterize the community-dwelling senior population (including those residing in assisted living and other senior housing outside of nursing home facilities) with respiratory illnesses in terms of the socio-economic and health characteristics that put them at heightened risk in the context of the pandemic. We then briefly summarize how certain current approaches to the pandemic may be exposing them to additional risk and conclude by putting forward concrete actions to be taken to better protect them.

A highly vulnerable sub-population

Part of what makes the population living at home with respiratory illness so vulnerable is that they have multiple additional risk factors in addition to their respiratory problems. Our analysis (Figure 1), which compares some of

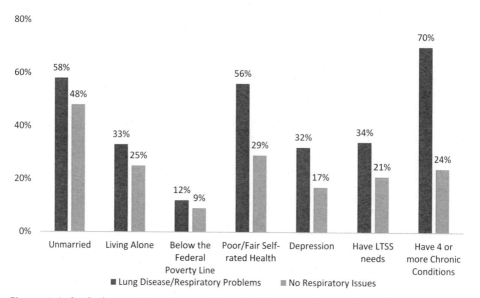

Figure 1. Individuals age 65 and over with and without respiratory issues by selected socio-demographic characteristics.

the key health and socio-demographic characteristics between groups with and without respiratory illnesses, shows that older adults living in non-institutional settings **with** respiratory illnesses are more likely to be unmarried and living alone and are 1.3 times more likely to be living below the poverty line.

Not surprisingly, older adults with chronic respiratory issues living on their own in the community also suffer from additional health issues that place them at high risk. They are about twice as likely to report that their health is fair or poor, twice as likely to report depression, 1.6 times as likely to need long-term services and supports (LTSS) in their homes, and 2.9 times more likely to have four or more chronic conditions (inclusive of, and often medically related to, their respiratory conditions) than are those without respiratory issues. This pattern of heightened risk is not surprising given that they tend to be somewhat older on average – age 77 versus age 74.

Given the profile of these individuals, the current strategy for dealing with the virus – social distancing – may be exacerbating other problems that already exist: namely, the problem of social isolation (Blumenthal et al., 2020). Specifically, 33% of individuals with respiratory illnesses live alone and we know from other research that many do not have Internet connections (Anderson & Perrin, 2017). There is a large body of literature documenting the negative health effects of social isolation (Holt-Lunstad et al., 2015). These effects have been considered more detrimental to health than smoking 15 cigarettes a day (Tate, 2018). Thus, while socially distancing or isolating individuals may be an appropriate short-term strategy to aid our health care system, over the long-term, it will likely lead to additional health-related issues for this population. As well, during the current pandemic non-urgent doctors' visits and chronic illness checkups are being significantly delayed or canceled. This means that even without contracting COVID-19, this population is facing increased health risks from reduced management of their existing respiratory disease (LTSS Center, 2020). Furthermore, for those with LTSS needs – roughly 34% of those with respiratory illnesses or 2.4 million people – there is an added risk: they are being cared for by front line home care workers who lack essential protective equipment amid national shortages, even basics such as hand sanitizers and gloves (Leland, 2020).

What can be done?

The coronavirus pandemic poses an elemental challenge to our society: How diligently will we respond to prioritize the safety and care of all groups who are at heightened risk, especially those older adults living at home with respiratory illnesses? We can meet this challenge in several ways, including the provision of additional testing, assessment, social support, and a focus on basic needs, as well as protection of the home care workers who care for them. Clearly, taking the actions we put forward below is not without challenges. There are continued shortages of tests, the front-line work force is already stretched caring for those who currently have symptoms of the illness, and not all care workers have personal protective equipment. Nevertheless, in order to minimize the potential harm for this group, taking these steps, at the earliest time possible, is both a public health and moral imperative.

Increasing testing

It is critically important that we prioritize older adults with known respiratory issues for coronavirus testing, wherever they live. Screening will save lives, as it will be possible to target resources to individuals who may be at the early stages of symptoms and illness onset, thus affording more potential for early intervention treatment options. Some states such as Massachusetts and Florida have targeted communities with higher populations of older adults and other at-risk individuals for random coronavirus testing among even among those who are asymptomatic as a way to track the virus and limit its spread. Screening those with known respiratory issues should fall under this same umbrella of targeted community testing efforts.

Conducting assessments

Healthcare providers such as physicians and hospital staff should proactively assess older adults' underlying medical and social conditions that pose a higher risk of death, should they contract COVID-19. This means proactively flagging all chronic conditions, particularly known respiratory issues, for all their patients' providers in order to encourage proper vigilance and early treatment.

Providing social support

Supportive services providers must reach out to this population using tele-health approaches in order to combat isolation and loneliness. A schedule of "check-ins" with isolated older adults is vital to provide social connection and meaningful interactions, either by way of telephone calls or, if the person has access, through video technologies that facilitate face-to-face interactions (e.g., Zoom, Facetime, Facebook Messenger video chat, Skype, etc.).

Meeting basic needs

Essential food and medicine must be delivered to these older adults in their homes so that they avoid potential exposure to the virus by going out, for the duration of time physical distancing needs to be practiced. This may be in the form of expanding already existing Meals on Wheels programs as well as coordinated efforts on the part of senior centers and/or food banks to reconfigure services to provide food delivery.

Protecting home care workers

Amid the national crisis of shortages of personal protective equipment (PPE), frontline workers providing LTSS to older adults in their homes lack essential protective equipment (Leland, 2020). These workers, and the people they dedicatedly care for, must be protected by prioritizing allocation of PPE to them (Beckman et al., 2020). In addition, this work force needs other protections: financial protections similar to those that were provided to 9/11 emergency responders; the ability to self-isolate and not come to work when sick; regular testing; and compensated respite days.

Conclusion

Even amidst the mounting reports of catastrophic transmission and fatality clusters within institutional settings, we must be proactive in monitoring and caring for the millions of older adults with preexisting respiratory disease living on their own in the community. Further, it is not only the pandemic-related illness that should be of concern to us. This group suffers a variety of health and social challenges that must be tended to even in the midst of this pandemic. There are already reports of individuals not using hospitals and emergency rooms when they should be doing so, due to fears about catching the virus, concerns about over-burdening front-line health workers, or a lack of transportation (Hearst Television, Inc., 2020). The multi-prong approach that we are advocating here should help to ameliorate these concerns and mitigate further risk. It is incumbent on us to work together with urgency to keep these vulnerable seniors safe.

Key points

- Seniors living in the community with respiratory illnesses are particularly vulnerable to COVID-19.
- This population suffers from multiple health and social risks and if exposed to the virus, are likely to face very high mortality rates.
- Current approaches for protecting this population are inadequate and may exacerbate the risks faced.
- What is needed is a focus on improved testing, better assessment, increased social supports, assurance that basic needs are being met, and protection for home care workers.

Disclosure statement

No potential conflict of interest was reported by the authors.

Funding

This work was supported by the Self Funded.

References

AARP. (n.d.). *Baby boomer facts on 50+ livable communities and aging in place.* AARP Livable Communities. Retrieved April 27, 2020, from http://www.aarp.org/livable-communities/info-2014/livable-communities-facts-and-figures.html

Anderson, M., & Perrin, A. (2017, May 17). *Technology use among seniors.* Pew Research Center: Internet, Science & Tech. https://www.pewresearch.org/internet/2017/05/17/technology-use-among-seniors/

Beckman, A. L., Gondi, S., & Forman, H. P. (2020, March 18). *How to stand behind frontline health care workers fighting coronavirus.* Health Affairs. https://www.healthaffairs.org/do/10.1377/hblog20200316.393860/full/

Begley, S. (2020, March 30). *What explains Covid-19's lethality for the elderly?* STAT Health. https://www.statnews.com/2020/03/30/what-explains-coronavirus-lethality-for-elderly/

Blumenthal, D., Jacobson, G., & Shah, T. (2020, April 3). The gaps in our social safety net. *The Hill.* Opinion. https://thehill.com/opinion/healthcare/491007-the-gaps-in-our-social-safety-net

Condon, B., & Herschaft, R. (2020, April 13). Nursing home deaths soar past 3,600 in alarming surge. *The Idaho News.* https://idahonews.com/news/coronavirus/nursing-home-deaths-soar-past-3600-in-alarming-surge

Hearst Television, Inc. (2020, April 23). *Gov. Baker urges people who need non-COVID-19 emergency care to seek it* [Video]. https://www.wcvb.com/article/gov-charlie-baker-urges-people-who-need-non-covid-19-emergency-care-to-seek-it/32255040

Holt-Lunstad, J., Smith, T. B., Baker, M., Harris, T., & Stephenson, D. (2015). Loneliness and social isolation as risk factors for mortality: A meta-analytic review. *Perspectives on Psychological Science, 10*(2), 227–237. https://doi.org/10.1177/1745691614568352

Institute for Social Research. (2020). *Health and retirement study.* Health and Retirement Study. https://hrs.isr.umich.edu/

Kaiser Family Foundation. (2019, June 3). *Total number of residents in certified nursing facilities.* The Henry J. Kaiser Family Foundation: State Health Facts. https://www.kff.org/other/state-indicator/number-of-nursing-facility-residents/

Leland, J. (2020, March 22). She had to choose: Her Epileptic patient or her 7-year-old daughter. *The New York Times.* https://www.nytimes.com/2020/03/22/nyregion/coronavirus-caregivers-nyc.html

LTSS Center. (2020, March 23). *COVID-19 is disrupting services for older adults living in community.* The LeadingAge LTSS Center @UMass Boston. https://www.ltsscenter.org/covid-19-is-disrupting-services-for-older-adults-living-in-community/

Mosk, M., Romero, L., Pecorin, A., & Freger, H. (2020, April 19). Inside nursing homes, coronavirus brings isolation and 7,300 deaths; Outside, families yearn for news. *ABC News.* https://abcnews.go.com/Health/inside-nursing-homes-coronavirus-brings-isolation-7300-deaths/story?id=70225836

Syre, S. (2020, April 6). *Institute talk: A conversation with Hospice Physician Joanne Lynn about nursing homes dealing with COVID-19.* University of Massachusetts Boston: The Gerontology Institute Blog. http://blogs.umb.edu/gerontologyinstitute/2020/04/06/insti tute-talk-a-conversation-with-hospice-physician-joanne-lynn-about-nursing-homes-deal ing-with-covid-19/

Tate, N. (2018, May 4). *Loneliness rivals obesity, smoking as health risk.* WebMD. https:// www.webmd.com/balance/news/20180504/loneliness-rivals-obesity-smoking-as-health-risk

Verity, R., Okell, L. C., Dorigatti, I., Winskill, P., Whittaker, C., Imai, N., Cuomo-Dannenburg, G., Thompson, H., Walker, P. G. T., Fu, H., Dighe, A., Griffin, J. T., Baguelin, M., Bhatia, S., Boonyasiri, A., Cori, A., Cucunubá, Z., FitzJohn, R., Gaythorpe, K., Hamlet, A., ... Ferguson, N. M. (2020). Estimates of the severity of coronavirus disease 2019: A model-based analysis. *The Lancet Infectious Diseases.* https://doi.org/10.1016/S1473-3099(20)30243-7

Weisman, R. (2020, April 26). *Assisted-living sites struggle with coronavirus in shadow of nursing home crisis—The Boston Globe.* The Boston Globe. https://www.bostonglobe.com/2020/04/26/metro/assisted-living-sites-struggle-with-covid-19-shadow-nursing-home-crisis/

Meeting the Transitional Care Needs of Older Adults with COVID-19

Mary D. Naylor ⓘ, Karen B. Hirschman ⓘ, and Kathleen McCauley

ABSTRACT

Older adults with COVID-19 who survive hospitalizations and return to their homes confront substantial health challenges and an unpredictable future. While understanding of the unique needs of COVID-19 survivors is developing, components of the evidence-based Transitional Care Model provide a framework for taking a more immediate, holistic response to caring for these individuals as they moved back into the community. These components include: increasing screening, building trusting relationships, improving patient engagement, promoting collaboration across care teams, undertaking symptom management, increasing family caregiver care/education, coordinating health and social services, and improving care continuity. Evidence generated from rigorous testing of these components reveal the need for federal and state policy solutions to support the following: employment/redeployment of nurses, social workers, and community health workers; training and reimbursement of family caregivers; widespread access to research-based transitional care tools; and coordinated local efforts to address structural barriers to effective transitions. Immediate action on these policy options is necessary to more effectively address the complex issues facing these older adults and their family caregivers who are counting on our care system for essential support.

The unprecedented response by health systems and government at all levels prompted by the emergence and rapid spread of the coronavirus has focused on the heroic efforts of hospital staff to save lives. In contrast, comparatively little attention has been paid to the care needs of the nine out of 10 adults who survive hospitalizations and return to their homes (Richardson et al., 2020). Most of these survivors are older adults who are coping with multiple chronic conditions and social vulnerabilities and whose health status is substantially complicated by the devastating impact of this virus (Richardson et al., 2020). For many, early evidence suggests that complex and long-term physical, functional, cognitive, and emotional negative health consequences will be the norm (Stam et al., 2020). However, the trajectories of healthcare needs of older adults with COVID-19 in the weeks and months following hospital discharge have yet to be identified. Nor are the challenges that their needs pose for family caregivers well understood. This essential knowledge will develop with time. In the nearer term, the core components of the Transitional Care Model demonstrated to effectively address the holistic needs of "at risk" older adults, coupled with early findings regarding the unique concerns of those with COVID-19, suggest a path for immediate practice and policy responses to caring for this population as they transition back from the hospital to the community.

A framework for immediate action

The Transitional Care Model is a care management strategy proven in multiple National Institutes of Health clinical trials to enhance health and quality of life and reduce health-care costs for diverse subgroups of hospitalized older adults to home. The evidence-based components of the Transitional Care model provide a framework to address the complex care needs of older adults with COVID-19 throughout episodes of acute illness (Naylor et al., 1994, 1999, 2004, 2014). These components include increasing screening, building trusting relationships, improving patient engagement, promoting collaboration across care teams, undertaking symptom management, increasing family caregiver care/education, coordinating health and social services, and improving care continuity.

Increasing screening

To assure the delivery of timely and effective transitional care services for older adults with COVID-19, the consistent use of a standardized screening tool to identify and communicate health and social factors that increase their risk for poor outcomes is necessary. Such a tool must provide a comprehensive assessment of the needs of older adults, including information on preexisting physical, behavioral health, and cognitive conditions, functional deficits, and social vulnerabilities such as low socioeconomic status. Risks unique to COVID-19 must include key symptoms (e.g., shortness of breath) and treatments (e.g., days on ventilators). Equally important are data about family caregivers (i.e., relatives, neighbors, or friends, hereafter referred at as caregivers) whose availability (e.g., ability and willingness to provide in-home support) and capacity (e.g., health status, knowledge, and skills) certainly impacts older adults' risks. Factors unique to this pandemic include data regarding caregivers' development of COVID-19 symptoms and their mental health responses to the crisis. Mechanisms to assure timely communication of screening findings with acute, primary, post-acute care and community-based staff involved in older adults' care are essential to enable these team members' to prioritize timing of contacts with patients at higher risk for adverse outcomes and position them with interventions targeting risk mitigation.

Building trusting relationships

Developing and maintaining trusting interpersonal relationships between older adults, caregivers and members of the care team are an important focus especially for the high proportion of socially disadvantaged older adults who are hospitalized with COVID-19 (Center for Disease Control, 2020), many of whom lack trust in the healthcare system (Guerrero et al., 2015). Given severe restrictions in hospital visitation policies coupled with substantially decreased in-person contact following discharge, care team members are increasingly relying on phones, texts, and video conferencing to communicate with older adults and their caregivers. While such modifications to care delivery are understandable, attention must be paid to assure that effective, culturally sensitive strategies are considered in the development of digital forms of communication. For example, engaging people who represent diverse racial and ethnic groups in the design of communication technologies will help to ensure that e-health literacy and language competency are addressed into these solutions (Barclay et al., 2014). Standards that promote the engagement of minorities in the creation of these solutions and foster the education of health professionals to deliver culturally sensitive digital care need to be advanced (Chang et al., 2004). Of critical importance is the role of a clinician who is the consistent point person in communications with older adults and their caregivers.

Improving patient engagement

Collectively, the severity of older adults' illnesses, limited in-person contact with caregivers, and overwhelmed hospital nurses and physicians have made identifying what matters to older adults and aligning plans of care with their preferences and values enormously difficult during this crisis. Indeed, these challenges highlight the importance of advance care plans that clearly describe older adults' goals of care. Public service messages should encourage immediate conversations between older adults, family caregivers, and primary care clinicians to develop advance care plans and to make sure those plans are documented in electronic health records. Given that most hospitalized older adults with COVID-19 are individuals confronting multiple other risks, special attention should be paid to their decision-making regarding the potential use of ventilators. Since early findings reveal that as many as half of the older adults placed on ventilators did not survive (Richardson et al., 2020), some might choose palliative versus curative care. Among those hospitalized who have not communicated goals of care, every effort should be made to connect with knowledgeable caregivers and assure that discussion of treatment options takes into consideration older adults' goals. Fostering engagement of older adults must extend throughout the entire illness episode to assure that changes in goals associated with worsening health status are clearly communicated.

Promoting collaboration across care teams

Achieving consensus on plans of care between members of the hospital, post-acute, and primary care teams is complicated under the best of circumstance, with challenges exacerbated during this pandemic. At the peak of the crisis, traditional investments made by hospital clinicians in discussing care plans with primary or post-acute providers were impossible. Clinicians' priorities were to stabilize patients and to transfer them as quickly as possible to make room for others. Even as the number of hospitalizations have declined, effective collaboration remains difficult. Given the expected spread of this disease for months and perhaps years to come, employment/redeployment of nurses who are not involved in the care of COVID-19 patients to assume a primary role in assuring high-quality collaboration among all team members should be a priority. As of early May, over 1.4 million of America's health-care workers, including nurses, lost their jobs (Sanger-Katz, 2020). While many of these positions will be restored, increased financial strain among hospitals may result in some longer-term unemployment. Additionally, many hospital nurses who have been serving on the front lines throughout this pandemic may benefit emotionally from role changes. On-line programs (e.g., *Foundations in Transitional Care*) exist to rapidly prepare nurses for these central roles. Federal programs established to mitigate the impact of COVID-19 on unemployment, especially among health-care workers, and health plans seeking to prevent breakdowns in care that result in costly hospital read-missions are likely to support this training.

Undertaking symptom management

Early identification and management of older adults' physical, emotional, and cognitive symptoms are especially tricky given limited evidence about the course of this disease and, for many, its ultimate human consequences. At hospital discharge, most adults with COVID-19 are physically and emotionally depleted; some also report cognitive deficits (Khullar, 2020; The New York Times, 2020). At the same time, these patients confront a largely unpredictable future in a context, for many, characterized by social isolation and financial distress. Little wonder that early reports of anxiety and depression are common among COVID-19 survivors (Horowitz, 2020; The New York Times, 2020). Health systems have responded by substantially increasing their outreach using telehealth and other virtual tools with a primary goal of assessing physical symptom changes. Monitoring needs to be extended to include assessment and effective management of cognitive deficits and mental health concerns as a failure to address these issues will have prolonged negative health consequences (Ohrnberger et al., 2017). Engaging and training community health workers to conduct such assessments and implement an early intervention for those with mild deficits, coupled with the increased use of social workers who can provide support for more severe challenges, are examples of strategies that have the potential to mitigate the impact of COVID-19 for this population.

In 2019, approximately 60,000 community health workers were providing a range of largely social support services in U.S. communities (U.S. Bureau of Labor Statistics, 2020). Evidence from other countries suggest these trained lay people also could play a major role in identifying mental health issues such as depression or anxiety and helping those with mild issues (Stanley et al., 2014). The Center for Medicare and Medicaid Innovation should support the testing of the effects of trained community health workers in identifying and managing the mental health challenges experienced by older adults with COVID-19 and their caregivers throughout challenging health-care transitions. Additionally, future efforts aimed at reducing unemployment in socially disadvantaged communities should target the expansion of community health workers.

Increasing family caregiver care/education

COVID-19 has placed a spotlight on the critical role of caregivers in assuring that the complex post-hospital care needs of older adults are addressed. Notably, preparing these "invisible caregivers" to meet expectations is occurring at a time when they are personally coping with the impact of this virus. Additionally, restrictions on visitations have prevented them from receiving teaching and instruction typically provided by hospital staff. In-person contact with home health-care teams, primary care providers, or care managers who generally provide similar guidance also is very limited. Thus, much of the preparation being provided to family caregivers is being delivered using telehealth. Caregivers confront the same set of challenges in receiving support through this mechanism as do older adults. Accessing telehealth, especially among disadvantaged populations, is hampered by limited Internet connectivity and access to technology (Yoon et al., 2020). Additionally, effective use of this mechanism in addressing the needs of culturally diverse subgroups, some of whom do not speak English, has not been demonstrated. Once again, rapid engagement of nurses and preparing them to identify caregivers' needs and support them during these very challenging times are essential.

Coordinating health and social services

Coordinating health and social services for older adults with COVID-19 has been challenged by failures to universally adopt commonsense solutions. For example, the Caregiver Advise, Record, Enable (CARE) Act, is a model state legislation designed, in part, to make sure the names of family caregivers who will assume primary responsibility for hospitalized older adults' care following transition to home are documented in their medical records. At times of crisis, immediate access to this basic information is central to effective transitions. As of 2019, 40 states and territories have enacted CARE Acts (Reinhard et al., 2019).

Another challenge to effective coordination has been the lack of consistent guidance to health-care facilities throughout this crisis. Early in the pandemic, for example, federal and state agencies strongly recommended that skilled nursing facilities (SNFs) refuse to accept COVID-19 patients (Center for Clinical Standards and Quality/Quality Safety & Oversight Group, 2020). By late April, some states reversed course and ordered SNFs to accept such patients (Schoch, 2020). Since then, some SNFs have decided to specialize in the care of COVID-19 residents. Others have instituted protocols that require clustering of infected residents in one area, assigning consistent staff to those residents for at least 14 days, and routinely testing all staff and residents to mitigate the spread of this deadly disease. Despite the availability of these protocols, SNFs in some regions still refuse to accept COVID-19 patients. Consequently, this group of patients require high-intensity, post-acute care in their homes (Werner & Van Houtven, 2020). This solution generally entails 24/7 telehealth support supplemented by in-home visits by nurses for services such as symptom management and intravenous infusions and therapists for post-acute rehabilitation. Faced with unsatisfactory alternatives for especially complex patients, clinicians continue to confront difficult transitional care decisions. Strong collaboration among leaders of local health-care organizations and policymakers is needed to remove this decision-making burden from clinicians and provide them with consistent and unified responses to challenges such as this.

The longer-term burden of coordinating care rests with their caregivers. In addition to monitoring older adults, making sure they receive their medications and other treatments, and communicating with multiple care team members, caregivers also are attempting to access food and other supplies while being asked to stay at home. For some, the financial burden associated with addressing older adults' needs, especially those caregivers affected by unemployment, only adds to their stress. Once again, engaging and training community health workers to collaborate with social workers to support these caregivers is essential to positive health outcomes for both older adults and their caregivers.

Improving care continuity

Given massive disruptions in the delivery of person-centered care following the rapid spread of COVID-19, the critical need for a single clinician to whom older adults and caregivers can confidently turn throughout vulnerable transitions cannot be overstated. The information overload accompanying this disease, for example, requires a trusted broker to assist these populations in accessing reliable and continually evolving knowledge regarding symptoms and treatments. Once again, rapid employment/redeployment of nurses to fill this role represents an immediate opportunity to address huge gaps in the area of care continuity.

Opportunities for policies to advance immediate action

Informed by this evidence-based framework, immediate implementation of targeted federal and state policy solutions would position a health and community-based care systems to respond more effectively to the enormous challenges encountered by older adults with COVID-19 throughout transitions from hospital to home. The following are among the key options federal and state policymakers should pursue:

- Support for rapid employment/redeployment and training of nurses, social workers, and community health workers to assume the transitional care roles described above.
- Investment in training and reimbursement of family caregivers to support them in assuming transitional care responsibilities.
- Universal adoption and implementation of the CARE Act.
- Investment in the design and implementation of public service messages (e.g., related to advance care planning), tools (e.g., standardized screening, effective communication using virtual technology), and strategies (e.g., addressing access to telehealth), all focused on improving care transitions.
- Support for local coordination to identify and address structural barriers to care transitions.

Conclusion

Increased understanding of the unique challenges facing older adults hospitalized with COVID-19 who transition to home is required. In the meantime, components of the evidence-based Transitional Care Model provide a framework for undertaking more immediate holistic responses to meeting the needs of this population. To more effectively address the complex issues confronting this population and support their family caregivers, immediate action on targeted policy solutions is needed.

Key points

- Little is known about the needs of older adults with COVID-19 after hospital discharge.
- Components of a transitional care model offer a framework for immediate response.
- Policies targeting training and support of key workforce members are a priority.
- Coordinated local efforts are needed to address barriers to care transitions.

Disclosure statement

No potential conflict of interest was reported by the authors.

ORCID

Mary D. Naylor PhD, RN, FAAN ⓘ http://orcid.org/0000-0001-9287-153X
Karen B. Hirschman PhD, MSW ⓘ http://orcid.org/0000-0003-4886-7765

References

Barclay, G., Sabina, A., & Graham, G. (2014). Population health and technology: Placing people first. *American Journal of Public Health*, *104*(12), 2246–2247. https://doi.org/10.2105/AJPH.2014.302334

Center for Clinical Standards and Quality/Quality Safety & Oversight Group. (2020). *Guidance for infection control and prevention of coronavirus disease 2019 (COVID-19) in nursing homes (REVISED)* (Ref: QSO-20-14-NH). David R. Wright (Director, Quality, Safety & Oversight Group); Centers for Medicare and Medicaid Services. https://www.cms.gov/files/document/qso-20-14-nh-revised.pdf

Center for Disease Control. (2020). *COVID view a weekly surveillance summary of U.S. COVID-19 activity (May 8, 2020)*. Centers for Disease Control and Prevention. Retrieved May 11, from https://www.cdc.gov/coronavirus/2019-ncov/covid-data/covidview/index.html

Chang, B. L., Bakken, S., Brown, S. S., Houston, T. K., Kreps, G. L., Kukafka, R., Safran, C., & Stavri, P. Z. (2004). Bridging the digital divide: Reaching vulnerable populations. *Journal of the American Medical Informatics Association*, *11*(6), 448–457. https://doi.org/10.1197/jamia.M1535

Guerrero, N., Mendes de Leon, C. F., Evans, D. A., & Jacobs, E. A. (2015). Determinants of trust in health care in an older population. *Journal of the American Geriatrics Society*, *63*(3), 553–557. https://doi.org/10.1111/jgs.13316

Horowitz, J. (2020, May 10). Surviving Covid-19 may not feel like recovery for some. *The New York Times*. https://www.nytimes.com/2020/05/10/world/europe/coronavirus-italy-recovery.html

Khullar, D. (2020, April 23). The challenges of post-COVID-19 care. *The New Yorker*. https://www.newyorker.com/science/medical-dispatch/the-challenges-of-post-covid-19-care

Naylor, M., Brooten, D., Jones, R., Lavizzo-Mourey, R., Mezey, M., & Pauly, M. (1994). Comprehensive discharge planning for the hospitalized elderly: A randomized clinical trial. *Annals Internal Medicine, 120*(12), 999–1006. https://doi.org/10.7326/0003-4819-120-12-199406150-00005

Naylor, M. D., Brooten, D., Campbell, R., Jacobsen, B. S., Mezey, M. D., Pauly, M. V., & Schwartz, J. S. (1999). Comprehensive discharge planning and home follow-up of hospitalized elders: A randomized clinical trial. *Journal of the American Medical Association, 281*(7), 613–620. https://doi.org/10.1001/jama.281.7.613

Naylor, M. D., Brooten, D. A., Campbell, R. L., Maislin, G., McCauley, K. M., & Schwartz, J. S. (2004). Transitional care of older adults hospitalized with heart failure: A randomized, controlled trial. *Journal of the American Geriatrics Society, 52*(5), 675–684. https://doi.org/10.1111/j.1532-5415.2004.52202.x

Naylor, M. D., Hirschman, K. B., Hanlon, A. L., Bowles, K. H., Bradway, C., McCauley, K. M., & Pauly, M. V. (2014). Comparison of evidence-based interventions on outcomes of hospitalized, cognitively impaired older adults. *Journal of Comparative Effectiveness Research, 3*(3), 245–257. https://doi.org/10.2217/cer.14.14

The New York Times. (2020, May 7). 'An Anvil sitting on my chest': What it's like to have Covid-19. *The New York Times.* https://www.nytimes.com/article/coronavirus-symptoms.html

Ohrnberger, J., Fichera, E., & Sutton, M. (2017). The dynamics of physical and mental health in the older population. *Journal of the Economics of Ageing, 9*(2017), 52–62. https://doi.org/10.1016/j.jeoa.2016.07.002

Reinhard, S., Young, H., Ryan, E., & Choula, R. (2019). *The CARE act implementation: Progress and promise.* AARP Public Policy Institute. https://www.aarp.org/content/dam/aarp/ppi/2019/03/the-care-act-implementation-progress-and-promise.pdf

Richardson, S., Hirsch, J. S., Narasimhan, M., Crawford, J. M., McGinn, T., & Davidson, K. W., & the Northwell COVID-19 Research Consortium. (2020, April 30). Presenting characteristics, comorbidities, and outcomes among 5700 patients hospitalized with COVID-19 in the New York City area. *Journal of the American Medical Association, 20*(323), 2052–2059.. https://doi.org/10.1001/jama.2020.6775

Sanger-Katz, M. (2020, May 8). Why 1.4 million health jobs have been lost during a huge health crisis. *The New York Times.* https://www.nytimes.com/2020/05/08/upshot/health-jobs-plummeting-virus.html

Schoch, D. (2020, April 21). *Nursing homes Balk at COVID patient transfers from hospitals: States pressure homes to take patients.* AARP. https://www.aarp.org/caregiving/health/info-2020/coronavirus-transfers-to-nursing-homes.html

Stam, H. J., Stucki, G., & Bickenbach, J. (2020). Covid-19 and post intensive care syndrome: A call for action. *Journal of Rehabilitation Medicine, 52*(4), jrm00044. https://doi.org/10.2340/16501977-2677

Stanley, M. A., Wilson, N. L., Amspoker, A. B., Kraus-Schuman, C., Wagener, P. D., Calleo, J. S., Cully, J. A., Teng, E., Rhoades, H. M., Williams, S., Masozera, N., Horsfield, M., & Kunik, M. E. (2014). Lay providers can deliver effective cognitive behavior therapy for older adults with generalized anxiety disorder: A randomized trial. *Depression and Anxiety, 31*(5), 391–401. https://doi.org/10.1002/da.22239

U.S. Bureau of Labor Statistics. (2020, March 31). *Occupational employment and wages, May 2019; 21-1094 community health workers.* U.S. Department of Labor. Retrieved May 18, from https://www.bls.gov/oes/current/oes211094.htm

Werner, R., & Van Houtven, C. (2020). In the time of Covid-19, we should move high-intensity postacute care home. *Health Affairs Blog.* https://www.healthaffairs.org/do/10.1377/hblog20200422.924995/full/

Yoon, H., Jang, Y., Vaughan, P. W., & Garcia, M. (2020). Older adults' Internet use for health information: Digital divide by race/ethnicity and socioeconomic status. *Journal of Applied Gerontology, 39*(1), 105–110. https://doi.org/10.1177/0733464818770772

The Unique Impact of COVID-19 on Older Adults in Rural Areas

Carrie Henning-Smith (ID)

ABSTRACT

Older adults in rural areas of the U.S. face unique risks related to COVID-19. Rural areas are older, on average, than urban areas, and have more underlying health conditions and fewer economic resources. Rural health care is more limited, as is access to technology and online connectivity. Altogether, this puts rural older adults at risk of not only the virus, but of not being able to meet their health care, social, and basic needs. Rural/urban inequities, combined with within-rural inequities in health, health care, and financial resources cause particular challenges to health and well-being from COVID-19 for some older adults.

Introduction

Many of the risk factors for COVID-19 are exacerbated in rural areas and rural older adults lie at the center of that. Rural areas have older populations (Pender et al., 2019), on average, and more people with underlying health conditions than suburban and urban communities (National Center for Health Statistics, 2018), both of which make rural communities and older adults living within them uniquely susceptible to the virus (Centers for Disease Control and Prevention, 2020). Rural residents, including older adults, have fewer financial resources to help them weather the economic impact of COVID-19, relative to urban residents (Pender et al., 2019). Rural areas also face persistent challenges related to health care capacity, including health care workforce shortages and hospital closures (Brown et al., 2011; The Cecil G. Sheps Center for Health Services Research, 2020). As a result, older adults living in rural areas may struggle to access the care they need, both for COVID-19 and other emergent and chronic health problems during the pandemic. This perspective identifies challenges posed by limited health care capacity for rural older adults in light of the COVID-19 pandemic. It also addresses the devasting economic impact of the pandemic for rural older adults and the difficulties posed for meeting rural older adults' social and emotional needs. The implications of within-rural inequities are discussed as well.

Health care capacity

Rural areas have persistent challenges to maintaining health care access of all types. Particularly relevant for COVID-19, more than 125 rural communities have seen their local hospital close in the past decade and many other rural communities have hospitals that struggle to make ends meet from month to month (The Cecil G. Sheps Center for Health Services Research, 2020). As social distancing requires cancelation of routine and elective procedures and appointments, the financial status of rural hospitals has become even more tenuous (Siegler, 2020).

Health care facilities within rural communities are less well-resourced and are struggling to access testing, personal protective equipment, and intensive care unit beds and necessary equipment to serve people most severely affected by the virus, many of whom will be older adults. As a result, many rural hospitals, including Critical Access Hospitals, find themselves needing to transfer rural residents with more serious cases of COVID-19 to larger facilities in urban areas for treatment (Diaz et al., 2020). Leaving one's community for care may be both frightening and disorienting, especially when visitors are not allowed. Long-term care facilities in rural areas also have long-standing challenges, including recruiting and retaining workforce (Brown et al., 2011) and disparities in quality of care relative to urban facilities (Bowblis et al., 2013). Health care workers face heightened risk of exposure to COVID-19 and rural facilities – including long-term care – do not always have a deep bench from which to pull in additional help. As COVID-19 has already spread to the majority of rural counties in the U.S. (Ullrich & Mueller, 2020), this raises important and concerning issues about the capacity of rural health care to serve older adults affected by the virus.

Economic impact

Further, the economic impact of this pandemic has the potential to be devastating in many rural communities. Rural areas recovered more slowly from the Great Recession of the late 2000's and already had lower median incomes and higher poverty rates than urban areas (Pender et al., 2019). Older adults in rural areas have higher poverty rates and fewer resources available to them compared to their counterparts in urban areas (Hash et al., 2015). A 2017 report from AARP and IMPAQ International found that more than one-third of older adults in rural areas had multiple unmet social needs, including food insecurity, inadequate transportation, loneliness, and strained financial resources (Pooler et al., 2017). Housing stock in rural areas is also older, and of poorer quality than housing stock in urban areas (White, 2015), which may be problematic if older adults, especially those living alone, are isolating themselves in their homes without visitors during the COVID-19 pandemic. Poorer quality housing is associated with higher risks of poor health outcomes for older adults, and safety issues (e.g., falls) may arise for older adults with functional limitations if they are navigating multiple floors or houses without appropriate safety features while isolating at home (Henning-Smith et al., 2018; White, 2015). Altogether, there is less of a cushion to absorb financial losses in rural areas, including among older adults. COVID-19 has already caused an economic crisis and recovery will likely be slow and difficult. For older adults in rural areas, many of whom were already living on the brink of making ends meet, economic disruption in their lives and in their communities could be particularly injurious.

Meeting basic needs – social and otherwise

COVID-19 also poses unique risks to the emotional and social well-being of older adults in rural areas. To protect against the worst of COVID-19, and to give our health care and other essential workers a fighting chance to endure this pandemic and provide timely care to those who need it, we must distance ourselves from one another as much as possible. This physical distancing is necessary to "flatten the curve", and yet is causing widespread feelings of isolation and loneliness. To counter this, an incredible amount of creatively and resourcefulness has been poured into finding ways to connect with one another virtually. While most people may be grateful for any and all tools to stay connected, it is important to recognize inequities in who has access to the technology and connectivity needed to foster social relationships online.

A recent Pew Research Center report showed that less than two-thirds of rural adults in the U.S. have broadband Internet at home (compared with three-quarters of urban adults); rural adults also have consistently lower rates of smartphone, computer, and tablet ownership (Perrin, 2019). Even when rural residents have access to the Internet, it is often at slower speeds with poorer connections, making synchronous activities like video-conferencing especially difficult (Kaur, 2020). Access to and use of online technology is also consistently lower among older adults than their younger counterparts, with rates especially low among adults age 80+ and those with lower incomes (Anderson & Perrin, 2017). As a result, older adults in rural areas are among the most likely to be left out of any creative, technologically-based adaptations to meet social and other needs during this crisis.

The University of Minnesota Rural Health Research Center (UMNRHRC) has shown that, while rural older adults have larger and stronger social networks (both friends and family) than their urban peers, they are also more likely to experience feelings of loneliness (Henning-Smith, Moscovice, et al., 2019). The reasons for these seemingly contradictory findings are complex, but likely relate to unique challenges in rural areas related to addressing social isolation, including geographic distances, transportation challenges, and financial constraints (Henning-Smith, Ecklund, et al., 2019). As people stay home to slow the spread of COVID-19, inequities in loneliness for rural older adults could be exacerbated, especially among those who are left out of opportunities to connect virtually. People living alone during this time face particular risks of isolation and loneliness (Lewis et al., 2020). The UMNRHRC recently released a study showing that living alone is more common in nonmetropolitan (rural) counties than in metropolitan (urban) counties, including among older adults (Henning-Smith et al., 2020). Given these differences, rural older adults face considerable barriers to meeting their social and emotional needs during this already frightening time.

Beyond social connectedness, there are new and complicated challenges to meeting one's basic daily needs in the era of COVID-19. Grocery shopping, running errands, accessing health care, and having assistance in the home all come with new risks. In urban areas, people with the financial means to do so have options to have groceries delivered. Rural areas are less likely to have the infrastructure in place for grocery delivery (Brandt et al., 2019). Rural areas also face constraints in accessing other resources virtually, including telehealth, given the aforementioned constraints on online connectivity. For older adults in rural areas who already had difficulty leaving home, and who rely on home-delivered meals, even brief social and wellness check-ins with their meal delivery drivers have become challenging (Gunderson, 2020). For older adults in remote rural locations, going without even those brief in-person interactions may be profoundly isolating – and potentially dangerous.

Within-rural inequities

Finally, beyond rural/urban inequities in health, health care, and the potential consequences of COVID-19, it is important to acknowledge the fact that not all rural areas and not all rural residents face the same level of risk. Rural older adults already living at or near the poverty line and those living far from health care providers and facilities will likely face the greater challenges in accessing the care they need in a timely manner. Transportation barriers and concerns about any out-of-pocket costs related to treatment – for COVID-19 or other health issues that emerge during this crisis – may prevent some rural older adults from getting the care they need quickly enough – or at all.

Rural areas also contain significant racial and ethnic diversity and rural counties with a majority of Black or Indigenous residents had higher rates of premature death, food insecurity, and unemployment and lower median incomes before COVID-19 (C. E. Henning-Smith et al., 2019). Today, those same counties are experiencing higher rates of mortality from COVID-19, as structural racism puts people of color and Indigenous folks at higher risk for adverse health outcomes (Kijakazi, 2020). Older adults living in those rural counties will likely face heightened risk of both the health and economic consequences of this pandemic, as will rural older adults of color across the country.

Conclusion

Older adults living in rural areas face particular risks and challenges related to COVID-19. While older adults are by no means universally susceptible to this virus, nor are they its only victims, they do face unique risks. In rural areas, the greater proportion of older adults, coupled with higher rates of underlying health conditions and more limited access to health care creates a volatile combination for COVID-19 risk. Preexisting rural/urban inequities related to health care capacity, economic security, access to technology, and social needs, together with within-rural inequities by socio-demographic characteristics together amount to heightened risk of illness and isolation for many older adults in rural areas. Further, rural hospitals and clinics, many of which were already teetering on the edge of financial solvency, are vulnerable to closure during this pandemic as they limit elective and routine procedures. Should any more of those close – or other social and economic infrastructure collapse in rural communities – the long-term impact for rural older adults will be felt well beyond COVID-19. Immediate action is needed to slow the spread of COVID-19, to support health care and other essential workers, and to protect those at highest risk from the virus. But, emerging from this on the other side, much more work is needed to address underlying inequities in access to health and wellbeing for rural older adults.

Key Points

- Older adults living in rural areas face unique risks from COVID-19.
- Rural areas are older, and have fewer economic and health care resources.
- Rural older adults have challenges to connecting online, increasing loneliness risk.
- Risk is not equally distributed among rural older adults.

Disclosure statement

No potential conflict of interest was reported by the author.

ORCID

Carrie Henning-Smith ⓘ http://orcid.org/0000-0002-0273-0387

References

Anderson, M., & Perrin, A. (2017). *Tech adoption climbs among older adults*. Pew Research Center. Retrieved from https://www.pewresearch.org/internet/wp-content/uploads/sites/9/2017/05/PI_2017.05.17_Older-Americans-Tech_FINAL.pdf

Bowblis, J. R., Meng, H., & Hyer, K. (2013). The urban-rural disparity in nursing home quality indicators: The case of facility-acquired contractures. *Health Services Research, 48*(1), 47–69. http://dx.doi.org/10.1111/j.1475-6773.2012.01431.x

Brandt, E. J., Silvestri, D. M., Mande, J. R., Holland, M. L., & Ross, J. S. (2019). Availability of grocery delivery to food deserts in states participating in the online purchase pilot. *JAMA Network Open, 2*(12), e1916444. http://dx.doi.org/10.1001/jamanetworkopen.2019.16444

Brown, D. K., Lash, S., Wright, B., & Tomisek, A. (2011). *Strengthening the direct service workforce in rural areas opportunities under the 2010 health reform law.* The National Direct Care Workforce Resource Center.

Centers for Disease Control and Prevention. (2020, April 15). *People who are at higher risk for severe illness*. U.S. Department of Health and Human Services. Retrieved April 20, 2020, from https://www.cdc.gov/coronavirus/2019-ncov/need-extra-precautions/people-at-higher-risk.html

Diaz, A., Chhabra, K. R., & Scott, J. W. (2020). The COVID-19 pandemic and rural hospitals—adding insult to injury. *Health Affairs Blog*. Retrieved from https://www.healthaffairs.org/do/10.1377/hblog20200429.583513/full/

Gunderson, D. (2020, March). Senior meal plans adjust, add deliveries as centers close amid COVID-19. *Minnesota Public Radio2*. Retrieved from https://www.mprnews.org/story/2020/03/20/senior-meal-plans-adjust-add-deliveries-as-centers-close-amid-covid19

Hash, K. M., Jurkowski, E. T., & Krout, J. A. (2015). *Aging in rural places: Policies, programs, and professional practice.* (K. M. Hash, E. T. Jurkowski, & J. A. Krout, Eds.). Springer Publishing Company.

Henning-Smith, C., Ecklund, A., Lahr, M., Evenson, A., Moscovice, I., & Kozhimannil, K. B. (2019). *Key informant perspectives on rural social isolation*. University of Minnesota Rural Health Research Center. Retrieved from https://rhrc.umn.edu/publication/key-informant-perspectives-on-rural-social-isolation-and-loneliness/

Henning-Smith, C., Schroeder, J., & Tuttle, M. (2020). *Rates of living alone by rurality and age*. University of Minnesota Rural Health Research Center. Retrieved from https://rhrc.umn.edu/publication/rates-of-living-alone-by-rurality-and-age/

Henning-Smith, C., Moscovice, I., & Kozhimannil, K. (2019). Differences in social isolation and its relationship to health by rurality. *The Journal of Rural Health, 35*(4), 540–549. http://dx.doi.org/10.1111/jrh.12344

Henning-Smith, C., Shippee, T., & Capistrant, B. (2018). Later-life disability in environmental context: Why living arrangements matter. *The Gerontologist, 58*(5), 853–862. http://dx.doi.org/10.1093/geront/gnx019

Henning-Smith, C. E., Hernandez, A. M., Hardeman, R. R., Ramirez, M. R., & Kozhimannil, K. B. (2019). Rural counties with majority black or indigenous populations suffer the highest rates of premature death in the US. *Health Affairs, 38*(12), 2019–2026. http://dx.doi.org/10.1377/hlthaff.2019.00847

Kaur, H. (2020, April 29). Why rural Americans are having a hard time working from home. *CNN*. Retrieved from https://www.cnn.com/2020/04/29/us/rural-broadband-access-coronavirus-trnd/index.html

Kijakazi, K. (2020). *COVID-19 racial health disparities highlight why we need to address structural racism*. Urban Institute. Retrieved from https://www.urban.org/urban-wire/covid-19-racial-health-disparities-highlight-why-we-need-address-structural-racism

Lewis, C., Shah, T., Jacobson, G., McIntosh, A., & Abrams, M. K. (2020). *How the COVID-19 pandemic could increase social isolation, and how providers and policymakers can keep us connected.* The Commonwealth Institute. Retrieved from https://www.commonwealthfund. org/blog/2020/how-covid-19-pandemic-could-increase-social-isolation-and-how-providers -and-policymakers

National Center for Health Statistics. (2018). *Health, United States, 2017: With special feature on mortality.* U.S. Department of Health and Human Services. Retrieved from https:// www.cdc.gov/nchs/data/hus/hus17.pdf

Pender, J., Hertz, T., Cromartie, J., & Farrigan, T. (2019). *Rural America at a glance, 2019 Edition.* U.S. Department of Agriculture. Retrieved from https://www.ers.usda.gov/publica tions/pub-details/?pubid=95340

Perrin, A. (2019). *Digital gap between rural and nonrural America persists.* Pew Research Center. https://www.pewresearch.org/fact-tank/2019/05/31/digital-gap-between-rural-and-nonrural-america-persists/

Pooler, J., Liu, S., & Roberts, A. (2017). *Older adults and unmet social needs.* AARP Foundation and IMPAQ International. Retrieved from https://endseniorhunger.aarp.org/ wp-content/uploads/2017/11/SDOH-among-older-adults-2017_IssueBrief_COR-Final.pdf

Siegler, K. (2020, April 9). *Small-town hospitals are closing just as coronavirus arrives in rural America.* National Public Radio. Retrieved from https://www.npr.org/2020/04/09/ 829753752/small-town-hospitals-are-closing-just-as-coronavirus-arrives-in-rural-america

The Cecil G. Sheps Center for Health Services Research. (2020). *128 rural hospital closures: January 2010 - present.* University of North Carolina. Retrieved from http://www.shepscen ter.unc.edu/programs-projects/rural-health/rural-hospital-closures/

Ullrich, F., & Mueller, K. (2020). *Confirmed COVID-19 cases, Metropolitan and Nonmetropolitan counties.* University of Iowa RUPRI Center for Rural Health Policy Analysis. Retrieved from https://rupri.public-health.uiowa.edu/publications/policybriefs/2020/COVID%20and% 20Hospital%20Beds.pdf

White, G. B. (2015, January). Rural America's silent housing crisis. *The Atlantic.* https://www. theatlantic.com/business/archive/2015/01/rural-americas-silent-housing-crisis/384885/

Families and Caregivers of Older Adults

The Demographics and Economics of Direct Care Staff Highlight Their Vulnerabilities Amidst the COVID-19 Pandemic

Beth Almeida, Marc A. Cohen, Robyn I. Stone, and Christian E. Weller

ABSTRACT

An estimated 3.5 million direct care staff working in facilities and people's homes play a critical role during the COVID-19 pandemic. They allow vulnerable care recipients to stay at home and they provide necessary help in facilities. Direct care staff, on average, have decades of experience, often have certifications and licenses, and many have at least some college education to help them perform the myriad of responsibilities to properly care for care recipients. Yet, they are at heightened health and financial risks. They often receive low wages, limited benefits, and have few financial resources to fall back on when they get sick themselves and can no longer work. Furthermore, most direct care staff are parents with children in the house and almost one-fourth are single parents. If they fall ill, both they and their families are put into physical and financial risk.

There are an estimated 3.5 million direct care staff providing care for the elderly, the disabled and those recovering from surgeries and other hospital stays in 2019, up from 3.4 million in 2018 (Bureau of Labor Statistics, 2020). Most of them help people in their homes, but many, including certified nursing assistants (CNAs), also work in residential assisted living facilities and nursing homes (Spetz et al., 2019). Next to family members and other unpaid caregivers, direct care staff provide the vast majority of hands-on assistance to these vulnerable populations (Campbell, 2017; Stone & Bryant, 2019). The continued work by direct care staff, who typically care for elderly patients and people with disabilities, is both essential in reducing the spread of the coronavirus and dangerous because of the personal risks that aides face.

Direct care staff play a critical role in the COVID-19 response

Direct care staff help with personal tasks such as cooking, eating, bathing and toileting. They also assist with running errands, including going shopping and taking people to the doctor. They are often part of a team of professionals that provide direct care and are often able to observe subtle changes in condition that assist care professionals in the management of chronic illnesses and functional decline (Reckrey et al., 2019). Direct care staff themselves are also an important source of emotional support for care recipients and their families (Butler et al., 2012; Franzosa et al., 2019; Reckrey et al., 2019; Rodat, 2014). For those receiving care at home, the presence of a consistent visit from members of a home care team can mean the difference between aging in place and perhaps having to move to an institutional setting (Spillman, 2016; Stone et al., 2017). The support provided by direct care staff in both home and institutional settings may also help keep people from having to make unnecessary trips to the emergency department or be admitted to a hospital unnecessarily – something particularly important at this time of crisis (Campbell, 2017; Feltner et al., 2014; Murtaugh et al., 2017).

Direct care staff possess the experience, education, and certification to undertake the multitude of these tasks. They have an average of more than two decades of labor market experience – a standard human capital measure[1]; almost half have at least some college education, and 34.6 percent report having a professional license or certification (Figure 1). This experience suggests that many direct care staff are well-situated to handle the emerging challenges of a pandemic and to provide ongoing care for population groups facing some of the highest health risks.

Direct care staff face economic and health risks with COVID-19

Direct care staff are often not rewarded for their qualifications and the demands of their job. The benefit of an additional year of education, for instance, for direct care staff is much smaller than for other workers (Osterman, 2017). Average hourly earnings were just 13.36 USD in 2019[2] with almost half of such staff – 48.2% – earning less than a living wage (Figure 1). Yet, even if working close to full time most of the year, 42.9% of direct care staff received some form of public assistance in 2019 (Figure 1). These economic vulnerabilities for direct care staff occur even as many works all year round, and 6.4% have more than one job (Figure 1). For many aides, continued work even amid emerging health risks, is both a professional commitment and an economic necessity.

These workers and their families already face substantial health and financial risks, which the pandemic only exacerbates. For instance, 14.2% of direct care

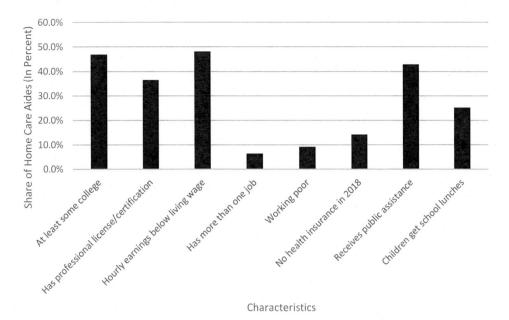

Figure 1. Select Economic Characteristics of Direct Care Staff, 2018/2019.
Notes: Direct care professionals include nursing, psychiatric, home health aides, and personal care aides from the CPS occupational codes 3600 and 4610. Monthly data are pooled for all months in 2019. Dollar values are in real 2018 dollars. Individual wage income and total family income are taken from the Annual Social and Economic Supplement (ASEC). Those data are collected in March of each year and refer to the previous 12 months and thus reflect mainly data received in 2018. Working poor is defined as having worked at least 27 weeks over the past year and having income below the official federal poverty line. Public assistance includes Medicaid, free and reduced school lunches, housing subsidies, food stamps and earned income tax credits. Wages are deflated using the Consumer Price Index for Clerical Workers (CPI-W) and income is deflated using the Consumer Price Index for Urban Consumers (CPI-U) from the Bureau of Labor Statistics. Wages Source is from Flood et al. (2018)

staff did not have health insurance in 2018 (Figure 1). Also, their health insurance often leaves them vulnerable to lack of health care and higher medical debt. More than a third of health-care support staff, mainly direct care staff, skipped health care such as follow up visits or going to the doctor when they were sick in 2018 (Figure 2). Further, a whopping 71.3% of health-care support staff, owed medical debt after an unexpected health-care emergency in 2018 (Figure 2). Moreover, most of these jobs lack paid sick leave, which means that aides may continue to work even if there is a risk that they might be infected.

The spreading virus and the associated health risks only serve to high-light other economic risks that the pandemic magnifies. Almost half of all direct care staff have children at home and nearly a quarter (23.9%) are single mothers with no other incomes to fall back on when they can no longer work (Figure 3). Caught between worries over the risk to their own health posed by their jobs and the need to care for their families, direct care staff experience even greater stress when they must find proper child

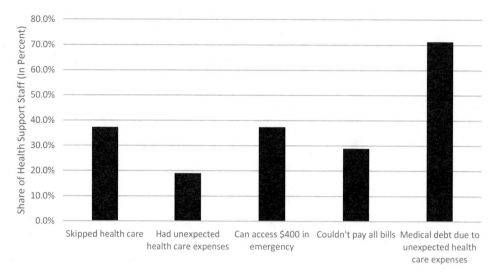

Figure 2. Financial Vulnerability of Health Support Staff, 2018.
Note: Source is Fed. (Federal Reserve, 2019). Skipping health care includes not going to doctor, not taking prescribed medicine, not going to follow up visit. The sample for medical debt includes only those who had unexpected health-care expenses in the previous year.

care when their kids cannot attend school. For those with children who depend on free or reduced school lunches – which is the case for 25.2% of direct care staff (Figure 3) – the situation becomes even more dire. Moreover, many direct care staff are themselves older, with more than a quarter, 26.5%, over the age of 55 years (Figure 3), which puts them at higher risk of experiencing severe health consequences if they become infected with the coronavirus. The pandemic can quickly put their own and their families' physical and financial health at risk.

Even as aides face substantial risks, they often have limited resources to fall back on in case of an emergency such as contracting COVID-19. In 2018, even before the crisis, 29.0 percent of these workers couldn't pay all of their bills and only 37.4 percent could come up with 400 USD in an emergency (Figure 2). Moreover, almost one-third are African-Americans, who have about one-tenth the wealth of whites at the median (Hanks et al., 2018). As well, more than half are single women (Figure 3), who typically have about half the wealth of single men (Weller and Tolson, 2017, 2018). The spreading virus and the associated health risks thus exacerbate the already widespread financial risks that direct care staff regularly face.

Conclusion

Those charged with the front-line responsibilities for keeping some of the most vulnerable people safe from the coronavirus and helping to stem the

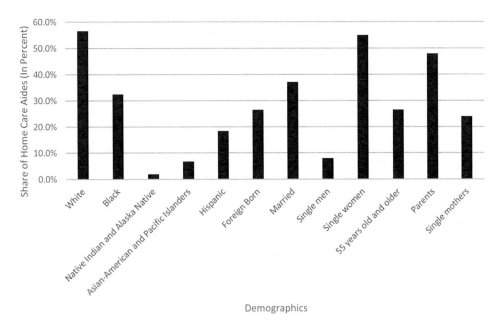

Figure 3. The Demographics of Direct Care Staff.
Note: Direct care staff include nursing, psychiatric, home health aides, and personal care aides from the CPS occupational codes 3600 and 4610. Monthly data are pooled for all months in 2019. Source is Flood et al. (2018).

flow of patients to already overburdened hospital intensive care units are themselves facing untenable risks. Without quick action focused on assuring adequate training in how to deal with the virus, providing the equipment necessary to protect against it, paying higher wages, providing health insurance, and ensuring other specific wrap-around services to meet direct care staff's own health care, child care, and other financial challenges, this financially exposed workforce will not be able to meet the growing need presented by the current pandemic. The result could be a greater spread of the virus itself, increased burdens on our acute care hospital system, and more lives lost.

Key Points

- An estimated 3.5 million direct care staff work mainly in people's homes.
- Direct care staff have substantial qualifications to perform their work.
- Almost half of all direct care staff earn less than a living wage.
- Often, direct care staff have no or only inadequate health insurance.
- More than half are parents, so contracting an infection puts their families at risk.

Notes

1. Experience is a standard human capital measure that together with formal educational attainment explains large share of wage differentials. Authors' calculations based on Flood et al. (2018).
2. Authors' calculations based on Flood et al. (2018).

Disclosure statement

No potential conflict of interest was reported by the authors.

References

Bureau of Labor Statistics. (2020). *Current population survey.* BLS.

Butler, S. S., Wardamasky, S., & Brennaning, M. (2012). Older women caring for older women: The rewards and challenges of the home care aide job. *Journal Women & Aging, 24*(3), 194–215. https://doi.org/10.1080/08952841.2012.639667

Campbell, S. (2017). U.S. home care workers: Key facts. *PHI National.* https://phinational.org/wp-content/uploads/2017/07/phi-home-care-workers-key-facts.pdf

Federal Reserve. (2019). *Survey of household economics and decisionmaking 2018.* Fed.

Feltner, C., Jones, C. D., Cené, C. W., Zheng, Z. J., Sueta, C. A., Coker-Schwimmer, E. J., Arvanitis, M., Lohr, K. N., Middleton, J. C., & Jonas, D. E. (2014). Transitional care interventions to prevent readmissions for persons with heart failure: A systematic review and meta-analysis. *Annals of Intern Medicine, 160*(11), 774–784. https://doi.org/10.7326/M14-0083

Flood, S., King, M., Rodgers, R., Ruggles, S., & Warren, J. R. (2018). Integrated Public Use Microdata Series, Current Population Survey: Version 6.0. Minneapolis, MN: IPUMS.

Franzosa, E., Tsui, E. K., & Baron, S. (2019). "Who's caring for US?": Understanding and addressing the effects of emotional labor in home health aides' well-being. *The Gerontologist, 59*(6), 1055–1064. https://doi.org/10.1093/geront/gny099

Hanks, A., Solomon, D., & Weller, C. E. (2018). *Systematic inequality: How America's structural racism helped create the black-white wealth gap.* CAP Report. Center for American Progress.

Murtaugh, C. M., Deb, P., Zhu, C., Peng, T. R., Barrón, Y., Shah, S., Moore, S. M., Bowles, K. H., Kalman, J., Feldman, P. H., Siu, A. L. (2017). Reducing readmissions among heart failure patients discharged to home health care: Effectiveness of early and intensive nursing services and early physician follow-up. *Health Services Research, 52*(4), 1445–1472. https://doi.org/10.1111/1475-6773.12537

Osterman, P. (2017). *Who will care for US?* Russell Sage Foundation.

Reckrey, J. M., Tsui, E. K., Morrison, R. S., Geduldig, E. T., Stone, R. I., Ornstein, K. A., & Federman, A. D. (2019). Beyond functional support: The range of health-related tasks performed in the home by paid caregivers in New York. *Health Affairs, 36*(6), 927–933. https://doi.org/10.1377/hlthaff.2019.00004

Rodat, C. (2014). *Training New York City home care aides: A landscape survey.* Report, PHI

Spetz, J., Stone, R. I., Chapman, S. A., & Bryant, N. (2019). Home and community-based workforce for patients with serious illness requires support to meet growing needs. *Health Affairs, 38*(6), 902–909. https://doi.org/10.1377/hlthaff.2019.00021

Spillman, B. (2016). *Does home care prevent or defer nursing home use? Report to the Department of Health and Human Services, Assistant Secretary of Planning and*

Evaluation, Aging, Long-Term, Contract *Contract HHSP23320095654WC.* Urban Institute. https://aspe.hhs.gov/sites/default/files/pdf/245701/preventNH.pdf

Stone, R., Wilhelm, J., Bishop, C. E., Bryant, N. S., Hermer, L., & Squillace, M. R. (2017). Predictors of intent to leave the job among home health workers: Analysis of the national home health aide survey. *The Gerontologist, 57*(5), 890–899. https://doi.org/10.1093/geront/gnw075

Stone, R. I., & Bryant, N. S. (2019). The future of the home care workforce: Training and supporting aides as members of home-based care teams. *Journal of the American Geriatrics Society, 67*(S2), S444–S448. https://doi.org/10.1111/jgs.15846

Weller, C., & Tolson, M. (2017). Women's Economic Risk Exposure and Savings. CAP Report, Washington. DC: Center for American Progress.

Weller, C., & Tolson, M. (2018). Do unpaid caregivers save less for retirement? *Journal of Retirement, 6*(2), 61–73. https://doi.org/10.3905/jor.2018.6.2.061

Amid the COVID-19 Pandemic, Meaningful Communication between Family Caregivers and Residents of Long-Term Care Facilities is Imperative

Edem Hado and Lynn Friss Feinberg

ABSTRACT

Older adults residing in long-term care facilities are especially vulnerable for severe illness or death from COVID-19. To contain the transmission of the virus in long-term care facilities, federal health officials have issued strict visitation guidelines, restricting most visits between residents and all visitors, including family members. Yet, many older adults rely on family care for social support and to maintain their health, well-being, and safety in long-term care facilities, and therefore need to stay connected to their families. The federal government, state and local leaders, and long-term care facilities should take further actions to enable the relationship between residents of long-term care facilities and families during the COVID-19 pandemic.

In describing the COVID-19 pandemic, Andrew Cuomo, Governor of New York, said the "coronavirus in a nursing home can be like fire through dry grass" (Harris et al., 2020). In the United States, more than 2 million Americans reside in long-term care facilities like nursing homes and assisted living residences (Kaiser Family Foundation, 2017; Ungar & Hancock, 2020). Nearly half (48%) of nursing home residents are living with Alzheimer's or other dementias, and among older adults in residential care settings, including assisted living facilities, 42% have some form of dementia (Alzheimer's Association, 2020).

Family and other unpaid caregivers – including relatives, partners, friends, and neighbors – are the most important source of emotional and practical support for older adults with chronic, disabling, or serious health conditions (National Academies of Sciences, Engineering and Medicine, 2016; Reinhard et al., 2019). This perspective thus highlights the reliance of long-term care facilities on family support and the importance of the family caregiver role with the COVID-19 pandemic. It argues that family caregivers can serve as crucial and trusted partners in the nation's strategy to curb the spread of the COVID-19 virus, and help the people they care for to cope with the stress and anxiety of this unprecedented situation (Centers for Disease Control and Prevention, 2020). Proactive solutions for maintaining the family caregiver role during the COVID-19 pandemic are proposed.

Residents of long-term care facilities rely on family support

Across the nation, family caregivers are often the critical factor that enables older adults and people with disabilities who need long-term services and supports (LTSS) – also known as long-term care – to live at home and in the community (Hado & Komisar, 2019). As an older adult's care coordinator and primary advocate, family caregivers oftentimes become the "eyes and ears" for the concerns and safety of the care recipient with complex care needs, including when their care recipient resides in a long-term care facility like a nursing home or assisted living facility. They help navigate the health and LTSS systems, facilitating communication with providers and discussing issues that require shared decision making (Sarkar & Bates, 2014; Wolff, 2012). They also commonly serve as surrogate decision-makers when the care recipient loses the capacity to make important decisions (National Academies of Sciences, Engineering and Medicine, 2016). Because of their crucial support role, family caregivers are in a unique position to better understand, articulate and support the emotional, social, and health needs of the care recipient (Reinhard et al., 2019). Across all ethnic groups, family care is the most preferred and trusted source of assistance for individuals who need help with activities of daily living (Whitlatch & Feinberg, 2007).

Family caregiver role grows with COVID-19

As the COVID-19 virus spreads across the country, residents of long-term care facilities are among the populations hardest hit by virus-related deaths (Barnett & Grabowski, 2020). To slow the spread of COVID-19 to vulnerable older adults in long-term care facilities, the federal Centers for Medicare & Medicaid Services (CMS), which regulates most skilled nursing homes, has issued strict guidelines on visitation to nursing homes (Centers for Medicare & Medicaid Services, 2020a). Most assisted living facilities, although not regulated by the federal government, are also limiting or halting visitors to their facilities.

Even if physical visits are not possible, the guidelines should not inhibit relationships and connections between residents and their family members and close friends, which are crucial to one's well-being – both physical and emotional. Family caregivers of nursing home residents, and those living in assisted living facilities, should monitor the health, well-being, and safety of their family members in long-term care facilities as closely as possible.

Despite the unique challenges that protecting vulnerable older adults from the coronavirus presents, the current surge in COVID-19-related deaths in long-term care facilities makes meaningful human and family connections all the more important. Residents and family members should be able to communicate and visit virtually, especially during times of stress – such as this one. The health impacts of social isolation are real and very serious (National Academies of Sciences, Engineering and Medicine, 2020; Tan, 2020).

Proactive solutions to meet the challenge

Enabling the relationship between the family and residents of long-term care facilities is especially challenging at this time, and necessitates action in multiple areas, including strengthening communication channels, activating family councils, and mobilizing gerontological social work students. At the same time, family caregivers must look out for their own safety and health.

Strengthening nursing home-family caregiver communication channels

In the updated guidelines, CMS is encouraging nursing homes to keep residents' loved ones informed about their care. CMS should strengthen this measure by requiring nursing homes to do so. It is vitally important to ensure timely communication with family caregivers, especially in light of the recent CMS recommendations on transferring or discharging residents between facilities based on COVID-19 status (Centers for Medicare & Medicaid Services, 2020b). Long-term care facilities should, to the fullest extent possible, inform family of any requirements and procedures for placement in alternative facilities. One way that facilities can achieve this is by assigning staff members as primary contacts for families (e.g., the designated family caregiver or representative) to facilitate regular communications with staff by telephone, e-mail or video. Facilities should also promote ways for family caregivers to stay in touch with residents – through, for example, regular phone calls and "virtual visitation" (e.g., Face Time, Skype, Zoom). This should include facilitating conversations with residents and their family caregivers about treatment options and putting advance care plans in place (Lynn, 2020).

State and local leaders can also play an important role. They should encourage specific communication workarounds for residents and families as they put in place visitation limitations. These might include processes for staff to facilitate phone calls, making video-enabled devices available to facilities, and requiring more frequent facility communication with families. A state's long-term care ombudsman may be able to help facilitate this effort (The National Consumer Voice for Quality Long-Term Care, 2016).

Activating family councils

Federal regulations give family caregivers of nursing home residents the right to be part of a family council and meet together on-site in the nursing home to advocate for residents and partner with staff to improve quality of care (The National Consumer Voice for Quality Long-Term Care, 2020). During the COVID-19 pandemic, facilities should facilitate alternative means of communication for family councils (using e-mail, Skype, or "phone trees") to exchange information and for family members to support one another and stay informed.

Mobilizing students and trainees

Because family visits are an essential method for monitoring quality of care, and because workforce shortages also pose key challenges for long-term care facilities now and in the foreseeable future (Gardner et al., 2020), a range of strategies will be needed by facilities to ensure that regular communication is provided to the family caregivers of residents. One potential strategy is to mobilize students and trainees such as gerontological social work students – also known as geriatric social work – to assist staff in long-term care facilities to maintain communication and provide social support. These students are trained in skills to promote active listening, communication, empathy, and critical thinking, among others. These and other students and trainees in the health professions could be assigned to call family caregivers of residents on a regular basis to keep them apprised of their family member's situation and infection control procedures in the facilities, and to lend support to these caregiving families.

Although beyond the scope of this article, other steps are urgently needed now to reduce the risks to older adults in long-term care facilities posed by the adverse consequences of COVID-19 for staff. These steps include universal testing of residents and staff, ensuring personal protective equipment for staff and residents, and providing paid sick leave as an employment benefit (Gardner et al., 2020; Glynn, 2020; Harris et al., 2020).

Family caregivers must maintain personal safety and take care of their health

During COVID-19, it is also critical that family caregivers manage their *own* health, stress, and well-being. It is especially important to address the feeling of helplessness and heightened anxiety about a care recipient living in a long-term care facility that is restricting the access of residents' families and friends to protect them from the spread of this disease. Joining online caregiver support groups can help foster the sharing of information, advice and encouragement.

Conclusion

The health, well-being, and safety of residents of long-term care facilities remains a top concern for families across the country, particularly during the COVID-19 pandemic. For many vulnerable older adults residing in nursing homes or assisted living facilities, family and friend involvement and connectivity are crucial factors that enable them to reside in a facility setting. Accordingly, the federal government, states, and long-term care facilities should ensure continuous and meaningful family engagement, communication, and inclusion in all settings of care, particularly in long-term care facilities.

Key Points

- Older adults in long-term care facilities are at greater risk for severe illness or death from COVID-19.
- Family caregivers are the most trusted allies and care coordinators for residents of long-term care facilities.
- Recent federal guidelines restricts family visitation in nursing homes, leading to greater isolation among residents.
- Lack of physical visitation should not inhibit ongoing family communication and engagement especially during the COVID-19 crisis.
- Federal government, state and local leaders, and long-term care facilities can take specific actions to enable meaningful communication between residents of long-term care facilities and families.

Disclosure statement

This article is based on a blog published by the AARP Public Policy Institute on April 7, 2020. No potential conflict of interest was reported by the authors.

References

Alzheimer's Association. (2020). 2020 Alzheimer's disease facts and figures. *Alzheimer's & Dementia, 16*(3), 391+. https://doi.org/10.102/alz.12068

Barnett, M. L., & Grabowski, D. C. (2020, March 24). Nursing homes are ground zero for COVID-19 pandemic. *JAMA Health Forum.* https://jamanetwork.com/channels/health-forum/fullarticle/2763666

Centers for Disease Control and Prevention. (2020). *Groups at higher risk for severe illness.* https://www.cdc.gov/coronavirus/2019-ncov/need-extra-precautions/groups-at-higher-risk.html

Centers for Medicare & Medicaid Services. (2020a). *CMS.gov: Guidance for infection control and prevention of coronavirus disease 2019 (COVID-19) in nursing homes (Revised).* Department of Health and Human Services. Retrieved April 13, 2020, from https://www.cms.gov/files/document/3-13-2020-nursing-home-guidance-covid-19.pdf

Centers for Medicare & Medicaid Services. (2020b). *CMS.gov: 2019 novel coronavirus (COVID-19) long-term care facility transfer scenarios*. Department of Health and Human Services. Retrieved April 14, 2020, from https://www.cms.gov/files/document/qso-20-25-nh.pdf

Gardner, W., States, D., & Bagley, N. (2020). The coronavirus and the risks to the elderly in long-term care. *Journal of Aging & Social Policy*, 1–6. https://doi.org/10.1080/08959420.2020.1750543

Glynn, S. J. (2020). *Congress must extend paid leave protections to all workers in next Coronavirus response bill*. Center for American Progress. https://www.americanprogress.org/issues/women/news/2020/03/24/482196/congress-must-extend-paid-leave-protections-workers-next-coronavirus-response-bill/

Hado, E., & Komisar, H. (2019). *Long-term services and supports*. AARP Public Policy Institute. https://www.aarp.org/content/dam/aarp/ppi/2019/08/long-term-services-and-supports

Harris, A. J., Leland, J., & Tully, T. (2020, April 11). Nearly 2,000 dead as Coronavirus ravages nursing homes in N.Y. region. *The New York Times*. https://www.nytimes.com/2020/04/11/nyregion/nursing-homes-deaths-coronavirus.html

Kaiser Family Foundation. (2017). *Total number of residents in certified nursing facilities: 2017*. https://www.kff.org/other/state-indicator/number-of-nursing-facility-residents/?currentTimeframe=0&sortModel=%7B%22colId%22:%22Location%22,%22sort%22:%22asc%22%7D

Lynn, J. (2020). Getting ahead of COVID-19 issues: Dying from respiratory failure out of the hospital. *Health Affairs*. https://www.healthaffairs.org/do/10.1377/hblog20200330.141866/full/

National Academies of Sciences, Engineering, and Medicine. (2016). *Families caring for an aging America*. National Academies Press. https://nam.edu/families-caring-for-an-aging-america/

National Academies of Sciences, Engineering, and Medicine. (2020). *Social Isolation and loneliness in older adults: Opportunities for the health care system*. National Academies Press. https://www.nap.edu/read/25663/chapter/1#ii

Reinhard, S. C., Feinberg, L. F., Houser, A., Choula, R., & Evans, M. (2019). *Valuing the invaluable: 2019 update*. AARP Public Policy Institute. https://www.aarp.org/ppi/info-2015/valuing-the-invaluable-2015-update.html

Sarkar, U., & Bates, D. W. (2014). Care partners and online patient portals. *Journal of the American Medical Association*, *311*(4), 357–358. https://doi.org/10.1001/jama.2013.285825

Tan, E. (2020, March 16). How to fight social isolation of coronavirus. *AARP*. https://www.aarp.org/health/conditions-treatments/info-2020/coronavirus-social-isolation-loneliness.html

The National Consumer Voice for Quality Long-Term Care. (2016). *Long-term care ombudsman program: What you must know*. https://ltcombudsman.org/uploads/files/library/long-term-care-ombudsman-program-what-you-must-know.pdf

The National Consumer Voice for Quality Long-Term Care. (2020). *Covid-19 and nursing homes: What residents and family need to know*. https://theconsumervoice.org/uploads/files/general/covid-19-consumer-fact-sheet.pdf

Ungar, L., & Hancock, J. (2020, April 9). COVID-19 crisis threatens beleaguered assisted living industry. *Kaiser Health News*. https://khn.org/news/covid-19-crisis-threatens-beleaguered-assisted-living-industry/

Whitlatch, C. J., & Feinberg, L. F. (2007). Family care and decision making. In C. Cox (Ed.), *Dementia and social work practice: Research and interventions*(pp. 129–147). Springer.

Wolff, J. (2012). Family matters in health care delivery. *Journal of the American Medical Association*, *308*(15), 1529–1530. https://doi.org/10.1001/jama.2012.13366

Intergenerational Relationships, Family Caregiving Policy, and COVID-19 in the United States

Jeffrey E. Stokes and Sarah E. Patterson

ABSTRACT

Families and intergenerational relationships are important sources of risk for COVID-19 infection, especially for older adults who are at high risk of complications from the disease. If one family member is exposed to the virus they could serve as a source of transmission or, if they fall ill, the resources they provide to others could be severed. These risks may be especially heightened for family members who work outside the home and provide care, or for those family members who care for multiple generations. Policies have the potential to help families bear the burden of these decisions. This essay argues that policies that address health, employment, and other social issues have implications for families, and that policies aimed at families and caregivers can affect the health, employment, and the general well-being of the nation.

Introduction

COVID-19 has spread globally within the period of a few short months, devastating populations and straining healthcare systems in Asia, Europe, and – more recently – the United States. The virus has demonstrated uneven risks for mortality across different population groups, with severest risks among older adults, those with preexisting conditions, and racial minority groups (Dowd et al., 2020). Yet one of the most treacherous aspects of COVID-19 is its ability to transmit from person-to-person even when carriers are asymptomatic or show very few indications of infection (Qian et al., 2020). This leads to another axis upon which COVID-19 may differentially impact certain population groups, which has received less attention in the media to date – that of family structure and intergenerational bonds (for an exception from Italy, see Balbo et al., 2020). Families are a central source of many social contacts and daily interactions – and thus a potential source of

Note: Authors contributed equally to this manuscript.

disease spread – particularly among some of the highest-risk groups for COVID-19 complications (Dorélien et al., 2020).

This perspective examines the implications of multigenerational family relationships for COVID-19 exposure and transmission, with a particular focus on the caregiving roles that "sandwich" generation adults often play, even as they remain active in the formal workforce. Both gender and racial disparities in these caregiving responsibilities, and the risks they pose during the present pandemic, are of central importance.

Caregiving and COVID-19

The United States offers less generous social welfare protections for families and caregivers than most other Organisation for Economic Cooperation and Development (OECD) nations (Colombo, Llena-Nozal, Mercier, & Tjadens, 2011). Social policies and programs that maximize these individual risks also compound racial and gender inequalities that accumulate across the life course (Harrington Meyer & Herd, 2007). Additionally, in part due to this lack of a strong social safety net, as well as due to financial losses during the Great Recession that severely harmed retirement and pension accounts (Newman, 2019), a substantial proportion of older adults remain in the workforce themselves (Toossi & Torpey, 2017). This combination of limited social welfare policies, insufficient retirement savings and support for older adults, and strong "family as caregiver" norms in the U.S. results in older Americans depending largely upon family members – typically spouses or adult children – to provide informal care. This is particularly the case among the oldest-old, those with physical limitations and disabilities, and racial and ethnic minority populations (Harrington Meyer & Herd, 2007).

Indeed, family members are the front-line caregivers in the United States, especially for older adults (Wolff et al., 2016). On average, in the U.S., informal care provided by working age adults for older adults is valued at 412 billion USD per year; that number rises to 522 billion USD when accounting for caregivers who are 65 and older (Chari et al., 2015). Even when institutionalized in a nursing home, older adults rely on "care convoys" made up of family members who provide additional care for them (Kemp et al., 2018).

COVID-19 may prevent critical family contact and care from occurring or could serve as a source of potential exposure for at-risk older adults. This may be especially true for families with "essential" workers, such as those in healthcare, law enforcement, or food/grocery industries, particularly if those workers must balance multiple care duties at work and at home (e.g., Van Houtven et al., 2020). Federal and state governments, alongside major private-sector employers, have encouraged the use of telework options during the COVID-19 pandemic (Hadden Loh & Fishbane, 2020). However, this is not possible for all workers, nor even permitted for those workers deemed "essential" (Hadden Loh & Fishbane, 2020).

Even under normal conditions, the stresses of caregiving – in addition to those of formal workforce participation – can be harmful for health and well-being, especially among the women who inordinately bear those responsibilities (Moen & DePasquale, 2017; Schulz, 2020). In fact, a long-standing literature has illustrated a multitude of negative consequences for caregivers, even including increased risk of mortality (Schulz & Beach, 1999). Despite increases in women's formal labor force participation over the course of the last half-century, the burden of informal carework remains highly gendered, with wives, daughters, and other women being more likely to provide any care – and to provide *more* care – to one or more family members than are men (Patterson & Margolis, 2019). "Essential" workers, in particular, are often caregivers for children or aging parents, and both caregiving burdens and such employment are clustered among women and racial/ethnic minority populations in the U.S. (Robertson & Gebeloff, 2020; Van Houtven et al., 2020). As a recent article in *The New York Times* noted, "One in three jobs held by women has been designated as essential … Nonwhite women are more likely to be doing essential jobs than anyone else." (Robertson & Gebeloff, 2020).

Multigenerational families and households and COVID-19

The age and family structure of population groups may also be important determinants of COVID-19 spread (Balbo et al., 2020). By sharing resources or providing care, multigenerational *families* – those that contain family members of various ages and generations – may be a heightened source of potential disease contact (Dowd et al., 2020). For instance, "sandwiched" caregivers, who provide care both for young children and for aging parents may be an especially important population to focus on for pinpointing and isolating spread because the rates of multigenerational care are highest among working age adults, whose caregiving roles can extend across generations (Patterson & Margolis, 2019). Additionally, an increasing number of Americans live in multigenerational *households*, wherein members of three or more generations live together under one roof, and they in particular may be at higher risk of disease transmission. Under such circumstances, the ability to engage in social distancing or self-quarantine among each generation is unlikely, if not impossible. Moreover, in coresident multigenerational families the eldest generation serves as an important care provider for young children, often in order to allow middle-generation parents to work outside the home (Harrington Meyer, 2020; Luo et al., 2012). Populations at high risk for complications from COVID-19, such as racial and ethnic minority older adults, are more likely to live with other family members, including grandchildren (Cross, 2018; Luo et al., 2012).

Multigenerational families and households are particularly important for understanding disease dispersion because COVID-19 generally presents as less severe among children and young adults, making it possible that infected children may transmit COVID-19 to their "sandwich" generation parents or grandparents before anyone is aware that they were even infected (Qian et al., 2020). This risk is particularly grave for racial and ethnic minority groups and lower-socioeconomic status populations, who are more likely to (a) have employment that is contingent, lower-paid, and unable to be performed from home; (b) rely on family networks to provide needed care, whether to young children and/or aging parents; and (c) have underlying health problems and other health disparities resulting from cumulative dis/advantage (Luo et al., 2012; Robertson & Gebeloff, 2020; Sarkisian et al., 2007; Sarkisian & Gerstel, 2004). Indeed, COVID-19 hotspots have emerged in municipalities with substantial racial and ethnic minority populations, large proportions of residents deemed "essential" employees, and high population density and prevalence of multigenerational households (e.g., Florida, 2020).

A thin safety net for families

While the U.S. lacks generous family and social welfare policies in general, those that specifically support family caregivers are even more slim. The U.S. does not have a formal federal system that supports caregivers, instead relying on piecemeal state policies, in stark contrast with other peer nations (Organisation for Economic Cooperation and Development, 2011). The widest reaching benefit – the Family and Medical Leave Act (FMLA) – grants only uncompensated time off, and only guarantees leave and the maintenance of group health benefits for 12 weeks, though it does apply to all employers in the U.S. The ability to take unpaid leave, however, is not practically available to all caregivers, many of whom may be unable to forego consistent income while providing care to loved ones, or for whom caregiving responsibilities persist over long periods of time.

Congress did pass the Recognize, Assist, Include, Support, and Engage (RAISE) Family Caregivers Act in 2018 to establish a national strategy to acknowledge and assist family caregivers through policy, infrastructure, and programming. Previously, the National Family Caregiver Support Program was established in 2000 and offers grants to states and territories in order to provide services to caregivers of an older adult, focusing on information and connections to services like respite care (e.g., planned or emergency care provided to caregivers) (see Administration for Community Living, n.d.).

Although an important step, more funding is needed to directly help family caregivers, who spend roughly 7,000 USD per year out-of-pocket on costs associated with caring for an older family member (Rainville et al., 2016). The current policy landscape thus leaves gaps in care needs, forcing many families to foot the bill themselves (if they can) for extra supports (e.g., respite care; Whittier et al., 2005). Caregivers of Black and Hispanic older adults in particular report challenges in accessing support services, but it is not clear what role the availability, affordability, and/or desirability of services offered play in these choices (Potter, 2018). Caregiving responsibilities and burdens may be intensified during COVID-19 when stay-at-home orders are in place, making access to available supports and services crucial yet difficult to obtain.

Moving forward: policy implications for family caregivers

Numerous state governments have imposed social distancing and stay-at-home guidelines for residents, with exceptions for "essential" workers and activities such as grocery shopping and exercise. Yet these guidelines may be limited in influence when it comes to working caregivers, especially those who are economically and socially marginalized, for whom the decision to stay home and protect loved ones from infection may at the same time be a decision to go without pay, forego health insurance coverage, and risk food insecurity or even eviction. For working caregivers, broad-based policies such as paid family and sick leave may be critical for helping families to physically distance when needed, in order to either quarantine or prevent further spread of the virus, while also balancing care roles (Schulz, 2020).

Although there is no federal policy to date, some states have or will soon be implementing paid leave for caregivers, including California, New Jersey, Rhode Island, New York, and Washington (National Partnership for Women & Families, 2019). California implemented a program in 2004 entitled the California Paid Family Leave Program (CA-PFL) and early analyses show that the program is effective in helping caregivers to continue work, especially for some particularly at-risk populations, including middle-aged working caregivers or the near-poor (Kang et al., 2019). This program also reduced the proportion of older adults that required care in nursing homes (Arora & Wolf, 2018). Keeping older adults out of nursing homes is particularly important for protecting against the spread of viral pathogens such as COVID-19, which has been particularly devastating within residential long-term care (Gardner et al., 2020).

We recommend that policy makers keep in mind that families and public health go hand-in-hand, and that policies aimed at workers, caregivers, and older adults can help advance life expectancy and reduce health inequities (Moen & DePasquale, 2017; Schulz, 2020). In such cases, the more universal and accessible these policies are, the more likely they are to benefit caregivers and families in need (e.g., Herd & Moynihan, 2019). Take income support in the context of the current crisis, for example. Unemployment benefits support those who are laid off, but not those who voluntarily quit in order to reduce the risk of infection for themselves and/or dependent family members, nor does it cover workers across all sectors (Badger & Parlapiano, 2020). Further, eligibility and application requirements to access unemployment benefits vary across states and can create barriers to obtaining benefits in a timely fashion (Badger & Parlapiano, 2020). Conversely, programs such as universal basic income, direct payments to caregivers, or stimulus checks like those proposed and passed in April, can help families provide basic goods like housing and food so that they can focus on their caregiving responsibilities, without restricting eligibility or requiring administrative burdens in order to access needed funds (for instance, those required to file for a dependent tax credit).

Unfortunately, even when supports are available, families are often unaware of them, unable to determine whether they qualify, or simply unable to complete the difficult and time-consuming documentation required (Herd & Moynihan, 2019). It is therefore critical that policies and programs implemented be as broad-based and accessible as possible, without the presence of onerous administrative burdens, in order to maximize the likelihood that benefits will actually accrue to the most marginalized and at-risk populations (Herd & Moynihan, 2019).

Conclusion

Family, caregiving, and intergenerational relationships are important sources of potential exposure to COVID-19 infection. In multigenerational families, the "sandwich" generation adults – especially women – are often care providers to young children and/or older parents, while also being engaged in the formal labor force. This is particularly true among racial and ethnic minority and lower-socioeconomic status populations, who are likelier to live in multigenerational households, and to work in "essential" professions that preclude distance-working alternatives. It is therefore crucial that policies aimed at protecting population health and those intended to support families and caregivers be designed as complementary, and implemented in conjunction with one another (Schulz, 2020). Individual organizations or managers can support workers who are balancing care responsibilities (Plaisier et al., 2015). However, policies set at the state and national levels can be much more effective at providing the support necessary to allow caregivers to forego formal work during critical periods in order to focus on caregiving, especially when these policies are free from administrative burdens (Herd & Moynihan, 2019). Intergenerational relationships, family structure, and public health are inseparable, and the most effective public policy regimes and interventions will be those that recognize these intersections and design policies accordingly.

Key Points

- Families and intergenerational relationships may be an underexplored source of risk for transmission of COVID-19.
- Women and racial minorities are particularly likely to be caregivers for one or more family members of older and younger generations.
- Policies aimed at health, employment, and social welfare should take the diversity of family structure and the importance of family caregiving into account.
- Policies aimed at families and caregivers have the potential to have a positive impact on reducing the spread of COVID-19 through helping family members to balance work and caregiving responsibilities.

Acknowledgments

This work was supported by the National Institute on Aging of the National Institutes of Health (T32AG000221). The content is solely the responsibility of the authors and does not necessarily represent the official views of the National Institutes of Health.

Disclosure statement

No potential conflict of interest was reported by the authors.

ORCID

Jeffrey E. Stokes http://orcid.org/0000-0002-3630-0959
Sarah E. Patterson http://orcid.org/0000-0002-5040-7576

References

Administration for Community Living. (n.d.). *Support to caregivers*. https://acl.gov/programs/support-caregivers

Arora, K., & Wolf, D. A. (2018). Does paid family leave reduce nursing home use? The California experience. *Journal of Policy Analysis and Management, 37*(1), 38–62. https://doi.org/10.1002/pam.22038

Badger, E., & Parlapiano, A. (2020, April 30). States made it harder to get jobless benefits. Now that's hard to undo. *The Upshot*. https://www.nytimes.com/2020/04/30/upshot/unemployment-state-restrictions-pandemic.html

Balbo, N., Billari, F. C., & Melegaro, A. (2020). The strength of family ties and COVID-19. *Contexts: Sociology for the Public*. https://contexts.org/blog/structural-shocks-and-extreme-exposures/#balbo

Chari, A. V., Engberg, J., Ray, K. N., & Mehrotra, A. (2015). The opportunity costs of informal elder-care in the United States: New estimates from the American time use survey. *Health Services Research*, *50*(3), 871–882. https://doi.org/10.1111/1475-6773.12238

Colombo, F., Llena-Nozal, A., Mercier, J., & Tjadens, F. (2011). Help wanted?: Providing and paying for long-term care. *OECD Health Policy Studies, OECD Publishing*. https://doi.org/10.1787/9789264097759-e

Cross, C. J. (2018). Extended family households among children in the United States: Differences by race/ethnicity and socio-economic status. *Population Studies*, *72*(2), 235–251. https://doi.org/10.1080/00324728.2018.1468476

Dorélien, A. M., Ramen, A., & Swanson, I. (2020). *Analyzing the demographic, spatial, and temporal factors influencing social contact patterns in US and implications for infectious disease spread*. [Unpublished manuscript] Humphrey School of Public Affairs, University of Minnesota. http://www.audreydorelien.com/wp-content/uploads/2020/04/ATUS_social_contact_latest.pdf

Dowd, J. B., Rotondi, V., Adriano, L., Brazel, D. M., Block, P., Ding, X., … Mills, M. C. (2020). Demographic science aids in understanding the spread and fatality rates of COVID-19. *PNAS*, *117*(18), 9696–9698. https://doi.org/10.1073/pnas.2004911117

Florida, R. (2020, April 3). The geography of coronavirus. *City Lab*. https://www.citylab.com/equity/2020/04/coronavirus-spread-map-city-urban-density-suburbs-rural-data/609394/

Gardner, W., States, D., & Bagley, N. (2020). The coronavirus and the risks to the elderly in long-term care. *Journal of Aging & Social Policy*, 1–6. https://doi.org/10.1080/08959420.2020.1750543

Hadden Loh, T., & Fishbane, L. (2020). *COVID-19 makes the benefits of telework obvious*. The Brookings Institute. https://www.brookings.edu/blog/the-avenue/2020/03/17/covid-19-makes-the-benefits-of-telework-obvious/

Harrington Meyer, M. (2020, May 1). Grandmothers at work during Coronavirus. *Lerner News Archive*. https://lernercenter.syr.edu/2020/05/01/grandmothers-at-work-during-coronavirus/?fbclid=IwAR3vUX8wFK_T5dIcw_vp0trgfM6_QrBnvpaAo7qywYBOS6lJT748YqmzX-Y

Harrington Meyer, M., & Herd, P. (2007). *Market friendly or family friendly? The state and gender inequality in old age*. Russell Sage Foundation.

Herd, P., & Moynihan, D. P. (2019). *Administrative burden: Policymaking by other means*. Russell Sage Foundation.

Kang, J. Y., Park, S., Kim, B. R., Kwon, E., Cho, J., & Pruchno, R. (2019). The effect of California's paid family leave program on employment among middle-aged female caregivers. *Gerontologist*, *59*(6), 1092–1102. https://doi.org/10.1093/geront/gny105

Kemp, C. L., Ball, M. M., Morgan, J. C., Doyle, P. J., Burgess, E. O., & Perkins, M. M. (2018). Maneuvering together, apart, and at odds: Residents' care convoys in assisted living. *Journals of Gerontology - Series B Psychological Sciences and Social Sciences*, *73*(4), e13–e23. https://doi.org/10.1093/geronb/gbx184

Luo, Y., LaPierre, T. A., Hughes, M. E., & Waite, L. J. (2012). Grandparents providing care to grandchildren: A population-based study of continuity and change. *Journal of Family Issues*, *33*(9), 1143–1167. https://doi.org/10.1177/0192513X12438685

Moen, P., & DePasquale, N. (2017). Family care work: A policy-relevant research agenda. *International Journal of Care and Caring*, *1*(1), 45–62. https://doi.org/10.1332/239788217X14866284542346

National Partnership for Women & Families. (2019). *The family and medical insurance leave act (The FAMILY Act)*. https://www.nationalpartnership.org/our-work/resources/economic-justice/paid-leave/family-act-fact-sheet.pdf

Newman, K. S. (2019). *Downhill from here: Retirement insecurity in the age of inequality.* Metropolitan Books.

Patterson, S. E., & Margolis, R. (2019). The demography of multigenerational caregiving: A critical aspect of the gendered life course. *Socius: Sociological Research for a Dynamic World, 5.* https://doi.org/10.1177/2378023119862737

Plaisier, I., Broese van Groenou, M. I., & Keuzenkamp, S. (2015). Combining work and informal care: The importance of caring organisations. *Human Resource Management Journal, 25*(2), 267–280. https://doi.org/10.1111/1748-8583.12048

Potter, A. J. (2018). Factors associated with caregivers' use of support services and caregivers' nonuse of services sought. *Journal of Aging & Social Policy, 30*(2), 155–172. https://doi.org/10.1080/08959420.2017.1414539

Qian, G., Yang, N., Ma, A. H. Y., Wang, L., Li, G., Chen, X., & Chen, X. (2020). A COVID-19 transmission within a family cluster by presymptomatic infectors in China. *Clinical Infectious Diseases, ciaa316,* 19–20. https://doi.org/10.1093/cid/ciaa316

Rainville, C., Skufca, L., & Mehegan, L. (2016, November). *Family caregiving and out-of-pocket costs: 2016 report.* AARP. https://doi.org/10.26419/res.00138.001

Robertson, C., & Gebeloff, R. (2020). How Millions of women became the most essential workers in America. *New York Times.* https://www.nytimes.com/2020/04/18/us/corona virus-women-essential-workers.html

Sarkisian, N., Gerena, M., & Gerstel, N. (2007). Extended family integration among Euro and Mexican Americans: Ethnicity, gender, and class. *Journal of Marriage and Family, 69*(1), 40–54. https://doi.org/10.1111/j.1741-3737.2006.00342.x

Sarkisian, N., & Gerstel, N. (2004). Kin support among blacks and whites: Race and family organization. *American Sociological Review, 69*(6), 812–837. https://doi.org/10.1177/000312240406900604

Schulz, R. (2020). The intersection of family caregiving and work: Labor force participation, productivity, and caregiver well-being. In S. J. Czaja, J. Sharit & J. B. James (Eds.), *Current and emerging trends in aging and work* (pp. 399–413). Springer.

Schulz, R., & Beach, S. R. (1999). Caregiving as a risk factor for mortality: The caregiver health effects study. *JAMA, 282*(23), 2215–2219. https://doi.org/10.1001/jama.282.23.2215

Toossi, M., & Torpey, E. (2017). *Older workers: Labor force trends and career options.* U.S. Bureau of Labor Statistics. Retrieved April 30, 2020, from https://www.bls.gov/careerout look/2017/article/older-workers.htm

Van Houtven, C. H., DePasquale, N., & Coe, N. B. (2020). Essential long-term care workers commonly hold second jobs and double- or triple-duty caregiving roles. *Journal of the American Geriatrics Society.* Advance online publication. https://doi.org/10.1111/jgs.16509

Whittier, S., Scharlach, A., & Dal Santo, T. S. (2005). Availability of caregiver support services: Implications for implementation of the national family caregiver support program. *Journal of Aging & Social Policy, 17*(1), 45–62. https://doi.org/10.1300/J031v17n01_03

Wolff, J. L., Spillman, B. C., Freedman, V. A., & Kasper, J. D. (2016). A national profile of family and unpaid caregivers who assist older adults with health care activities. *JAMA Internal Medicine, 176*(3), 372. https://doi.org/10.1001/jamainternmed.2015.7664

Bereavement in the Time of Coronavirus: Unprecedented Challenges Demand Novel Interventions

Deborah Carr ⓘ, Kathrin Boerner, and Sara Moorman

ABSTRACT
COVID-19 fatalities exemplify "bad deaths" and are distinguished by physical discomfort, difficulty breathing, social isolation, psychological distress, and care that may be discordant with the patient's preferences. Each of these death attributes is a well-documented correlate of bereaved survivors' symptoms of depression, anxiety, and anger. Yet the grief experienced by survivors of COVID-related deaths is compounded by the erosion of coping resources like social support, contemporaneous stressors including social isolation, financial precarity, uncertainty about the future, lack of routine, and the loss of face-to-face mourning rituals that provide a sense of community and uplift. National efforts to enhance advance care planning may help dying patients to receive care that is concordant with the preferences of them and their families. Virtual funeral services, pairing bereaved elders with a telephone companion, remote counseling, and encouraging "continuing bonds" may help older adults adapt to loss in the time of pandemic.

More than 75,000 people in the U.S. have died of COVID-19 as of May 6, 2020, with fatalities climbing daily (Centers for Disease Control and Prevention, 2020). COVID-related deaths can strike anyone, although this risk rises dramatically with age. Older adults ages 65 years and older make up 16% of the U.S. population, yet account for 31% of all cases, 45% of hospitalizations, 53% of ICU admissions, and 80% of deaths associated with COVID-19. Oldest-old persons are especially vulnerable; the COVID-related death rate for people ages 85+ is three times higher than among persons ages 65 to 84 (CDC COVID-19 Response Team, 2020).

While daily statistics focus on the decedents, less attention is paid to the loved ones they leave behind. In this Perspective, we argue that COVID-related fatalities embody the attributes of a "bad death," making them particularly devastating for bereaved kin, whose grief may be compounded by their own social isolation, lack of practical and emotional support, and high-stress living situations marked by financial precarity, worries about their own or other family members' health, confinement to home, and the loss of routine and activity that once structured their days. New models of support must be implemented to meet the emotional needs of bereaved persons in the wake of COVID-19.

COVID-19 fatalities epitomize "bad deaths"

"Bad" or poor quality deaths are marked by physical discomfort, difficulty breathing, social isolation, psychological distress, lack of preparation, being treated without respect or dignity, and the receipt of unwanted medical interventions or being deprived of treatments one desires (Krikorian et al., 2020). "Good deaths," conversely, are distinguished by physical comfort, emotional and spiritual well-being, preparation on the part of patient and family, being surrounded by loved ones in a peaceful environment, being treated with respect and dignity, and receiving treatments concordant with one's wishes (Gawande, 2014; Steinhauser et al., 2000). Due to the excessive burden on the health care system, deaths thus far from Coronavirus have exemplified "bad deaths."

Roughly three-quarters of all COVID-related deaths take place in hospitals or nursing homes, although surveys consistently show that more than three-quarters of older adults would prefer to die at home (Centers for Disease Control and Prevention, 2020). Physical and cognitive aspects of COVID-19 deaths, including discomfort, difficulty breathing, lack of awareness, and reliance on mechanical ventilation are hallmarks of a "bad death" (Steinhauser et al., 2000). Because of the highly contagious nature of the virus, hospital and nursing home rules now prevent all patients from having visitors. As such, they are dying in isolation, separated from their loved ones; the best case scenario is that staff members facilitate family conversations via phone or video chat apps (Wakam et al., 2020). For those dying in over-crowded or overwhelmed facilities, bodies may not be treated with the dignity they would ordinarily receive, as beleaguered staff quickly make beds available for patients, with dead bodies "piling up" in hallways or refrigeration trucks (Young et al., 2020).

Why "bad deaths" are so difficult to grieve

Death context predicts survivors' symptoms of depression, anger, anxiety, and risk of complicated grief. Bereaved family members have heightened psychological symptoms when they did not have an opportunity to say "good bye" to the decedent, when the decedent was in pain, when the death was unexpected, when they perceive that the death was unjust and could have been prevented, when the death occurred in an ICU or hospital rather than at home, and the treatments received were intrusive or discordant with the patient's preferences (e.g., Carr, 2003; Chi & Demiris, 2017; Wright et al., 2010). Dying patients' moves from home to hospital in their final days are a source of distress to family members both during the transition and after the death (Coleman, 2003).

"Bad deaths" are distressing because they challenge notions of an idealized death, they prevent family members from having meaningful conversations and resolving "unfinished business," they trigger pain in seeing a loved one suffer, and they may make family members feel guilty that they could not protect their loved one from the devastating situation (e.g., Carr, 2003; Li et al., 2019). Bereaved persons who believe their loved one's death came too quickly, too young, or unjustly due to a lack of appropriate care, may experience anger and a desire to cast blame, in order to make sense of or seek retribution for their loss (Carr, 2009; Neimeyer, 2000).

Bad deaths are distressing under normal circumstances, yet the pandemic has created a context in which the pain of loss is amplified by concurrent stressors. These stressors include social isolation, financial precarity, health concerns, worries about other family members, deaths of other friends and family, and anxiety about one's own mortality (World Health Organization, 2020). This accumulation of stressors within a relatively short time period can overwhelm one's capacity to cope (Folkman, 2011).

Social and emotional support from friends and family are essential for bereaved persons' adjustment to loss (Ha, 2008). However, most older adults are now self-quarantining, so their loved ones must offer support remotely, which may not adequately meet bereaved elders' emotional and physical needs (Peek et al., 2014). Additionally, the persons upon whom older adults rely may be beset with their own struggles regarding family relationships, financial security, employment, and other losses which undermine their capacity to support their aged bereaved relatives. Many of the face-to-face interactions that support older adults as they mourn, including funeral services and religious rituals like sitting shiva, are prohibited in most U.S. states, forcing families to turn to remote memorial services (Pauly, 2020; Waters, 2020). As such, the pain of loss is compounded by co-occurring stressors, and the erosion of supports, coping resources, and rituals that are essential to bereaved persons' well-being.

Proposed practices

The best way to mitigate against survivor grief is to alter the quality of deaths experienced by those dying of Coronavirus, although such solutions will be impossible in the short and intermediate term in the absence of major invest-ments in the health care systems caring for the dying (Murthy et al., 2020). However, efforts to increase rates of advance care planning (ACP), including living wills and durable power of attorney for health care (DPAHC) designations, may help to ensure that more COVID-19 patients can convey their treatment preferences to health care providers, even if they lack decision-making capacity at the moment a decision is required. Many health and palliative care organizations like Respecting Choices (2020), Compassion in Choices (2020), and Center to Advance Palliative Care (2020) have created documents to assist with ACP and guides for effective end-of-life conversations.

Small-scale interventions may be effective in mitigating bereavement symptoms, at least in the immediate aftermath of loss. (Major investments in social programs and infrastructures will be required in the longer term, a topic beyond the scope of this brief essay). Health care workers can share respectful digitized photos of the decedent's face to provide evidence of the death and protect against the pain of ambiguous loss (Boss, 2009; Wang et al., 2020). Virtual memorial services and celebrations of the decedent's life have become the norm, yet older adults may require assistance in learning to download and use streaming services; the bereaved person's kin and support personnel like social workers or home health aides could provide this guidance. More generally, family members could encourage older adults to talk about the kind of memorial service they want for themselves someday, helping them to celebrate their loved one's life in a way that accords with their wishes.

Both professionals and volunteers can be enlisted to help bereaved older adults cope in the immediate aftermath of the loss. Supports typically provided by hospice workers could be deployed remotely to bereaved persons, such as counseling via telephone or web-based telemedicine. Community programs that connect volunteers with isolated older adults for daily telephone calls could provide special training for volunteers who are assigned to work with bereaved persons, or could recruit bereaved persons to serve as the contact for the newly bereaved, similar to the highly effective Widow to Widow program (Naylor, 2020; Silverman, 2004).

However, such programs should recognize that older persons value close ties with fewer confidants rather than many ties with fleeting acquaintances, so every effort should be made to ensure continuity of relationships (Charles & Carstensen, 2010). Additionally, practitioners who provide remote counseling to older adults must be careful to discern whether the patient's distress symptoms are grief reactions to the loss, which will fade over time, versus more serious symptoms of long-standing depression that one suffered prior to the loss. The latter require more intensive treatments, as persons with underlying depression are particularly vulnerable in times of crisis (Bonanno, 2004). For some older adults, financial insecurity may increase anxiety and require material assistance. Both professional and lay support persons also should recognize the importance of and encourage "continuing bonds" (Klass et al., 2014). Encouraging the bereaved person to recall positive memories and share stories of the decedent, to write down their memories, and to think about the conversations they might have with the decedent may provide a source of uplift and inspiration. Remembering that grief is the "price we pay for love" may provide a glimmer of solace during these bleak times (Parkes, 2014).

Conclusion

The COVID-19 pandemic has dramatically altered how older adults live, die, and mourn. Persons dying of the virus spend their final days in hospitals and nursing facilities, separated from their families. Their bereaved kin must mourn the loss without the comforting embrace of loved ones, or the support of mourners who show their respect for the deceased at funerals. The symptoms of grief, sadness, and anger experienced by bereaved family members will ultimately diminish, a reflection of human resilience in the face of loss (Bonanno, 2004). The recovery process will require innovative modes of support from professionals, family members, and community volunteers who come together to nurture the most vulnerable in their time of need.

Key Points

- COVID-19 deaths exemplify "bad" deaths: discomfort, difficulty breathing, social isolation, and treatments discordant with one's wishes.
- "Bad deaths" are especially distressing because they violate cultural expectations for a peaceful death, and involve awareness of a loved one's suffering.
- Distress associated with bereavement is compounded by older adults' social isolation, co-occurring stressors, and loss of face-to-face mourning rituals.
- Virtual memorial services, telephone support groups, and other innovations may provide short-term support for survivors of COVID-19 deaths.
- National efforts to promote advance care planning may help dying patients to receive care concordant with their wishes.
- Programs targeting the grief of older bereaved persons must take into account their distinctive needs, preferences, and anxieties.

Disclosure statement

No potential conflict of interest was reported by the authors.

ORCID

Deborah Carr ⓘ http://orcid.org/0000-0002-8175-5303

References

Bonanno, G. A. (2004). Loss, trauma, and human resilience: Have we underestimated the human capacity to thrive after extremely aversive events? *American Psychologist, 59*(1), 20–28. https://doi.org/10.1037/0003-066X.59.1.20

Boss, P. (2009). *Ambiguous loss: Learning to live with unresolved grief.* Harvard University Press.

Carr, D. (2003). A "good death" for whom? Quality of spouse's death and psychological distress among older widowed persons. *Journal of Health and Social Behavior, 44*(2), 215–232. https://doi.org/10.2307/1519809

Carr, D. (2009). Who's to blame? perceived responsibility for spousal death and psychological distress among older widowed persons. *Journal of Health and Social Behavior, 50*(3), 359–375.

CDC COVID-19 Response Team. (2020). Severe outcomes among patients with coronavirus disease 2019 (COVID-19)—United States, February 12–March 16, 2020. *MMWR, 69*(12), 343–346. https://doi.org/10.15585/mmwr.mm6912e2

Center to Advance Palliative Care. (2020). *CAPC COVID-19 response resources.* New York: Center to Advance Palliative Care. Retrieved April 28, 2020, from. https://www.capc.org/toolkits/covid-19-response-resources/.

Centers for Disease Control and Prevention. (2020). *Cases of coronavirus disease (COVID-19) in the U.S.* CDC. Retrieved April 25, 2020, from https://www.cdc.gov/coronavirus/2019-ncov/cases-updates/cases-in-us.html

Charles, S. T., & Carstensen, L. L. (2010). Social and emotional aging. *Annual Review of Psychology, 61*(1), 383–409. https://doi.org/10.1146/annurev.psych.093008.100448

Chi, N. C., & Demiris, G. (2017). Family caregivers' pain management in end-of-life care: A systematic review. *American Journal of Hospice and Palliative Medicine*, *34*(5), 470–485. https://doi.org/10.1177/1049909116637359

Coleman, E. A. (2003). Falling through the cracks: Challenges and opportunities for improving transitional care for persons with continuous complex care needs. *Journal of the American Geriatrics Society, 51*(4), 549–555. https://doi.org/10.1046/j.1532-5415.2003.51185.x

Compassion in Choices. (2020). *COVID-19: Advance care planning.* Portland, OR: Compassion in Choices. Retrieved April 28, 2020, from. https://compassionandchoices.org/resource/covid-19-advance-care-planning/.

Folkman, S. (2011). Stress, health, and coping: An overview. In *The Oxford handbook of stress, health, and coping,* ed. by S. Folkman, (pp. 3–11). New York: Oxford University Press.

Gawande, A. (2014). *Being mortal: Medicine and what matters in the end.* Macmillan.

Ha, J. H. (2008). Changes in support from confidants, children, and friends following widowhood. *Journal of Marriage and Family, 70*(2), 306–318. https://doi.org/10.1111/j.1741-3737.2008.00483.x

Klass, D., Silverman, P. R., & Nickman, S. (2014). *Continuing bonds: New understandings of grief.* Taylor & Francis.

Krikorian, A., Maldonado, C., & Pastrana, T. (2020). Patient's perspectives on the notion of a good death: A systematic review of the literature. *Journal of Pain and Symptom Management, 59*(1), 152–164. https://doi.org/10.1016/j.jpainsymman.2019.07.033

Li, J., Tendeiro, J. N., & Stroebe, M. (2019). Guilt in bereavement: Its relationship with complicated grief and depression. *International Journal of Psychology, 54*(4), 454–461. https://doi.org/10.1002/ijop.12483

Murthy, S., Gomersall, C. D., & Fowler, R. A. (2020). Care for critically ill patients with COVID-19. *JAMA, 323*(15), 1499–1500. https://doi.org/10.1001/jama.2020.3633

Naylor, D. (2020, April 26). Project HELLO to help R.I. seniors feel connected. *Providence Journal*. Retrieved April 26, 2020 from /20200426/project-hello-to-help-ri-seniors-feel-connected

Neimeyer, R. A. (2000). Searching for the meaning of meaning: Grief therapy and the process of reconstruction. *Death Studies, 24*(6), 541–558. https://doi.org/10.1080/07481180050121480

Parkes, C. M. (2014). *The price of love: The selected works of Colin Murray Parkes*. Routledge.

Pauly, M. (2020, March 23) *Virtual memorials and no hugs: The funeral industry prepares for coronavirus*. Mother Jones. Retrieved April 26, 2020, from https://www.motherjones.com/coronavirus-updates/2020/03/coronavirus-funerals/.

Peek, S. T., Wouters, E. J., Van Hoof, J., Luijkx, K. G., Boeije, H. R., & Vrijhoef, H. J. (2014). Factors influencing acceptance of technology for aging in place: A systematic review. *International Journal of Medical Informatics, 83*(4), 235–248. https://doi.org/10.1016/j.ijmedinf.2014.01.004

Respecting Choices. (2020). *COVID-19 resources*. Oregon, WI: Respecting Choices. Retrieved April 28, 2020, from. https://respectingchoices.org/covid-19-resources/.

Silverman, P. R. (2004). *Widow to widow: How the bereaved help one another*. Routledge.

Steinhauser, K. E., Christakis, N. A., Clipp, E. C., McNeilly, M., McIntyre, L., & Tulsky, J. A. (2000). Factors considered important at the end of life by patients, family, physicians, and other care providers. *JAMA, 284*(19), 2476–2482. https://doi.org/10.1001/jama.284.19.2476

Wakam, G. K., Montgomery, J. R., Biesterveld, B. E., & Brown, C. S. (2020, April 14). Not dying alone—modern compassionate care in the Covid-19 pandemic. *New England Journal of Medicine* (April 14, 2020). https://doi.org/10.1056/NEJMp2007781

Wang, S. S., Teo, W. Z., Yee, C. W., & Chai, Y. W. (2020). Pursuing a good death in the time of COVID-19. *Journal of Palliative Medicine*. https://doi.org/10.1089/jpm.2020.0198

Waters, M. (2020). The surprising intimacy of the live-streamed fneral. *The New York Times* (April 2, 2020).

World Health Organization. (2020, March 18). *Mental health and psychosocial considerations during the COVID-19 outbreak* (No. WHO/2019-nCoV/MentalHealth/2020.1).

Wright, A. A., Keating, N. L., Balboni, T. A., Matulonis, U. A., Block, S. D., & Prigerson, H. G. (2010). Place of death: Correlations with quality of life of patients with cancer and predictors of bereaved caregivers' mental health. *Journal of Clinical Oncology, 28*(29), 4457–4464. https://doi.org/10.1200/JCO.2009.26.3863

Young, R., Carpenter, J., & Murphy, P. P. (2020, April 14). Photos show bodies piled up and stored in vacant rooms at Detroit hospital." *CNN*.

Local and Community Responses

Fast-track Innovation: Area Agencies on Aging Respond to the COVID-19 Pandemic

Traci L. Wilson ⓘ, Marisa Scala-Foley, Suzanne R. Kunkel, and Amanda L. Brewster

ABSTRACT
Millions of older Americans depend on services provided by Area Agencies on Aging to support their nutritional, social, and health needs. Social distancing requirements and the closure of congregate activities due to COVID-19 resulted in a rapid and dramatic shift in service delivery modes. Area Agencies on Aging were able to quickly pivot due to their long-standing expertise in community needs assessment and cross-sectoral partnerships. The federal Coronavirus relief measures also infused one billion dollars into the Aging Network. As the pandemic response evolves, Area Agencies on Aging are poised to be key partners in a transformed health system.

Introduction

The nation's 622 Area Agencies on Aging (AAAs) are community-centered organizations that currently serve more than 11 million adults aged 60 years and older per year.[1] Established in 1973 under the Older Americans Act, AAAs plan, coordinate, and deliver social, nutritional, and long-term services and supports that help older adults live independently in their own homes. From the outset of the COVID-19 pandemic, which has been particularly challenging for older adults, AAAs had to quickly make major adjustments to meet the growing and shifting needs of the population they serve. As confirmed cases of COVID-19 spread across the US, states began to impose restrictions on social gatherings in March 2020. Even before states issued stay-at-home orders for the general public, federal and state governments implemented measures to limit the spread of COVID-19 to older adults, such as restricting visitors to nursing homes (Centers for Medicare & Medicaid Services [CMS], 2020a) and closing down the in-person services offered by

---

This article has been republished with minor changes. These changes do not impact the academic content of the article.

AAAs including congregate meals, evidence-based wellness classes, and other group social activities. Examples of new modes of service delivery quickly emerged in the network of AAAs.

In this *Perspective*, we discuss how AAAs' rapid response to COVID-19 was enabled by their long-standing expertise in assessing and meeting community needs, their cross-sectoral partnerships, and an infusion of federal funding for a network that was positioned to respond when needed. We also argue that the AAAs' roles in reducing potentially avoidable health care use and spending takes on critical importance during the pandemic. We conclude that AAAs are a key partner to ensure continuity of care in the COVID-19-transformed health system, in particular through their ability to manage and support transitions from hospital or nursing facility to home.

A rapid shift to meet older adults' basic needs

Meal provision is one example of AAAs rapid response as COVID-19 profoundly altered daily life. Prior to the pandemic, the most recent national data about AAA (2017) services showed that 1.5 million older adults regularly attended congregate meal sites to meet their nutritional and social needs, receiving over 76 million meals at these community sites. In addition, more than 860,000 older adults received nearly 144 million home-delivered meals funded by the Older Americans Act (AGID, 2017). When congregate meals were no longer an option for those millions of older adults who had been going out into their communities to share a meal with others, AAAs shifted resources to meet the skyrocketing requests for home-delivered meals (Brewster et al., 2020).

One challenge AAAs faced to meet this increased service demand was a dwindling volunteer pool. For meal delivery and other services, AAAs often rely on volunteers, many of whom are older adults themselves and at higher risk of complications from COVID-19. To overcome this sudden shortage in volunteers, the methods and modalities used to deliver services had to change. Strategies included delivering shelf-stable or frozen meals to reduce the number of trips, offering drive-through meal collection, and redeploying staff. For example, at Elder Services of the Merrimack Valley, a Massachusetts AAA, staff redeployed from providing in-person program delivery to conducting telephonic wellness checks and delivering meals. Like many AAAs, they reported an increase in referrals due to social distancing and COVID-19 concerns.

The legislated community-centered mission of AAAs set the stage for this kind of response. Their position as a hub for community-based service planning and coordination requires AAAs to routinely assess and respond to the needs of older adults in their areas. This role keeps AAAs in touch with their communities and makes them attentive to evolving situations that can influence the needs and well-being of the older adults in their communities. In addition to this long-held responsibility for monitoring and supporting the needs of older adults in their areas, two other factors enabled AAAs' to quickly shift their work in response to COVID-19.

First was an infusion of new federal funding that acknowledged the life-sustaining importance of the services provided by the Aging Network. As part of the three initial coronavirus response bills, the federal government invested over one billion dollars in the Aging Network. The Families First Coronavirus Response Act, which was signed into law on March 18, 2020, included 250 USD million designated to the Administration for Community Living (ACL) to support Older Americans Act nutrition services (Dawson & Long, 2020). The Coronavirus Aid, Relief, and Economic Security (CARES) Act on March 27 allocated 955 USD million to ACL, of which 820 USD million was earmarked for activities authorized under the Older Americans Act, including 200 USD million for Title III B home and community-based services, 480 USD million for Title III C nutrition services including home-delivered meals, 20 USD million for nutrition and related services for Native American Aging Programs under Title VI, 100 USD million for support services for family caregivers under Title III E, and 20 USD million for Title VII elder rights protection activities (Wexler et al., 2020).

A second factor that enabled the AAAs' agile response was the existence of partnerships, collaborations, and contracting relationships between AAAs, health care entities, and other service providers in their communities. Previous research has shown that AAAs are often local leaders in connecting health care and social service organizations (Brewster et al., 2019). Their long-standing experience at the intersection of health and social care has resulted in AAAs becoming a key partner in managed- and integrated-care systems. Seventy-four percent of AAAs report a partnership with a hospital or health system, and 62% have a partnership with a health plan or managed care organization (National Association of Area Agencies on Aging, 2020).

Contracting between health care and social service organizations represents a formalized partnership, and provides an opportunity for more people to receive supportive services and for AAAs and other community-based organizations to be compensated for this work. The most recently available data shows that 42% of AAAs have a contract with a health care entity to provide services, and that the most common services provided through contracts are case management (55%), care transitions (46%), and nutrition programs (40%) (Kunkel et al., 2018, 2017). Recognizing that AAAs may play an important role in integrating health and social services, the Older Americans Act reauthorization, Supporting Older Americans Act (2020), added clarifying language that states: "Nothing in this Act shall restrict an area agency on aging from providing services not provided or authorized by this Act, including through – (1) contracts with health care payers ... "

What now? Building on AAA-health care partnerships

Now that the initial crisis response has created a "new normal", AAAs are shifting attention to additional ways their expertise can meet new COVID-19 related demands and opportunities. As of May 1, 2020, some states are beginning to "reopen" in various ways. The next 12–18 months will bring a continuation of social distancing to minimize risk of transmission, in particular for those most susceptible to serious illness. What does this mean for our systems of support for older adults in the community?

By providing services that help older adults remain safe and independent in their own homes, AAAs help these individuals limit their potential exposure to SARS-CoV-2. Previous research suggests that AAA partnerships help to prevent unnecessary hospitalizations and nursing home admissions (Brewster et al., 2018, 2020), locations that can increase risk of exposure. In the COVID-19 era, reducing unnecessary admissions has taken on even more importance than before for several reasons. First, as health systems prepared for a possible surge of COVID-19 cases, they sought to free as many beds as possible; this may be required again in the future as the number of COVID-19 cases ebb and flow in different regions. Second, the usual chain of care transitions may need to be adjusted to address concerns about introducing COVID to the facility. Skilled nursing facilities may refuse or be reluctant to admit new consumers for this fear. The resulting lack of skilled beds can create a backlog that slows down release from the hospital to rehabilitation.

As one means to address this situation, the Centers for Medicare & Medicaid Services (CMS) have instituted the Hospital Without Walls initiative which, among other flexibilities, allows hospitals to bill for outpatient services that are provided in temporary expansion sites, including patients' homes (CMS, 2020b). Delivering hospital services in patients' homes and other non-health care settings requires strong partnerships between health care entities and community-based service providers. In many regions, AAAs are logical partners to provide remote monitoring, case management and care coordination, meal services, discharge planning, and care transitions services (Aging and Disability Business Institute, 2020).

One example of a AAA providing these services is the Council on Aging of Southwestern Ohio (COA), a AAA that provides care management and home and community-based services for over 25,000 individuals in the Cincinnati region. Beginning in 2012, COA provided care transitions with funding from the CMS Community-based Care Transitions Program (CCTP). When CCTP funding ended, COA built on this experience and launched their FastTrack Home care transitions program in 2017, which is now in place in skilled nursing facilities and most large hospitals in Cincinnati, Ohio. The program provides an in-person pre-discharge assessment to determine the type, frequency, and duration of in-home support services needed. A care manager works with the individual and family to set up and manage the services, which might include meal delivery, transportation to medical appointments, and homemaking.

The Council on Aging of Southwestern Ohio has responded to the COVID-19 crisis by adapting its FastTrack Home model to support patients leaving skilled nursing facilities and hospitals encountering a surge in demand. Faced with challenges of limiting in-person contact and meeting increased demand, COA has implemented the following emergency-response innovations to the FastTrack Home model:

- Changing the referral and coaching model by establishing telephonic coaching protocols, dropping hospital coaching presence and adding an intake queue;
- Ramping up capacity by shifting staff resources and training, and expanding days of operation to seven days a week;
- Developing provider guidance and protocols to ensure services continue to be provided safely and in alignment with guidelines from the Centers for Disease Control and Prevention;
- Expanding home-delivered meals availability to seven days a week; and
- Adapting services that are especially needed by those coming out of the hospital in the following ways: Durable Medical Equipment (deliver pre-assembled equipment so installer does not need to enter the home), Emergency Medical Response Systems (switch to GPS/wireless devices that do not require installation), and transportation to primary care appointments (drivers have PPE and sanitize hard surfaces after each trip).

Conclusion

The pandemic crisis highlights the importance of meeting social needs to support community health and has increased awareness of the value of services that AAAs provide. AAAs were designed as locally-responsive organizations to assess and plan for community needs. Since their inception, they have repeatedly demonstrated that they can design, adapt, and innovate in response to government mandates, community demand, health care partner needs, and emergency situations. The federal COVID-19 response has included a huge infusion of funding into the Aging Network to provide nutrition, home and community-based services, and support for caregivers. The examples shared in this article demonstrate not only the critical role that AAAs play in meeting older adults' basic needs, but also in their ability to rapidly adapt and innovate to meet situational and delivery challenges.

Key Points

- Area Agencies on Aging (AAAs) quickly adapted services to meet the basic needs of older adults during COVID-19.
- AAAs responded by offering innovative service provision and delivery during the pandemic.
- AAAs leveraged expertise in community needs assessment and planning, supplemented by federal relief.
- AAAs are a key partner to ensure continuity of care in a transformed health system.

Note

1. AAAs were established in a 1973 amendment to the Older Americans Act (OAA) of 1965, and given a very specific role in their communities. The most recent reauthorization of OAA signed into law on March 25, the Supporting Older Americans Act of 2020 (Robertson, 2020), reaffirms the initial enabling legislation that gave the Aging Network the community-centered mandate to design and deliver services that best meet the needs of older adults in their local area with agility, flexibility and adherence to shared underlying principles. For background on the role and evolution of the OAA and AAAs, see (Applebaum et al., 2018; Kunkel, 2019).

Disclosure statement

No potential conflict of interest was reported by the authors.

Funding

This work was supported by The John A. Hartford Foundation [2018-0195] and The SCAN Foundation [19-010].

ORCID

Traci L. Wilson DPhil http://orcid.org/0000-0002-7010-728X

ORCID

Traci L. Wilson DPhil http://orcid.org/0000-0002-7010-728X

References

AGID. (2017). *Profile of state OAA programs.* https://agid.acl.gov/StateProfiles/Profile/Pre/?id=109&topic=0

Aging and Disability Business Institute. (2020, May). *Hospital without walls- new opportunities for CBOs.* https://www.aginganddisabilitybusinessinstitute.org/resources/hospital-without-walls-new-opportunities-for-cbos/

Applebaum, R., Kunkel, S., & Hudson, R. B. (2018). The life and times of the aging network. *Public Policy & Aging Report, 28*(1), 39–43. https://doi.org/10.1093/ppar/pry007

Brewster, A. L., Kunkel, S. R., Straker, J. K., & Curry, L. A. (2018). Cross-sectoral partnerships by area agencies on aging: associations with health care use and spending. *Health Affairs, 37* (1), 15–21. https://doi.org/10.1377/hlthaff.2017.1346

Brewster, A. L., Wilson, T. L., Frehn, J., Berish, D., & Kunkel, S. R. (2020). Linking health and social services through area agencies on aging is associated with lower health care use and spending. *Health Affairs (Project Hope), 39*(4), 587–594. https://doi.org/10.1377/hlthaff.2019.01515

Brewster, A. L., Wilson, T. L., Kunkel, S. R., Markwood, S., & Shah, T. (2020, April 8). *To support older adults amidst the COVID-19 pandemic, look to area agencies on aging.* Health Affairs. https://www.healthaffairs.org/do/10.1377/hblog20200408.928642/full/

Brewster, A. L., Yuan, C. T., Tan, A. X., Tangoren, C. G., & Curry, L. A. (2019). Collaboration in health care and social service networks for older adults: Association with health care utilization measures. *Medical Care, 57*(5), 327–333. https://doi.org/10.1097/MLR. 0000000000001097

Centers for Medicare & Medicaid Services. (2020a, March 13). *CMS announces new measures to protect nursing home residents from COVID-19 | CMS.* https://www.cms.gov/newsroom/press-releases/cms-announces-new-measures-protect-nursing-home-residents-covid-19

Centers for Medicare & Medicaid Services. (2020b). *Hospitals: CMS flexibilities to fight COVID-19.* https://www.cms.gov/files/document/covid-hospitals.pdf

Dawson, L., & Long, M. (2020, March 23). *The families first coronavirus response act: Summary of key provisions.* The Henry J. Kaiser Family Foundation. https://www.kff.org/coronavirus-covid -19/issue-brief/the-families-first-coronavirus-response-act-summary-of-key-provisions/

Kunkel, S. R. (2019). Building on the past, securing the future: Area agencies on aging and older americans act reauthorization. *Public Policy & Aging Report, 29*(2), 52–55. https://doi.org/ 10.1093/ppar/prz009

Kunkel, S. R., Lackmeyer, A. E., Straker, J. K., & Wilson, T. L. (2018). *Community-based organizations and health care contracting: Building and strengthening partnerships.* Oxford, OH: Scripps Gerontology Center, Miami University. https://www.miamioh.edu/cas/aca demics/centers/scripps/research/publications/2018/11/community-based-organizations-and-health-care-contracting-building-and-strengthening-partnerships.html

Kunkel, S. R., Straker, J. K., Kelly, E. M., & Lackmeyer, A. E. (2017). *Community-based organizations and health care contracting.* Oxford, OH: Scripps Gerontology Center, Miami University. https://www.miamioh.edu/cas/academics/centers/scripps/research/publi cations/2017/12/Community-based-organizations-and-health-care-contracting.html

National Association of Area Agencies on Aging. (2020). *National survey of area agencies on aging: 2019 results.* Washington, DC: National Association of Area Agencies on Aging. Forthcoming.

Robertson, L. (2020, March 25). *A renewed commitment to our nation's older adults [Text].* HHS.Gov. https://www.hhs.gov/blog/2020/03/25/renewed-commitment-our-nation -s-older-adults.html

Supporting Older Americans Act. (2020). Supporting Older Americans Act, H.R. 4334, 116th Cong. Retrieved from https://www.congress.gov/bill/116th-congress/house-bill/4334/text

Wexler, A., Dawson, L., Long, M., Freed, M., Ramaswamy, A., & Ranji, U. (2020, April 9). *The coronavirus aid, relief, and economic security act: Summary of key health provisions.* The Henry J. Kaiser Family Foundation. https://www.kff.org/coronavirus-covid-19/issue-brief /the-coronavirus-aid-relief-and-economic-security-act-summary-of-key-health-provisions/

Local Government Efforts to Mitigate the Novel Coronavirus Pandemic among Older Adults

Jacqueline L. Angel and Stipica Mudrazija

ABSTRACT

As the coronavirus crisis spreads swiftly through the population, it takes a particularly heavy toll on minority individuals and older adults, with older minority adults at especially high risk. Given the shockingly high rates of infections and deaths in nursing homes, staying in the community appears to be a good option for older adults in this crisis, but in order for some older adults to do so much assistance is required. This situation draws attention to the need for benevolent intervention on the part of the state should older adults become ill or lose their sources of income and support during the crisis. This essay provides a brief overview of public support and the financial and health benefits for older individuals who remain in the community during the pandemic. It reports the case example of Austin, Texas, a city with a rapidly aging and diverse population of almost a million residents, to ask how we can assess the success of municipalities in responding to the changing needs of older adults in the community due to COVID-19. It concludes with a discussion of what governmental and non-governmental leadership can accomplish in situations such as that brought about by the current crisis.

As the coronavirus crisis sweeps through nursing homes, our nation is reminded that where we live and with whom we live matters, especially for those of advanced age. Death rates from COVID-19 are highest among older adults, especially among those with underlying medical conditions. During the global pandemic individuals in most countries are confined to their residencies if possible, but this may be challenging for older adults due to dramatic changes in family living arrangements for aging Americans over the past half century. According to the U.S. Census Bureau, the fraction of people ages 65 years and over living alone has increased substantially in recent decades, and it now represents about 30% of individuals in this age group (U.S. Census Bureau, 2019). Living alone no doubt increases with age due to the loss of a spouse. In the U.S., about half of older women (45%) age

75 and above live alone (The Administration of Community Living, 2018). European countries in large part mirror these trends (Mudrazija et al., 2020).

Given the shockingly high rates of infections and deaths in nursing homes, remaining in the community appears to be a good option for older adults in this crisis, but in order for some older adults to do so much assistance is required. This essay argues that while living arrangements depend on one's circumstances and personal desires, the role of policies, both at the national and local levels, is also critical, especially in the context of promoting socially desirable outcomes and providing the resources necessary to achieve them. Communities in the U.S. – whether rural, urban barrios, or suburbs – may be ill-equipped to deal with aging populations and those at highest risk during COVID-19. The swift-spreading coronavirus public health crisis has caught many southern states off guard. These include Alabama, Florida, Georgia, Mississippi, and Texas, all of which have yet to expand Medicaid (Kaiser Family Foundation, 2020). Cities hit the hardest by the epidemic such as Atlanta, Georgia, and New Orleans, Louisiana scramble to mobilize resources to save lives, disproportionately in African American communities, amid already overwhelmed hospitals and public health services (Brooks, 2020).

We begin with a brief overview of living arrangements in the U.S. and the history of public support for keeping older adults within the community as long as possible in later life. We then take a close look at Texas, which, at 17.7%, had the highest uninsured rate in the country in 2018 (Keith, 2019). In many states, older residents – pre-retirement age, immigrants, and adult caregivers – lack easy access to a health care provider and thus, are unable to get tested for the virus during this crisis. By example, we present a case study of Austin, Texas, a city of almost a million residents with a rapidly aging and diverse population, to gauge the preparedness of the City in responding to the needs of older adults in the community during COVID-19. Austin is the first municipality in Texas to receive official approval for implementation of an Age-Friendly Action Plan, a World Health Organization and AARP initiative that enables people of all ages to stay at home for as long as possible (City of Austin Commission on Seniors Working Group, 2016). We end with a discussion of what the role of governmental and non-governmental leadership can accomplish in situations such as that brought about by the current crisis.

Living arrangements in the U.S

In the 20th-century, wealth generated by a vibrant post-World War II economy coupled with falling poverty rates made it possible for older adults to afford to live alone across most developed countries. Aside from having more income to support independence, many social norms associated with aging in recent years have altered the lives of older adults. Most individuals have developed an expectation of privacy, craving autonomy and independence when they reach old age. Similarly, most older adults prefer to continue living safely in their community and their home for as long as they can, as opposed to residing in a nursing home even in the event of cognitive decline (Evans et al., 2019; Portacolone et al., 2019). Home is not only an asset, but also a place to which a person is emotionally attached (Mudrazija & Butrica, 2017). The sense of belonging to a community where one lived for a substantial part of his or her life is generally very strong. Such values reflect an ardent preference toward living in one's own home as opposed to moving in with children or an assisted living facility. For most home owners it represents a major fraction of a family's total wealth and probably the largest portion of what they can leave to future generations (Mudrazija & Angel, 2014).

In the U.S., however, living arrangements are not uniform across racial and ethnic groups. Although currently only 20% of older adults age 65 years and over are members of a racial/ethnic minority group, projections show that aging African Americans, Hispanics, and Asians will account for 42% of the population by 2050 (Angel, 2018). Social scientists have long established that older minority American households are far more complex than the majority households. This complexity can be attributed to marked differences in marital dissolution and migration patterns, greater socioeconomic disadvantage, and a legacy of cultural preferences in kin solidarity (Himes et al., 1996). Low-income African Americans and Mexican Americans have a greater propensity than non-Hispanic whites to form joint households in response to changing needs for financial or health assistance (Cohn & Passel, 2016). In Europe, living in extended-family households that include relatives such as grandchildren, nephews, and adult children's spouses are the most common arrangement for people 60 and older (Ausubel, 2020).

In light of the global pandemic, however, new pressing considerations related to living arrangements are emerging. The pandemic has shown how close quarters and institutional settings have not fared well, which will impact how we age in the future (Horowitz & Bubola, 2020). Growing old in a nursing home is now a grim but clear reality for some of the nation's frailest, infirmed, and vulnerable older adults that places them at considerably greater risk from COVID-19 (Stockman et al., 2020), While shelter-in-place orders have worked to reduce the spread of the virus within the community, home has become a dangerous place for those who live with family in close quarters. Essentially, the family household has become a disease vector for many older adults alongside clusters of residents in nursing homes (Horowitz & Bubola, 2020). It is abundantly clear that the COVID virus outbreak is adding peril to the vulnerable populations already at-risk, sounding an alarm for aging policies that promote supportive services and programs that enable older adults to stay in their homes as the shelter-in-place orders linger.

Public support for aging in the community

A recent cross-national study compared the income and wealth profiles of the population aged 60 years and above for those living alone in the U.S. and 19 European countries. The data from the Health and Retirement Survey (HRS) and Survey of Health, Aging and Retirement in Europe (SHARE) revealed that living alone is far more common in old-age welfare systems like Germany, Sweden, Denmark, and Switzerland, partly because of generous social support and spending (Mudrazija et al., 2020). On the other hand, a lack of adequate public support in less generous welfare states such as the U.S., Greece, and Italy tended to constrain the ability of many low-income older adults without a partner to continue living independently.

In later years of the life course, where and with whom one lives greatly influences the quality of one's life. Yet a person's living arrangements are not solely the result of individual choices. The options from which an older person can choose are determined by his or her economic and social resources, as well as by his or her state of health. As a result, living arrangements and levels of independence vary greatly among the elderly. Gender differences in living arrangements magnify group disparities in care options as people age in place. For example, data from the largest and longest running study of older Mexican-Americans in the Southwestern United States show that women are more likely to live longer than other racial/ethnic groups of women and men. Consequently, they are at high risk of dependency on family and "fictive kin" partly because of limited options in formal community-based long-term care services and supports (Angel et al., 2018; Rote et al., 2017).

Many communities in the U.S. – rural, urban ethnic barrios, and suburbs – are underserved. Municipalities struggle fiscally in light of increasing demographic pressures to promote aging in place – with all of the services and supports that are needed – for their older residents while also attracting younger generations required to ensure continued economic prosperity and social vitality (Torres-Gil & Angel, 2019). In conjunction with the fact that many families face daunting challenges to provide care during COVID-19, other arrangements must be considered. These include semi-formal organizations consisting of community-based resources that family caregivers can call upon during the virus outbreak. Resources range from informal, unpaid care from family members and others, formal governmental agencies that provide eldercare services and, in between, non-governmental organizations. Examples of the latter include faith-based organizations, synagogues, and congregations that increasingly serve as vital sources of assistance to families caring for elders at risk for infection or who live alone and have no family support.

According to the Administration on Community Living, access to state-sponsored services like the state Area Agencies on Aging (AAA) and Aging and Disability Resource Centers is critical for older adults and their families. These local agencies offer an important support system for older adults 60 and over, including distributing information, providing assistance, helping to manage services, and giving access to publicly-funded programs like Medicaid. State AAAs may also receive grant funding, based on their share of the population age 70 and over, to administer the National Family Caregiver Support Program (NFCSP) program, which links services to caregivers 18 years and older, regardless of the age of the care recipient. However, few community-based programs have adequate funding to operate effectively given the need in low-resource communities. This lack of resources poses a challenge during regular operations but especially during crises like COVID-19.

Case example: Austin, Texas

Austin, Texas is the fastest-growing big city in America. Projections show that from 2015 to 2030 Travis County's population (within which Austin is situated) will grow by more than 20% to 1.3 million residents (City of Austin, 2015). The city's rapid expansion is the result of growth in every age group, but nowhere is that surge more pronounced than among seniors 55 and older (Angel, 2016). The Austin metropolitan area leads the nation in the growth rate of people ages 55 to 64, and has the second highest growth rate of those 65 and older (Aging Services Council of Central Texas, 2019). The population of individuals 65 and older in Travis County is projected to almost double between 2015 and 2040 (Neely, 2017). In ten years, one out of five Austin residents will be 65 or older (City of Austin, 2015). The needs of the older low-income population present unique challenges to policymakers in Travis County in light of COVID-19.

Austin is administered by an eleven-member city council consisting of ten council members elected by a geographic district plus a mayor elected at large who is Steve Adler. The City employs about 13,500 staff in more than 40 departments that offer a wide range of services (City of Austin, 2020). For example, Austin Public Health (APH) offers extensive public health services from health education programs to enforcing regulations that protect everyone from injury and illness (City of Austin, 2020).

After the declaration of the novel coronavirus global pandemic by the World Health Organization on March 11, 2020 (Branswell & Joseph, 2020), APH collaborated effectively with the Department of State Health Services, Centers for Disease Control and Prevention (CDC), and local and regional public health and healthcare agencies to develop a COVID-19 response plan in accordance with new CDC guidelines (Centers for Disease Control, 2020). APH is adjusting operations, modifying work schedules and programs, to continue providing services to residents while ensuring public health and safety in response to the coronavirus outbreak. As part of the strategy, senior residents are given special attention because of known sources of vulnerability to aging in place amid the crisis. Currently, APH's epidemiologists are actively investigating clusters of COVID-19 cases in Austin-Travis County as part of efforts to contain COVID-19. On March 30th, Austin Public Health announced a new plan for nursing home residents that tested positive for COVID-19 but do not require hospitalization. To keep the virus from spreading, two "isolation facilities" containing 100 beds total were set up in Travis and Williamson Counties to treat older residents who typically reside in nursing or assisted living facilities.

In addition, APH created a Senior Task Force to mobilize interagency guidance to assess gaps in service delivery and housing supports. Austin City Mayor Steve Adler gives daily briefings to educate the public. These provide consistent public messaging regarding the goals to protect residents' health by complying with stay at home and shelter orders that would contain the spread of the virus infection. Adherence to social distancing and washing hands have been emphasized as key mitigating strategies to save the lives of senior residents. Given the high risk among older adults in large public spaces, the City also issued a Mayoral declaration on March 16, 2020 closing all three senior activity centers. In addition, the City has partnered with local businesses and voluntary organizations to build capacity to produce more masks.

Led by APH, a cross-department Senior Task Force engages in daily dialogue to assess service gaps in changing needs for assistance and to identify unmet services and supports. Three of the ten members of the Austin City Council sit on this Task Force. In terms of public education and outreach, the City's Information Technology Department created a new web page with links to provide updated and vital COVID-19 information linked to the Travis County Dashboard (TCD), fostering transparency of confirmed COVID-19 cases and deaths (see www.austintexas.gov/covid19). Up-to-date Stay at Home Order Information and specific requirements are available on the TCD. For other Corona-related questions that cannot be answered by what is on the TCD, residents can call 3-1-1, the exchange for police non-emergency inquiries (see https://www.austintexas.gov/department/311). Additionally, APH works alongside Austin-Travis County Emergency Operation Center's newly created social services branch Task Forces in their ongoing COVID-19 response efforts to address the needs of the frailest and most vulnerable older adults in the community, including those with behavioral health problems and the homeless population (see http://austintexas.gov/news/austin-travis-county-creates-social-service-branch-emergency-response-efforts).

As the virus takes its course, the City of Austin uses the data report on the TCD to gauge benchmarks for containment of the virus, which is achieved after a sustained reduction in cases for at least two weeks. Importantly, the

Dashboard's home page also includes a self-assessment tool to assess COVID-19 symptoms. Seniors, caregivers, and others can pre-register for free testing, and schedule a no-cost, drive-through test at a local Austin Public Health facility. A Hotline number for the uninsured was set up by Central Health, a public entity funded by local taxes, for treatment at one of seven neighborhood health clinics (known as Federally Qualified Health Centers) in the City of Austin (Health Resources and Services Administration, 2018). A medical team triages all callers and makes appropriate recommendations while answering patient questions related to COVID-19.

Some City Council members also hold virtual Town Halls to assess the needs of District residents, provide updates posted on Facebook, and publish monthly newsletters. Senior issues are highlighted and panelists at the virtual Town Halls represent local grocery stores and nonprofit organizations, such as Meals on Wheels Central Texas, Drive a Senior West Austin, and the municipal government's Aging Services Council of Central Texas. These organizations are adapting to serve senior clients in the midst of the pandemic. Like counterparts around the country, grocery stores are holding senior-only store hours to minimize older adult's exposure to the coronavirus. Meals on Wheels Central Texas has adopted many programs, including the Pets Assisting the Lives of Seniors (PALS) service that supplies pet food and veterinary care (Texas, M. O. W. C., 2020). The Aging Services Council of Central Texas provides a list of special services related to COVID-19, opportunities to work for a nonprofit organization by volunteering at home or in the field as well as donate money to help support seniors age in place (Aging Services Council of Central Texas, 2020)

To facilitate aging-in-place, APH is working to align public and private organizations to address food insecurity. The Central Texas Food Bank, a nonprofit organization, currently serves around 1,600 seniors a month through the Healthy Options Program for the Elderly (HOPE) in partnership with Meals on Wheels Central Texas. In response to COVID-19, the Food Bank partnered with H-E-B, a Texas-based supermarket chain that offers food delivery service, and Capital Metro to deploy Help-at-Home kits that consist of pantry staples, such as peanut butter, rice, soup, and canned vegetables to the City of Austin's Metro-Access, a shared-ride service for seniors and people whose disabilities prevent them from riding other Austin bus and rail services (CapMetro, 2020). H-E-B instituted senior grocery delivery through the Favor App or Website (https://favordelivery.com/) for those 60 and older. Same day delivery is available 11 a.m-7 p.m. (H-E-B, 2020)

Drive-a-Senior West Austin (DSWA) now offers free grocery delivery services and prescription delivery services for clients. Similarly, Randall's Grocery gives the option of free delivery for prescriptions during this time. DSWA recently launched operation of an emergency food pantry delivery service to seniors 60 and older. The emergency response will be sustained until the end of 2020 and seniors, who are at the highest risk of death from the disease, will be encouraged to stay home much longer than the general public once orders are lifted (Drive a Senior Austin West, 2020).

While most state and local governments struggle to keep the outbreak at bay with shrinking budgets, the City of Austin shines a glimmer of hope on ways of doing this well. At the same time, the extent to which City officials, along with non-governmental partners, can manage the epidemic and economic damage alone has yet to be gauged. Current federal government efforts lag behind local municipalities in providing the real help low-income workers and their families need in the absence of adequate federal and state support. As the City of Austin has shown, it takes a smart deployment of resources by coordinating efforts of various agencies and departments that provide services to seniors. This coordination involves housing, social welfare programs, food access, transportation, and other supports critical for older adults to live independently. Such services are essential for those of limited and moderate means.

Notwithstanding these efforts, other vexing issues loom as COVID-19 lives on. According to the Aging Services Council of Central Texas, there are currently limited or no transportation services that will take seniors to testing sites. Many seniors worry about safe access to a local doctor's office or hospital. Seniors also lack access to reliable technical devices, and many do not understand how to use devices if given access, nor can they afford the additional cost of Wi-Fi. Social isolation is a major concern, especially for seniors living alone. Our seniors need contact from the community, during the pandemic and beyond (Austin City Council, 2020).

Conclusion

The range of actions taken by Austin's local government in partnership with nonprofits and for-profit businesses represents a successful example of how local authorities can facilitate life in the community for seniors. While these services have been introduced in response to the COVID-19 pandemic, at least some of them could and should stay in place permanently as they meaningfully improve the quality of life for seniors who live in the community.

Long-term, as the virus lingers, the pandemic accentuates in particular the risks for those seniors living without family and social support. This situation is avoidable with proper preparation. Austin, by example, is a template for a city's preparedness planning for an aging population under extraordinary circumstances and are likely to be useful in the future. While young and hip, the City is rapidly becoming older and more diverse which demands effective implementation of aging-in-place policies. The City is confronting many new challenges in addressing the needs of residents aging and living alone during the Corona virus outbreak. Isolated seniors and those with no relatives and a fragile social network are particularly at high risk of disability and death without a safety net. The rising cost of living, lack of affordable housing options, and need for support in retirement is a major concern and has given rise to shared living arrangements – co-residence and multigenerational households – placing many seniors, especially among immigrant families, precariously at high exposure to the virus given the small spaces that are shared most. For many cities, strengthening social resilience is vital for recovery. With strong partnerships and civic leaders, cities and the nation can rise to the challenge of enhancing livability for all in these difficult times.

Key points

- Helping older adults age safely in the community is far more important than ever in viral pandemic.
- Living alone is more common in municipalities that have generous old-age social support.
- Effective response to COVID-19 requires coordination among the local polity and private and not-for-profit organizations.
- COVID-19 presents fiscal and administrative challenges to sustaining livable communities for older residents who face the greatest barriers to sheltering in place.

Disclosure statement

No potential conflict of interest was reported by the authors.

References

The Administration of Community Living. (2018). *2017 profile of older Americans*. Retrieved May 5, 2020, from https://acl.gov/sites/default/files/Aging%20and%20Disability%20in%20America/2017OlderAmericansProfile.pdf

Aging Services Council of Central Texas. (2019). *Demographics of Aging Austin*. Retrieved May 8, 2020, from https://www.agingservicescouncil.org/stats

Aging Services Council of Central Texas. (2020). *Special services related to COVID-19 for central Texas*. Retrieved May 9, 2020, from https://www.agingservicescouncil.org/

Angel, J. L. (2016). *A better life for low-income elders in Austin*. The University of Texas at Austin. Retrieved May 1, 2020, from https://repositories.lib.utexas.edu/handle/2152/44507

Angel, J. L. (2018). Aging policy in a majority-minority nation. *Public Policy & Aging Report*, *28*(1), 19–23. https://doi.org/10.1093/ppar/pry005

Angel, J. L., Caldera, S., & Angel, R. J. (2018). *Medicaid long-term community care in California and Texas: A growing fiscal challenge in a new Era* (Vol. 4). Springer Nature.

Austin City Council. (2020). *Virtual town hall with council member alison alter*. Retrieved May 1, 2020, from https://nwaca.org/wp-content/uploads/2020/04/Overview-Seniors-Food-Access-Town-Hall.pdf

Ausubel, J. (2020). *Older people are more likely to live alone in the U.S. than elsewhere in the world*. Pew Research Center. Retrieved April 20, 2020, from https://www.pewresearch.org/ fact-tank/2020/03/10/older-people-are-more-likely-to-live-alone-in-the-u-s-than-elsewhere -in-the-world/

Branswell, H., & Joseph, A. (2020). WHO declares the Coronavirus outbreak a pandemic. *Stat*. Retrieved May 7, 2020, from https://www.statnews.com/2020/03/11/who-declares-the -coronavirus-outbreak-a-pandemic/

Brooks, R. A. (2020). African Americans struggle with disproportionate COVID death toll. *National Geographic*. Retrieved April 26, 2020, from https://www.nationalgeographic.com/ history/2020/04/coronavirus-disproportionately-impacts-african-americans/

CapMetro. (2020). CapMetro in the community. *Metro*. Retrieved May 9, 2020, from https:// capmetro.org/helpathomekits/

Centers for Disease Control. (2020). *Coronavirus disease 2019 (COVID-19)*. Retrieved May 7, 2020, from https://www.cdc.gov/coronavirus/2019-ncov/communication/guidance-list. html?Sort=Date%3A%3Adesc

City of Austin. (2015). *A demographic snapshot of Austin rotary club of Austin Westlake* (slide #36). Retrieved May 1, 2020, from http://www.austintexas.gov/edims/document.cfm?id= 286534

City of Austin. (2020). *Human resources*. Retrieved May 7, 2020, from http://austintexas.gov/ department/human-resources

City of Austin Commission on Seniors Working Group. (2016). *Age-friendly AustinAction plan: Executive summary*. Retrieved May 8, 2020, from http://www.austintexas.gov/edims/ document.cfm?id=260993

Cohn, D. V., & Passel, J. S. (2016). *A record 60.6 million Americans live in multigenerational households*. Pew Research Center. Retrieved July 8, 2016, from http://www.pewresearch. org/fact-tank/2016/08/11/a-record-60-6-million-americans-live-in-multigenerational-households/

Drive a Senior Austin West. (2020). *DAW Austin West*. Retrieved May 5, 2020, from https:// driveasenior.org/austin-west/

Evans, I. E. M., Llewellyn, D. J., Matthews, F. E., Woods, R. T., Brayne, C., & Clare, L. (2019). Living alone and cognitive function in later life. *Arcives of Gerontology and Geriatrics*, *81* (March–April), 222–233. https://doi.org/10.1016/j.archger.2018.12.014

Health Resources and Services Administration. (2018). *Federally qualified health centers*. Retrieved May 5, 2020, from https://www.hrsa.gov/opa/eligibility-and-registration/health-centers/fqhc/index.html

H-E-B. (2020). H-E-B and favor team up to support seniors. *Favor*. Retrieved May 5, 2020, from https://blog.favordelivery.com/h-e-b-and-favor-team-up-to-support-seniors -61f4ab4ad3ac

Himes, C., Hogan, D., & Eggebeen, D. (1996). Living arrangements of minority elders. *Journals of Gerontology. Series B, Psychological Sciences and Social Sciences*, *51*(1), S42– 48. https://doi.org/10.1093/geronb/51B.1.S42

Horowitz, J., & Bubola, E. (2020, April 24). *Isolating the sick at home, Italy stores up family tragedies*. *The New York Times*. Retrieved April 26, 2020, from https://www.nytimes.com/ 2020/04/24/world/europe/italy-coronavirus-home-isolation.html

Kaiser Family Foundation. (2020). *Status of state medicaid expansion decisions*. Retrieved May 7, 2020, from https://www.kff.org/medicaid/issue-brief/status-of-state-medicaid-expansion -decisions-interactive-map/

Keith, K. (2019). Uninsured rate rose in 2018, says Census Bureau report. *Health Affairs Blog*. Retrieved May 7, 2020, from https://www.healthaffairs.org/do/10.1377/hblog20190911. 805983/full/.

Mudrazija, S., & Angel, J. L. (2014). Diversity and the economic security of older Americans. In *The new politics of old age policy* (Vol. 3, pp. 138–154). Johns Hopkins University Press.

Mudrazija, S., Angel, J. L., Cipin, I., & Smolic, S. (2020). Living alone in the United States and Europe: The impact of public support on the independence of older adults. *Research on Aging*, 42(5–6), 150–162. https://doi.org/10.1177/0164027520907332

Mudrazija, S., & Butrica, B. A (2017). Homeownership, Social Insurance, and Old-Age Security in the United States and Europe. Center for Retirement Research at Boston College (CRR WP 2017-15). Boston, MA: Center for Retirement Research.

Neely, C. (2017, April 12). Five takeaways from Austin demographer's analysis of growing senior population. *Communit Impact Newspaper*. Retrieved May 8, 2020, from https://communityimpact.com/austin/city-county/2017/04/12/5-takeaways-from-austin-demographer-analysis-growing-senior-population/.

Portacolone, E., Rubinstein, R. L., Covinsky, K. E., Halpern, J., & Johnson, J. K. (2019). The precarity of older adults living alone with cognitive impairment. *The Gerontologist*, 59(2), 271–280. https://doi.org/10.1093/geront/gnx193

Rote, S., Angel, J. L., & Markides, K. (2017). Neighborhood context, dementia severity, and Mexican American caregiver wellbeing. *Journal of Aging and Health*, 29(6), 1030–1055. https://doi.org/10.1177/0898264317707141

Stockman, F., Richtel, M., Ivory, D., & Smith, M. (2020, April 17). 'They're Death Pits': Virus claims at least 7,000 lives in U.S. nursing homes. *The New York Times*. Retrieved April 26, 2020, from https://www.nytimes.com/2020/04/17/us/coronavirus-nursing-homes.html

Texas, M. O. W. C. (2020). *PALS: Greater Austin pet food and veterinary care assistance for pets of seniors*. Retrieved May 5, 2020, from https://www.mealsonwheelscentraltexas.org/programs/pals?gclid=Cj0KCQjwncT1BRDhARIsAOQF9Lk1tsyvpVnC77w5cw9RCRLRLC705mdgkcOLL0bamvugJFE7e7PFZlAaAuxxEALw_wcB

Torres-Gil, J. F., & Angel, J. L. (2019). *The politics of a majority-minority nation: Aging, diversity and immigration*. Sage Publishing.

U.S. Census Bureau. (2019). *Historical living arrangements of adults*. Retrieved April 25, 2020, from https://www.census.gov/data/tables/time-series/demo/families/adults.html

A Framework for Aging-Friendly Services and Supports in the Age of COVID-19

Geoffrey J. Hoffman ⓘ, Noah J. Webster, and Julie P. W. Bynum

ABSTRACT

COVID-19 has revealed gaps in services and supports for older adults, even as needs for health and social services have dramatically increased and may produce a cascade of disability after the pandemic subsides. In this essay, we discuss the perfect storm of individual and environmental risk factors, including deconditioning, reductions in formal and informal care support, and social isolation. We then evaluate opportunities that have arisen for strengthening person-centered services and supports for older adults, through in-home acute and primary medical care, aggressive use of video telehealth and social interaction, and implementation of volunteer or paid intergenerational service.

Introduction

The COVID-19 pandemic has drastically reduced activity levels and altered social and physical environments, limiting the spaces in which we typically operate. For many of us, this has been accompanied by feelings of dependency while waiting for help plus resignation to the unknown. These threats to autonomy are not novel for all, however. Gradual or sudden loss of independence is the lived experience of many older Americans. It is likely that the pandemic has particularly amplified this risk for older adults, given their clinical vulnerability to COVID-19 and the potentially harmful effects of prolonged quarantine and orders to shelter-in-place.

In addition, the pandemic has dramatically altered the environments older adults inhabit. These changes include restricted access to usual health care (e.g., medication management, fittings for new medical equipment) and daily activities (e.g., shopping at grocery stores), but also vital access to informal care from family and friends (e.g., social support systems) as well as acute and post-acute care needs (e.g., rehabilitation services after surgery or an injury). Furthermore, the longer this emergency lasts, the greater the likelihood for deconditioning, or physiological change due to sedentary behavior, that can harm long-term physical functioning. Therefore, we may see surges in mobility problems and injury once recommendations to shelter-in-place have been lifted. Combined with the negative effects of reduced social engagement, these changes may drive a surge in disability and injury and psychological and cognitive decline that outstrips the capabilities of the nation's health and long-term care systems to manage the increased demand for services.

A multi-pronged approach should address this potential disability crisis, through innovative supports for older adults' social and physical environments. To this end, we present a conceptual discussion of disability, environmental, and social risk factors that are exacerbated during a pandemic, then introduce a framework for addressing these risks.

Laying the groundwork

Disability is a process that begins with a biomedical or physiological abnormality and progresses to bodily impairments (e.g., sensory or visual issues) affecting physical, mental, or social functioning. If unchecked, impairment harms "fundamental physical and mental actions" (e.g., ability to get up from a chair, use of stairs) (Fauth et al., 2007) and may lead to disability, or a gap between "a person's intrinsic capabilities and the demands created by the social and physical environment" (Jette, 2006). Environmental factors (Verbrugge & Jette, 1994) increase or impede "feedback loops" in which cognitive, sensory, and functional impairments lead to new injuries or conditions, accelerating disablement.

When environmental demands increase, greater individual capability (physical, mental, and social functioning) is required to avoid maladaptive behaviors or negative affect (Lawton, 1989). Reduced stimulation (mobility, social contact) and supports (medication management, wellness checks, instrumental support) are characteristics of sub-optimal environments, in which demands can exceed individuals' functional capacity (Jette, 2006; Lawton, 1974). More than poor health, a poor fit between capability and environment can cause disability (Heckhausen & Schulz, 1999). Simultaneously, drastic changes in capability and demand, such as the rapid deconditioning and physical and social environment restrictions under COVID-19, require immediate and sustained attention to the fit between person and environment, to optimize health.

Older individuals' social resources are critical for health (Litwin & Shaul, 2019; Webster et al., 2015). A resource-poor social environment can result in social isolation (objective reduction in contact with others) or loneliness (subjectively felt isolation), which have strong negative influences on well-being (Cornwell & Waite, 2009), functional capacity (Luo et al., 2012), and even mortality (Holt-Lunstad et al., 2010). As many as one-quarter of community-dwelling older adults report having restricted social resources. While generally considered beneficial, in some cases social interactions can be detrimental to well-being (Birditt et al., 2020; Villalonga-Olives & Kawachi, 2017), e.g., when increased care demands result in tension and conflict between caregivers and care recipients.

In the U.S., management of older adult function involves informal and formal care structures comprised of primary and acute care and a set of services loosely designated as the long-term services and supports (LTSS) system. As many as 45 million unpaid caregivers provide informal support for older individuals. Nursing home care represents a fraction of LTSS; under state Medicaid programs, community-based services for several million Americans include homemaker, home health aide, adult day health care, and respite care (Watts, 2020) offered by a large direct care workforce (PHI, 2012). Area Agencies on Aging (AAAs) offer other LTSS locally, including Meals on Wheels, congregate meals, and adult day health care. Some state Medicaid programs allow beneficiaries to direct their own care (Disability Rights California, 2008) in consumer-directed programs (Foster et al., 2007; Simon-Rusinowitz et al., 2014). Medicare, the largest insurer of U.S. older adults, does not typically cover LTSS, but offers reimbursement for primary care beneficial to older adult well-being as well as acute care and shorter-term supports, such as post-acute rehabilitative care (that can prevent longer-term disability) administered in outpatient clinics or skilled nursing facilities, and at home by home health providers. Medicaid also supplements primary and acute care reimbursement from Medicare for low-income older adults. Current and future access to services and supports is under threat with COVID-19, with likely reductions in informal and formal caregiving and community programming (e.g., senior centers use) under shelter-in-place rules, and potential budget cuts to AAA and state Medicaid budgets due to local, state, and national budget constraints as a result of the pandemic. More recently, Medicare reimbursement models (e.g., bundled care payments) have substantially reduced spending for post-acute care that may particularly affect at-risk older adults with functional limitations.

Immediate challenges: perfect storm of knowns and unknowns

The pandemic has reduced informal caregiving support (Cahan et al., 2020) while increasing objective and subjective social isolation and reducing access to primary care and wellness checks. The impact of COVID-19 on formal LTSS has been particularly severe, with the highest mortality rates in the U.S. among older adults in nursing homes (Nadolny & Kwiatkowksi, 2020).

Access to Medicaid nursing home and paid home care services has likely been curtailed given potential reluctance of direct care workers to enter older adults' homes and because the risks of infection are greatest for low-income and African-American communities who disproportionately represent the direct care workforce. With states already cutting Medicaid budgets, access to these services will decrease even more. Those with post-acute care needs will particularly suffer. The demand for such care, provided in inpatient and outpatient settings by physical and occupational therapists and other providers for those recently experiencing strokes, heart failure, fall injuries, or with hip surgery, will likely skyrocket, far outstripping availability; demand for skilled nursing facility beds may double current U.S. capacity levels while outpatient post-acute care needs may surge to 10 million patients (Arora & Fried, 2020).

Other impacts are less certain. While recent regulatory changes expanded telehealth (Centers for Medicare and Medicaid Services (CMS, 2020a, 2020b), including new Medicare support from occupational and physical therapists (CMS, 2020b) and initiation of Medicaid home health services through telehealth (CMS, 2020a), the breadth of service adoption is uncertain. The extent to which the pandemic has deconditioned individuals is uncertain as well, though its potential impact is severe. Older adults have been more likely to self-isolate than other groups (Stone, 2020), affecting their emotional health, diet, exercise, and cognitive stimulation and creating vulnerability to new illnesses and injuries plus difficulties with self-care for existing ones (Steinman et al., 2020).

These person-environment threats and LTSS and post-acute care budgetary uncertainties create a perfect storm. Person-level deconditioning can create novel disability risks and exacerbate existing ones. Reductions or elimination of social and other environmental supports due to sheltering-in-place orders and looming state budget cuts limit opportunities to recondition and optimize functioning. Foregone care in the formal care system is unlikely to be supplanted by overburdened informal caregivers that has been diminished under shelter-in-place orders and available primary care and LTSS may be distributed or experienced inequitably due to differing generosity levels (eligibility criteria and community-based benefits) of state Medicaid programs and varying baseline resource levels (income, social network strength, familiarity and comfort with virtual technology). Responding to these person (deconditioning) and environment (medical, instrumental, and social support) challenges will require strengthened LTSS that restructure how services and supports are offered.

Proposed pandemic framework for addressing disablement

We propose comprehensive targeting of disablement, under the framework of an improved person-environment fit that is designed to address social and physical environmental risks both during and after the current pandemic. First, programs should prioritize and facilitate safe and patient-centered in-home primary and acute care and LTSS delivery. Second, policymakers should address social risk, through enhanced virtual supports and bridging of the digital divide. Third, intergenerational programming should be broadly incorporated into LTSS. Fourth, aging-friendly physical and social infrastructures should be implemented to promote supportive, socially cohesive communities.

Prioritizing in-home and consumer-directed care

The pandemic offers an opportunity to further rebalance the delivery mix in the U.S. health care system that prioritizes hospital-based medical care over longer-term health care management within the home. Hospital systems and the U.S. Department of Veterans Affairs (VA) healthcare system have successfully utilized in-home primary medical care and hospital-at-home care for highly at-risk older adults (Danielsson & Leff, 2019; Edes & Burris, 2014). Given fears of contagion and the need to reserve hospital capacity for COVID-19 cases, where appropriate, careful implementation of post-acute care at home involving daily interactions with an interdisciplinary medical team that includes physical and occupational therapists could expand access to care, potentially improving patient mobility and reducing hospital admissions among older patients sheltering-in-place (Werner & Van Houtven, 2020); this approach could also address home safety, medication, and clinical needs that are difficult to assess by providers outside the home. Home health agencies will need to increase their capabilities to support excess post-acute care demands, which will require expansion of their workforce (Arora & Fried, 2020).

Like telehealth, these post-acute care innovations would require changes to law, including new reimbursements for intensive rehabilitative services delivered at home under Medicare and Medicaid and changes in regulations regarding service eligibility. For instance, CMS should consider relaxing its "homebound" requirement and the exclusion from the home health benefit of individuals requiring more than part-time or intermittent post-acute care. This would benefit non-homebound individuals unable to access rehabilitative services in outpatient settings. While these changes would require safety protocols to avoid spreading infections to patients at home (and to providers making home visits), and would not apply to frail, vulnerable older adults, such enhancements of post-acute home health and skilled nursing care would broadly improve disability prevention and address concerns that at-risk older patients are currently avoiding care due to fear of infection, contributing to an unseen epidemic of excess deaths.

The coming disability cascade could also encourage states without consumer-directed care programs to adopt them and for states with such programs to expand their scope, to ensure that family members can offer caregiving support rather than seek out employment opportunities. Finally, telehealth expansions should be reconfigured after the pandemic, to regularly support conditioning and physical function, to improve inadequate population-based prevention efforts for older adults (e.g., to prevent fall injuries).

Expanding virtual support and bridging the digital divide

The current public health emergency has also illustrated welfare benefits from increased use of technology, with lessons for supporting older adults. Internet communication technologies (ICTs, e.g., computers, tablets, smart phones) help older adults stay socially connected, reducing social isolation and loneliness (Cotten et al., 2013), particularly for those with functional limitations (Sims et al., 2017). Although beneficial for telehealth, social interactions, and increasing access to vital medical and social resources, ICTs remain inaccessible to many older adults, due to resource, information, or usability constraints (Anderson & Perrin, 2017). To maximize the potential of ICTs, policymakers should address widespread gaps in access to video telehealth technology. This would include broad dissemination and reimbursement of technological (rather than durable) medical equipment (e.g., video tablets) under Medicare's Part B, building on the Veterans Health Administration's success delivering video telehealth technology to clinically vulnerable veterans (Zulman et al., 2019). Supports for the technology's use could be supplemented through consumer-directed family care programs and intergenerational supports.

Increasing intergenerational programming and bridging the age divide

The massive expansion of in-home health and long-term care required to address the pandemic's disability cascade can benefit from intergenerational service. Intergenerational programs provide bidirectional benefits and are popular: they can involve younger individuals who provide companionship to older adults, offering caregivers respite (Belman, 2018; Guerrero et al., 2017), as well as older adult volunteerism in schools (Fried et al., 2013) that improves cognition and functioning as well as younger adult educational performance and attitudes toward aging and behaviors toward older adults (Guerrero et al., 2017; Radford et al., 2018). Relationship-building and intergenerational supports can be strengthened through use of ICTs (Antonucci et al., 2017), with younger individuals assisting older adults with usability and access, while providing social support. This low-cost service could augment existing formal and informal supports, promote person-environment fit with enhanced social interaction, while meshing with ICTs and other home care programming.

Building an aging-friendly physical and social infrastructure

Many communities require additional external supports to develop aging-friendly environments, even as social capital and cohesion may naturally form in others during times of crisis. Supports from trusted organizations that work and interact with community-dwelling older adults on a regular basis (e.g., senior centers, AAAs) can help connect supply (e.g., interested and available children not in school during COVID-19) with demand (e.g., older adults in need of help to go grocery shopping), as could social media platforms (such as Nextdoor). Such interventions can lead to the development of social capital and cohesion within communities that have lasting impact beyond the pandemic. Medicaid and other agencies could reimburse development of aging-friendly communities adopting intergenerational approaches, while Medicare could promote social risk management through reimbursement reforms. This promotion could include transitioning hospitals to more holistic, socially supportive care across settings (e.g., developing broader relationships with community providers). Better connections between acute, post-acute, and community providers prior to COVID-19 might have helped the health care system keep better track of the most vulnerable patients and reduced excess mortality. These largely community-driven, government-supported solutions could be the best bet for scaling up supports for aging given market failures in providing integrated health and long-term care.

Conclusion

The COVID-19 public health emergency has introduced new threats to a beleaguered health and long-term care system, threatening to decondition and severely heighten disability risks for older adults. Novel approaches to scale up supports and services are required to supplement ruptured formal and informal caregiving and social interactions. We propose a pandemic disability intervention framework that relies on reimagined clinical and community supports involving broadly increased in-home acute and primary care, massive dissemination of telehealth technology and support for vulnerable older adults, and intergenerational exchanges. Together, with support from local and national organizations supporting aging, these policies can rebuild resilient aging-friendly communities and structures and promote a sense of societal cohesion.

Key Points

- COVID 19-related sheltering-in-place will decondition and socially isolate older adults;
- A cascade of disability may ensue and overwhelm the health and long-term care systems;
- In-home care, virtual care and connection, and intergenerational exchanges are indicated

Disclosure statement

No potential conflict of interest was reported by the authors.

ORCID

Geoffrey J. Hoffman ⓘ http://orcid.org/0000-0002-3583-6532

References

Anderson, M., & Perrin, A. (2017). *Technology use among seniors.* Pew Research Center. https://www.silvergroup.asia/wp-content/uploads/2017/07/Technology-use-among-seniors-_-Pew-Research-Center.pdf

Antonucci, T. C., Ajrouch, K. J., & Manalel, J. A. (2017). Social relations and technology: Continuity, context, and change. *Innovation in Aging, 1*(3), igx029. https://doi.org/10.1093/geroni/igx029

Arora, V. S., & Fried, J. E. (2020). *How will we care for coronavirus patients after they leave the hospital? By building postacute care surge capacity.* Health Affairs Blog. https://www.healthaffairs.org/do/10.1377/hblog20200408.641535/full/

Belman, O. (2018). *USC students to provide low-cost caregiving for seniors with Alzheimer's and dementia.* USC Leonard Davis School of Gerontology. https://gero.usc.edu/2018/02/12/usc-students-provide-low-cost-caregiving-seniors-alzheimers-dementia/

Birditt, K. S., Sherman, C. W., Polenick, C. A., Becker, L., Webster, N. J., Ajrouch, K. J., Antonucci, T. C., & Neupert, S. (2020). So close and yet so irritating: Negative relations and implications for well-being by age and closeness. *Journals of Gerontology Part B: Psychological Sciences and Social Sciences, 75*(2), 327–337. https://doi.org/10.1093/geronb/gby038

Cahan, E. M., Fuller, T., & Shah, N. R. (2020). *Protecting healthcare's family caregivers amidst the COVID-19 pandemic.* Health Affairs Blog. https://www.healthaffairs.org/do/10.1377/hblog20200421.666035/full/

CMS. (2020a). *COVID-19 Frequently Asked Questions (FAQs) for state Medicaid and Children's Health Insurance Program (CHIP) agencies.* Centers for Medicare & Medicaid Services. https://www.medicaid.gov/state-resource-center/downloads/covid-19-faqs.pdf

CMS. (2020b). *Medicare telemedicine health care provider fact sheet.* Centers for Medicare & Medicaid Services. https://www.cms.gov/newsroom/fact-sheets/medicare-telemedicine-health-care-provider-fact-sheet

Cornwell, E. Y, & Waite, L. J. (2009). Social disconnectedness, perceived isolation, and health among older adults. *Journal Of Health and Social Behavior, 50*(1), 31-48. https://doi.org/10.1177/002214650905000103

Cotten, S. R., Anderson, W. A., & McCullough, B. M. (2013). Impact of internet use on loneliness and contact with others among older adults: Cross-sectional analysis. *Journal of Medical Internet Research, 15*(2), e39. https://doi.org/10.2196/jmir.2306

Danielsson, P., & Leff, B. (2019). Hospital at home and emergence of the home hospitalist. *Journal of Hospital Medicine, 14*(6), 382–384. https://doi.org/10.12788/jhm.3162

Disability Rights California. (2008). *In-Home Supportive Services: Nuts & bolts manual.* Disablilty Rights California. http://www.disabilityrightsca.org/pubs/PublicationsIHSSNutsandBolts.htm

Edes, T., & Burris, J. F. (2014). Home-based primary care: A VA innovation coming soon. *Physician Leadership Journal, 1*(1), 38–40, 42. https://www.ncbi.nlm.nih.gov/pubmed/26211195

Fauth, E. B., Zarit, S. H., Malmberg, B., & Johansson, B. (2007). Physical, cognitive, and psychosocial variables from the Disablement Process Model predict patterns of independence and the transition into disability for the oldest-old. *The Gerontologist, 47*(5), 613–624. https://doi.org/10.1093/geront/47.5.613

Foster, L., Dale, S. B., & Brown, R. (2007). How caregivers and workers fared in Cash and Counseling. *Health Services Research, 42*(1p2), 510–532. https://doi.org/10.1111/j.1475-6773.2006.00672.x

Fried, L. P., Carlson, M. C., McGill, S., Seeman, T., Xue, Q.-L., Frick, K., Tan, E., Tanner, E. K., Barron, J., Frangakis, C., Piferi, R., Martinez, I., Gruenewald, T., Martin, B. K., Berry-Vaughn, L., Stewart, J., Dickersin, K., Willging, P. R., & Rebok, G. W. (2013). Experience Corps: A dual trial to promote the health of older adults and children's academic success. *Contemporary Clinical Trials, 36*(1), 1–13. https://doi.org/10.1016/j.cct.2013.05.003

Guerrero, L. R., Jimenez, P., & Tan, Z. (2017). TimeOut@UCLA: An intergenerational respite care and workforce development program. *Journal of Intergenerational Relationships, 15*(3), 290–294. https://doi.org/10.1080/15350770.2017.1329599

Heckhausen, J., & Schulz, R. (1999). The primacy of primary control is a human universal: A reply to Gould's (1999) critique of the life-span theory of control. *Psychological Review, 106*(3), 605–609. https://doi.org/10.1037/0033-295X.106.3.605

Holt-Lunstad, J., Smith, T. B., Layton, J. B., & Brayne, C. (2010). Social relationships and mortality risk: A meta-analytic review. *PLoS Medicine, 7*(7), e1000316. https://doi.org/10.1371/journal.pmed.1000316

Jette, A. M. (2006). Toward a common language for function, disability, and health. *Physical Therapy, 86*(5), 726–734. https://doi.org/10.1093/ptj/86.5.726

Lawton, M. P. (1974). Social ecology and the health of older people. *American Journal of Public Health, 64*(3), 257–260. https://doi.org/10.2105/AJPH.64.3.257

Lawton, M. P. (1989). Three functions of the residential environment. *Journal of Housing for the Elderly, 5*(1), 35–50. https://doi.org/10.1300/J081V05N01_04

Litwin, H., & Shaul, A. (2019). The effect of social network on the physical activity-cognitive function nexus in late life. *International Psychogeriatrics, 31*(5), 713–722. https://doi.org/10.1017/S1041610218001059

Luo, Y., Hawkley, L. C., Waite, L. J., & Cacioppo, J. T. (2012). Loneliness, health, and mortality in old age: A national longitudinal study. *Social Science and Medicine, 74*(6), 907–914. https://doi.org/10.1016/j.socscimed.2011.11.028

Nadolny, T. L., & Kwiatkowksi, M. (2020, May 1). "Our patients are dropping like flies': 16,000 dead from COVID-19 in U.S. Nursing Homes. *USA Today.* https://www.usatoday.

com/story/news/investigations/2020/05/01/coronavirus-nursing-homes-more-states-pressured-name-facilities/3062537001/

PHI. (2012). *Growing demand for direct-care workers*. Retrieved from www.PHInational.org)

Radford, K., Gould, R., Vecchio, N., & Fitzgerald, A. (2018). Unpacking Intergenerational (IG) programs for policy implications: A systematic review of the literature. *Journal of Intergenerational Relationships, 16*(3), 302–329. https://doi.org/10.1080/15350770.2018.1477650

Simon-Rusinowitz, L., Schwartz, A. J., Loughlin, D., Sciegaj, M., Mahoney, K. J., & Donkoh, Y. (2014). Where are they now? Cash and Counseling successes and challenges over time. *Care Management Journal, 15*(3), 104–110. https://doi.org/10.1891/1521-0987.15.3.104

Sims, T., Reed, A. E., & Carr, D. C. (2017). Information and communication technology use is related to higher well-being among the oldest-old. *The Journals Of Gerontology. Series B, Psychological Sciences And Social Sciences, 72*(5), 761–770. https://doi.org/10.1093/geronb/gbw130

Steinman, M. A., Perry, L., & Perissinotto, C. M. (2020). Meeting the care needs of older adults isolated at home during the COVID-19 pandemic. *JAMA Internal Medicine*. https://doi.org/10.1001/jamainternmed.2020.1661

Stone, A. (2020, April 29). Baby boomers were blasé about the coronavirus? Why did we believe that? *New York Times*. https://www.nytimes.com/2020/04/29/opinion/sunday/coronavirus-baby-boomers.html

Verbrugge, L. M., & Jette, A. M. (1994). The disablement process. *Social Science and Medicine, 38*(1), 1–14. https://doi.org/10.1016/0277-9536(94)90294-1

Villalonga-Olives, E., & Kawachi, I. (2017). The dark side of social capital: A systematic review of the negative health effects of social capital. *Social Science and Medicine, 194*, 105–127. https://doi.org/10.1016/j.socscimed.2017.10.020

Watts, M. O. (2020). *Medicaid Home and Community-Based Services enrollment and spending*. Kaiser Family Foundation. https://www.kff.org/report-section/medicaid-home-and-community-based-services-enrollment-and-spending-issue-brief/

Webster, N. J., Antonucci, T. C., Ajrouch, K. J., & Abdulrahim, S. (2015). Social networks and health among older adults in Lebanon: The mediating role of support and trust. *Journals of Gerontology Part B: Psychological Sciences and Social Sciences, 70*(1), 155–166. https://doi.org/10.1093/geronb/gbu149

Werner, R. M., & Van Houtven, C. H. (2020). *In the time of Covid-19, we should move high-intensity postacute care home*. Health Affairs. Retrieved from https://www.healthaffairs.org/do/10.1377/hblog20200422.924995/full/

Zulman, D. M., Wong, E. P., Slightam, C., Gregory, A., Jacobs, J. C., Kimerling, R., Blonigen, D. M., Peters, J., & Heyworth, L. (2019). Making connections: Nationwide implementation of video telehealth tablets to address access barriers in Veterans. *JAMIA Open, 2*(3), 323–329. https://doi.org/10.1093/jamiaopen/ooz024

When Going Digital Becomes a Necessity: Ensuring Older Adults' Needs for Information, Services, and Social Inclusion During COVID-19

Bo Xie ⓘ, Neil Charness, Karen Fingerman, Jeffrey Kaye, Miyong T. Kim, and Anjum Khurshid

ABSTRACT
Older adults are in triple jeopardy during COVID-19: compared with younger people, older adults are (1) more likely to develop serious conditions and experience higher mortality; (2) less likely to obtain high quality information or services online; and (3) more likely to experience social isolation and loneliness. Hybrid solutions, coupling online and offline strategies, are invaluable in ensuring the inclusion of vulnerable populations. Most of these solutions require no new inventions. Finding the financial resources for a rapid, well-coordinated implementation is the biggest challenge. Setting up the requisite support systems and digital infrastructure is important for the present and future pandemics.

Introduction

Older adults and people with underlying health conditions are at high risk from COVID-19, particularly those age 80 years and above who experience the highest mortality rate (Centers for Disease Control and Prevention, 2020a). To protect high-risk populations, CDC recommends that older adults should "stay home as much as possible" (Centers for Disease Control and Prevention, 2020b), and that nursing homes should "restrict all visitation except for certain compassionate care situations, such as end of life situations" and "restrict all volunteers and non-essential healthcare personnel" (Centers for Disease Control and Prevention, 2020c). Senior centers are being closed as well (National Council on Aging, 2020).

Though necessary during this pandemic, these measures risk further isolating older adults who are already suffering social isolation. Indeed, in 2019, 24% of men and 44% of women aged 75 years and older lived alone (United States Census Bureau, 2019). About 25% of older adults experience social isolation – that is, they have few social contacts throughout the week by virtue of living alone and low participation in outside groups or socializing (Cudjoe et al., 2020). Social isolation is a significant risk factor for loneliness, which is a subjective feeling and desire for greater contact with social partners. Although social isolation and loneliness do not always co-occur (e.g., one can feel "alone in a crowd"), they are both significant risk factors for negative health outcomes (Cacioppo & Cacioppo, 2014; Courtin & Knapp, 2017; Hayashi et al., 2020; National Academies of Sciences, Engineering and Medicine, 2020). Social distancing during a Stay At Home order or concerns about contracting the coronavirus may increase older adults' social isolation and their feelings of loneliness.

While going digital is now a necessity more than ever before, it alone is insufficient in reaching vulnerable populations like older adults. Over the past few decades, we have witnessed the increasing adoption of information technology to disseminate information and resources and to communicate with others. However, older adults' adoption and use of technology lags that of younger cohorts. While Internet use has increased exponentially over the past two decades, still 27% of older adults age 65+ in the U.S. are offline (Anderson, Perrin, Jiang, & Kumar, 2019). Nationally, 81% of American adults own a smartphone and 73% subscribe to home broadband, but these numbers drop down to 53% and 59%, respectively, among older Americans age 65+ (Anderson, 2019). Only 15% of older adults age 65+ mostly go online via their smartphone, the lowest rate of all American adult age groups (Anderson, 2019). Even among older adults who are online, the majority (73%) say they would need help setting up and using new electronic devices (Anderson & Perrin, 2017). Older adults do continue to watch television at a high rate and may obtain relevant information about public health crises in that manner (Gardner et al., 2014; Mares & Woodard, 2006), but television remains a passive technology for information and communication. It does not enable the two-way communication of telehealth portals, direct communication with social services via e-mail, social interactions with family and friends via social media, or search engines that facilitate information seeking via the Internet.

As such, older adults' eHealth literacy, or the ability to access, assess, and use health information to make informed healthcare decisions (Norman & Skinner, 2006, tends to be low and requires extensive assistance (Xie, 2011). Further, caregivers of older adults tend to be similarly disadvantaged, particularly those who are nonwhite, of lower education, and without regular health care (Bangerter et al., 2019).

In short, older adults are in triple jeopardy during this crisis: compared with younger people, older adults are (1) more likely to develop COVID-19 and experience higher mortality; (2) less likely to obtain high quality information or obtain food, supplies, and services online; and (3) more likely to experience social isolation and loneliness. Moreover, older adults from ethnic or racial minority groups are suffering a disproportionate burden during the COVID-19 pandemic, with higher rates of experiencing the disease, hospitalization, and death (Centers for Disease Control and Prevention, 2020d). Combined, this situation requires hybrid solutions, coupling online and offline health informatics strategies to addressing these challenges.

Hybrid informatics solutions

Health care is an information-intensive business where timely, accurate, and relevant information can be the difference between life and death. Informatics solutions can be invaluable in the prevention and management of COVID-19 and managing other health problems older adults experience during this outbreak. It is critical that researchers, educators, and practitioners find creative ways to extend the reach of informatics into every aspect of society, including work and personal lives. However, we must also acknowledge that informatics solutions alone are insufficient in reaching vulnerable populations. Government agencies, for-profit and nonprofit organizations, and community volunteers are required to ensure the accessibility and usability of effective solutions and interventions, both high-tech and low-tech (Xie et al., 2020). Toward this end, we recommend the following hybrid solutions to help address the challenges that older adults face during COVID-19.

Health information

Digital health information can spread rapidly via social media. Such information can help the public and healthcare workers alike obtain timely information that authoritative sources are unable to provide (Stephens et al., 2018; Xie et al., 2019), thereby improving management of a crisis. However, misinformation and disinformation spread fast as well. In rapidly developing situations like a pandemic, being able to discern misinformation and disinformation from high quality information is of critical importance. No sources, whether traditional print media, broadcast media (television, radio), or online media services, are immune to potential conscious or unconscious bias that can imperil the full understanding of ongoing public health crises.

To be effective, digital public health campaigns also need to be linguistically and culturally attuned to a diverse population of older adults, including those with disabilities. Given that vulnerable populations of older adults (e.g., those over age 80, ethnic or racial minorities, with less education, and fewer resources) tend to have insufficient eHealth literacy, we recommend the following solutions:

(1) Develop informatics tools that enable local organizations to identify needs and create appropriate digital content that matches the eHealth literacy levels of older adults (John A. Hartford Foundation, 2020), and explore timely and effective strategies to disseminate such content to older adults, their family members and caregivers, and healthcare providers;

(2) Develop usable (Czaja et al., 2019) intergenerational tools to support family members and other caregivers of older adults to be more effective in providing them with health information (Czaja et al., 2017);

(3) Develop digitally delivered training and interventions to improve older adults' eHealth literacy that are scalable and can be deployed rapidly;

(4) Develop informatics tools that are operational with basic technologies like telephones and that work with low or intermittent Internet availability;

(5) Train community health workers to be information and cultural brokers as well as technological brokers for socially isolated ethnic minority older adults. With the major influx of consumer information technology into everyone's daily lives, older adults in ethnic minority communities with limited resources often find themselves intimidated by the expanded choices or skeptical about unfamiliar approaches. Thus, they do not obtain the optimal benefits that these technology-incorporated features provide, including those of various mHealth interventions. Given the strengths of community health workers in community outreaching such as brokering culture, evidence-based practices, and language in many disadvantaged communities, they may be the ideal technological brokers, acting as strong bridges between the "digital touch" and "human touch". The use of community health workers with proper training and coordination can be a viable means of reducing health disparities among members of underserved populations in this new technological era.

(6) Promote informatics tools that allow older adults, or their authorized caregivers, easy access to their electronic medical records from multiple providers on a single mobile or online platform in accord with the 21st Century Cures Act, to be expedited by the Office of the National Coordinator for Health IT.

In short, it is important to explore hybrid ways – that may entail both high-tech and low-tech strategies (and balancing digital and personal touches) – to deliver trustworthy information to older adults, family care-givers, and healthcare providers to enhance preparedness and prevention of COVID-19 and manage daily lives. Older adults are not a homogenous population; thus, it is also important to consider their diversity in language, literacy levels, and cultural norms in developing informatics solutions. Active engagement and involvement of caregivers and older adults from diverse communities will be essential to the development of informatics tools.

Services

With proper coordination between health systems and testing sites, telehealth services can aid large-scale screening for the virus (Hollander & Carr, 2020). Telehealth can also help meet older adults' needs for routine healthcare services. Prior to COVID-19, Medicare had already been paying for tele-health, however only on a limited basis. On March 17, 2020, the Centers for Medicare and Medicaid Services (CMS) has broadened the coverage of telehealth, enabling Medicare beneficiaries to receive a broader range of healthcare services at home (Centers for Medicare & Medicaid Services, 2020). This policy change alone may not ensure prompt telehealth adoption given that telehealth has not been mainstreamed in our routine health systems (Smith et al., 2020). However, in just over two months health systems that have not had large volumes of telehealth encounters have seen extraordinary (>300%) increases in telehealth visits (Garrity, 2020). At one of the author's affiliated health system (OHSU Health Care), 69% of outpatient visits were conducted as remote digital visits during April 2020. These recent developments are encouraging; still, training and resources are important to ensure the least tech-savvy adult population have the necessary hardware, software, Internet connectivity, or eHealth literacy, to be able to actually use the broadened range of telehealth services.

Beyond health care, accessing food and household supplies during COVID-19 can be challenging for anyone due to closures of restaurants and crowded grocery stores. It is especially challenging for older adults due to closures of senior centers (where many older adults could get free meals) and due to inexperience with online shopping. Many older adults depend on social services such as Meals on Wheels for their food. These services may be more limited during a crisis. It is important to explore hybrid solutions that connect older adults in need of these services with their families, neighbors, local organizations, and community volunteers. Specific solutions for improving access to health care, food, and other services include:

(1) Guidance from healthcare providers for older adult patients to ensure that they are aware of and able to use telehealth services;

(2) Support from Internet service providers to ensure older adults' access to the equipment and connectivity necessary to use telehealth services, which may include arranging to offer Internet hotspots in neighborhoods with low income older adults;

(3) Training to improve older adults' eHealth literacy, particularly their use of telehealth services and online shopping; this should include training about cybersecurity to ease privacy concerns (Xie et al., 2012) and mitigate fraud (Gavett et al., 2017);

(4) Informatics solutions that connect older adults with their families, friends, and communities who can provide necessary training and support to ensure older adults' service needs are met. Examples of such solutions may include an intergenerational mobile app where older adults can use voice to record their grocery list, and this list would then be processed, either automatically by a vendor's system or manually by a younger family member to put into an online order or an application that allows older adults to ask for help from their neighbors for groceries or transportation;

(5) Currently, many vendors' online shopping windows open at midnight and are typically all taken within an hour if not sooner (e.g., Amazon Fresh, Walmart), which creates an additional barrier to older adults. Already, grocery stores nationwide are providing "protected time slots" for older adults to shop in store. Online vendors should follow this facilitated access practice to ensure older adults' online purchasing of groceries and other essential items (it is worth noting that, over the past several weeks as we developed this paper, we have seen vendors getting more experienced in overcoming this bottleneck and providing better online shopping services);

(6) Informatics solutions to help older adults identify and connect with community-based organizations that provide social services based in their zip code. Some of these applications are already in operation with varied coverage across the country but they need to be connected to local public health and social service agencies to be effective for older adults.

Social interaction

During COVID-19, as we practice "social distancing" and reduce visits to older adults, we need to also mitigate older adults' social isolation and loneliness. To use more precise language, older adults should experience "physical distancing" rather than "social distancing". In fact, we believe that all informatics solutions for older adults must incorporate, and emphasize, the *social* aspect. Specific recommendations include:

(1) Develop informatics tools like apps for mobile devices and intelligent voice assistants that promote intergenerational interactions among family members;

(2) Help older adults stay connected with friends they typically interact with at senior centers or churches, which may no longer be desirable or even feasible when many of these facilities are closed. Virtual gathering spaces have existed for years; however, they were typically considered inferior to in-person interactions, especially among older adults. During COVID-19, it is the opposite. Initiatives exist – for example, the Institute for Successful Longevity [ISL] at Florida State University has launched a Zoom initiative to help older adults fight social isolation (Institute for Successful Longevity (ISL) at Florida State University, 2020). More resources need to be channeled into the design, development, and implementation of these virtual gathering spaces, particularly spaces aimed at older adults;

(3) Develop informatics tools that enable older adults to continue to contribute to society. Many older adults remain active and desire to continue making positive contributions in retirement. Informatics tools can help older adults stay active by, for example, enabling their (virtual) participation in volunteering and community engagement, as illustrated in the ISL initiative (ISL, 2020);

(4) Provide hybrid solutions for those who are more digitally literate to help those who are less literate. For instance, digitally-connected people could arrange videoconferencing meetings and provide non-Internet connected people with phone-in numbers (ISL, 2020). In this respect, training community health workers' who have deep knowledge of and integration within resource-limited communities to be effective health information messengers can be a viable strategy.

Looking to the future

The recommendations proposed here address the current COVID-19 crisis and have implications for future pandemics. Most of these solutions do not require new inventions or technology. Finding the financial resources for a rapid, well-coordinated implementation is the biggest challenge. As a first step, it is important to identify an entity responsible for coordinating the efforts. This is no easy task, and it will require much deliberation to find the right entity or entities that can be efficient during a crisis while at the same time ensuring equity and inclusion. Public health departments clearly should play a major role in preventing and managing pandemics, which is the "Public Health 3.0" framework promoted by Dr. Karen DeSalvo and others, but any meaningful discussions about this topic should involve stakeholders in both the public and private sectors at all levels – federal, state, regional, local, and across national borders.

A hybrid solution may work best in this regard: specific informatics initiatives should come from the community level, because community organizers understand the unique needs of their residents, know the local resources available, and can move quickly. Meanwhile, community organizers should coordinate with agencies like the Area Agencies on Aging that have a state and federal mission (and state and federal funding) to support community need, and specifically support for aging and disabled individuals. For infrastructure needs, the federal government is an important piece of the puzzle, particularly in enabling Internet access in rural communities (e.g., through funding via FCC and USDA programs). Private agencies (e.g., Meals on Wheel), have always played an important role in serving older Americans. In light of COVID-19, when much information, services, and social interactions are forced to move online, there is an increasing need for funding to facilitate these agencies' ability to deliver digital technology to older adults.

Traditional clinical trials needed to develop medications to combat a virus can themselves expose more people to infection. Digital technologies may enable clinical trials to be conducted entirely remotely using telemedicine, digital sensors and devices that monitor vital functions, and point of care home-testing. Digital technologies may more quickly and efficiently identify the course of an epidemic (McNeil, 2020; Yasinski, 2020). For example, in a norovirus outbreak in a retirement community, those with infection could be identified by their activity passively monitored at home (Campbell et al., 2011). Opportunities such as these will require support for evidence-based research to ensure that promising approaches translate to the real-world of aging in place. Open-source, federal efforts have begun in this realm to enable researchers across the US to incorporate these models and methods into their research (Center for Research and Education on Aging and Technology Enhancement [CREATE], https://create-center.ahs.illinois.edu/; Collaborative Aging Research Using Technology [CART] Initiative, https://www.ohsu.edu/collaborative-aging-research-using-technology). More of these efforts are needed.

The length of the current pandemic and thus the duration of self-isolation is unknown, possibly ranging from a few months to well into the next year. Unfortunately, this is unlikely to be the last pandemic or health-related crisis that we will endure. Setting up the systems and digital infrastructure for the present and the future is an important goal. Hopefully, the lessons learned now will be well-taken, and there is much more that can be achieved with the assistance of digital technologies, both at a personal level as well as for public health.

Key Points

- Older adults require special attention from policy makers, tech companies, and other professions during COVID-19;
- Going digital alone is insufficient in reaching vulnerable populations like older adults;
- Coupling online and offline strategies are invaluable in addressing the challenges older adults face;
- Rapid, well-coordinated implementation of the requisite support systems and digital infrastructure are important for the present and future pandemics.

Acknowledgments

We would like to thank the editor and anonymous reviewers for their constructive feedback on our manuscript, and Dr. Zhiyong Lu for his constructive feedback on an earlier version of this manuscript.

Funding

BX is supported in part by NIH grants [R21AG052761] and [R21AG052060]; NC is supported in part by NIH grants [4 P01-AG 17211], [R21-AG061431], [1R01-AG064529]; NIDILRR grant [90REGE0012-01-00]; KF is supported in part by NIH grant [R01AG046460]; JK is supported in part by NIH grants [P30-AG008017], [P30-AG024978], [U2C-AG0543701]; Department of Veteran Affairs [IIR 17-144].

ORCID

Bo Xie ⓘ http://orcid.org/0000-0002-6016-6008

References

Anderson, M., & Perrin, A. (2017). Tech adoption climbs among older adults. Pew Research Center. https://www.pewresearch.org/internet/2017/05/17/tech-adoption-climbs-among-older-adults/

Anderson, M. (2019). Mobile technology and home broadband 2019. Pew Research Center. https://www.pewresearch.org/internet/2019/06/13/mobile-technology-and-home-broadband-2019/

Anderson, M., Perrin, A., Jiang, J., & Kumar, M. (2019). Who's not online in 2019? Pew Research Center. https://www.pewresearch.org/fact-tank/2019/04/22/some-americans-dont-use-the-internet-who-are-they/

Bangerter, L. R., Griffin, J., Harden, K., & Rutten, L. J. (2019). Health information–seeking behaviors of family caregivers: Analysis of the health information national trends survey. *JMIR Aging, 2*(1), e11237. https://doi.org/10.2196/11237

Cacioppo, J. T., & Cacioppo, S. (2014). Older adults reporting social isolation or loneliness show poorer cognitive function 4 years later. *Evidance Based Nursing, 17*(2), 59–60. https://doi.org/10.1136/eb-2013-101379

Campbell, I. H., Austin, D., Hayes, T. L., Pavel, M., Riley, T., Mattek, N., & Kaye, J. (2011). Measuring changes in activity patterns during a norovirus epidemic at a retirement community. *Conference proceedings: Annual international conference of the IEEE engineering in medicine and biology society* (pp. 6793–6796). Boston, MA. https://doi.org/ 10.1109/iembs.2011.6091675

Center for Research and Education on Aging and Technology Enhancement.University of Illinois, Urbana-Champaign. Centers for Disease Control and Prevention. (2020a). CDC media telebriefing: Update on COVID-19. Centers for Disease Control and Prevention. https://www.cdc.gov/media/releases/2020/t0309-covid-19-update.html.

Centers for Disease Control and Prevention. (2020b). Coronavirus disease 2019 (COVID-19): If you are at higher risk. Centers for Disease Control and Prevention. https://www.cdc.gov/coronavirus/2019-ncov/specific-groups/high-risk-complications.html

Centers for Disease Control and Prevention. (2020c). Interim additional guidance for infection prevention and control for patients with suspected or confirmed COVID-19 in nursing homes. Centers for Disease Control and Prevention. https://www.cdc.gov/coronavirus/2019-ncov/healthcare-facilities/prevent-spread-in-long-term-care-facilities.html

Centers for Disease Control and Prevention. (2020d). COVID-19 in racial and ethnic minority groups. Centers for Disease Control and Prevention. https://www.cdc.gov/coronavirus/2019-ncov/need-extra-precautions/racial-ethnic-minorities.html

Centers for Medicare & Medicaid Services. (2020). Medicare telemedicine health care provider fact sheet. Centers for Medicare & Medicaid Services. https://www.cms.gov/newsroom/fact-sheets/medicare-telemedicine-health-care-provider-fact-sheet.

Courtin, E., & Knapp, M. (2017). Social isolation, loneliness and health in old age: A scoping review. *Health & Social Care in the Community, 25*(3), 799–812. https://doi.org/10.1111/hsc.12311

Cudjoe, T. K. M., Roth, D. L., Szanton, S. L., Wolff, J. L., Boyd, C. M., & Thorpe, R. J. J. (2020). The epidemiology of social isolation: National health and aging trends study. *The Journals of Gerontology: Series B, 75*(1), 107–113. https://doi.org/10.1093/geronb/gby037

Czaja, S. J., Boot, W. R., Charness, N., & Rogers, W. A. (2019). *Designing for older adults: Principles and creative human factors approaches* (3rd ed.). CRC Press.

Czaja, S. J., Boot, W. R., Charness, N., Rogers, W. A., & Sharit, J. (2017). Improving social support for older adults through technology: Findings from the PRISM randomized control trial. *The Gerontologist, 58*(3), 467–477. https://doi.org/10.1093/geront/gnw249

Gardner, B., Iliffe, S., Fox, K. R., Jefferis, B. J., & Hamer, M. (2014). Sociodemographic, behavioural and health factors associated with changes in older adults' TV viewing over 2 years. *International Journal of Behavioral Nutrition and Physical Activity, 11*(1), 102–111. https://doi.org/10.1186/s12966-014-0102-3

Garrity, M. (2020). Telehealth visits up 312% in New York, causing major lag times. *Becker's Hospital Review*. Becker's Healthcare. https://www.beckershospitalreview.com/telehealth/telehealth-visits-up-312-in-new-york-causing-major-lag-times.html

Gavett, B. E., Zhao, R., John, S. E., Bussell, C. A., Roberts, J. R., & Yue, C. (2017). Phishing suspiciousness in older and younger adults: The role of executive functioning. *PLoS One, 12*(2), e0171620. https://doi.org/10.1371/journal.pone.0171620

Hayashi, T., Umegaki, H., Makino, T., Huang, C. H., Inoue, A., Shimada, H., & Kuzuya, M. (2020). Combined impact of physical frailty and social isolation on rate of falls in older adults. *The Journal of Nutritoin, Health & Aging, 24*(3), 312–318. https://doi.org/10.1007/s12603-020-1316-5

Hollander, J. E., & Carr, B. G. (2020). Virtually perfect? Telemedicine for COVID-19. *New England Journal of Medicine, 382*(18), 1679–1681. https://doi.org/10.1056/NEJMp2003539

Institute for Successful Longevity (ISL) at Florida State University. (2020). ISL launches Zoom initiative to help older adults fight social isolation. Florida State University. https://isl.fsu.edu/article/isl-launches-zoom-initiative-help-older-adults-fight-social-isolation

John A. Hartford Foundation. (2020). Coronavirus disease (COVID-19) resources for older adults, family caregivers and health care providers. John A. Hartford Foundation. https://www.johnahartford.org/dissemination-center/view/coronavirus-disease-covid-19-resources-for-older-adults-family-caregivers-and-health-care-providers

Mares, M. L., & Woodard, E. H. (2006). In search of the older audience: Adult age differences in television viewing. *Journal of Broadcasting & Electronic Media, 50*(4), 595–614. https://doi.org/10.1207/s15506878jobem5004_2

McNeil, D. G. J. (2020). Can smart thermometers track the spread of the coronavirus? *The New York Times*, March 18 https://www.nytimes.com/2020/03/18/health/coronavirus-fever-thermometers.html

National Academies of Sciences, Engineering and Medicine. (2020). *Social isolation and loneliness in older adults: Opportunities for the health care system.* The National Academies Press.

National Council on Aging. (2020). COVID-19 resources for senior centers. National Council on Aging. https://www.ncoa.org/news/ncoa-news/national-institute-of-senior-centers-news/covid-19-resources-for-senior-centers/

Norman, C. D., & Skinner, H. A. (2006). eHealth literacy: Essential skills for consumer health in a networked world. *Journal of Medical Internet Research, 8*(2), e9–e9. https://doi.org/10.2196/jmir.8.2.e9

Smith, A. C., Thomas, E., Snoswell, C. L., Haydon, H., Mehrotra, A., Clemensen, J., & Caffery, L. J. (2020). Telehealth for global emergencies: Implications for coronavirus disease 2019 (COVID-19). *Journal of Telemedicine and Telecare*. https://doi.org/10.1177/1357633x20916567

Stephens, K. K., Li, J., Robertson, B. W., Smith, W. R., & Murthy, D. (2018). Citizens communicating health information: Urging others in their community to seek help during a flood. In K. Boersma & B. Tomaszewski (Eds.), *Proceedings of the 15th international ISCRAM conference*. Rochester, NY: May.

United States Census Bureau. (2019). Historical living arrangements of adults. United States Census Bureau. https://www.census.gov/data/tables/time-series/demo/families/adults.html

Xie, B. (2011). Effects of an e-health literacy intervention for older adults. *Journal of Medical Internet Research, 13*(4), e90. https://doi.org/10.2196/jmir.1880

Xie, B., He, D., Mercer, T., Wang, Y., Wu, D., Fleischmann, K. R., Zhang, Y., Yoder, L. H., Stephens, K. K., Mackert, M., & Lee, M. K. (2020). Global health crises are also information crises: A call to action. *Journal of the Association for Information Science and Technology (JASIST)* https://doi.org/10.1002/asi.24357

Xie, B., Watkins, I., Golbeck, J., & Huang, M. (2012). Understanding and changing older adults' perceptions and learning of social media. *Educational Gerontology, 38*(4), 282–296. https://doi.org/10.1080/03601277.2010.544580

Xie, B., Zhou, L., Yoder, L., Johnson, K., Garcia, A., & Kim, M. (2019). Ebola-related health information wanted and obtained by hospital and public health department employees: Effects of formal and informal communication channels. *Disaster Medicine and Public Health Preparedness*. https://doi.org/10.1017/dmp.2019.45Published

Yasinski, E. (2020). Can social media inform public health efforts? *The Scientist*. https://www.the-scientist.com/news-opinion/can-social-media-inform-public-health-efforts–66891

Economic Risks to Older
Workers and Retirees

Older Workers on the COVID-19-Frontlines without Paid Sick Leave

Teresa Ghilarducci and Aida Farmand

ABSTRACT

The rapid spread of COVID-19 has left many workers around the world – workers in food distribution, truckers, janitors, and home and personal health care workers – deeply concerned about contracting the virus from exposure at work. In particular, older workers in frontline occupations are vulnerable to illness and to the deadly and debilitating effects of COVID-19, especially with inadequate protective gear and inadequate sick leave. In the absence of strong unions, which ensure that employers provide workers with accurate information, robust training, adequate equipment, and paid leave in the event of quarantines or illness, the COVID-19 pandemic highlights the need for additional legislation to shore up worker protections and provide paid sick leave.

The rapid spread of COVID-19 has left food distribution, transportation, janitorial, and home and personal health care workers around the world deeply concerned about their risk of contracting disease through exposure at work. In the United States, older people in the front lines providing essential services and fighting COVID-19 are in a particularly bad situation because they are much more likely to work than older adults in other nations (Ghilarducci & Novello, 2017). In addition, older workers constitute a larger share of the workforce in some frontline industries than they do in the workforce as a whole (Blewett et al., 2019).

As we adapt to the COVID-19 pandemic we are finding that some workers are particularly vulnerable to the financial and logistical hardships of stay-at-home orders and other restrictions. These include low-income workers in grocery stores, bars and restaurants, parents who must now educate young children or share workspaces and computers with older children, and those in medical, service, retail, and transportation jobs. But older workers in frontline occupations face particular risks. Research shows that older workers are more vulnerable to illness and to the deadly and debilitating effects of COVID-19 (Riou et al., 2020). They are also vulnerable socio-economically.

Historically, unions have tried to ensure that employers provide workers accurate information, robust training, adequate equipment, and paid leave in the event of quarantines or illness, but their influence has declined: only 13 percent of older workers were union members in 2019 (Flood et al., 2020).

This perspective highlights the comparative dearth of paid sick leave among older frontline workers in the COVID-19 crisis. Congress passed a comprehensive stimulus bill in the third week of March 2020, the Coronavirus Preparedness and Response Supplemental Appropriations Act. (2020). However, this legislation is lacking in several respects given the challenges faced by older workers on the frontlines, including insufficient worker protection and paid sick leave.

Paid sick leave and frontline older workers in COVID-19

Paid sick leave is critical to the health of older workers and to the public more generally. To determine which workers have access to paid sick leave, U.S. researchers must look to the Center for Disease Control (CDC). The fact that the CDC, which is charged with monitoring the nation's public's health, keeps some of the best numbers on paid sick leave underlines the importance of paid sick leave to public health.

Older workers have less access to paid sick days than younger workers. In 2018, 40% of workers aged 50 years and older lacked paid sick days, compared to 38% of workers under age 50 (see Table 1). Forty percent is a considerable share of the older working population, especially given the relatively high proportion of older workers who work in the health, personal care, and distribution infrastructure industries. Paid sick days are particularly uncommon in certain jobs requiring frequent contact with patients, which can have important public health implications. Indeed, 50% of older workers in healthcare support occupations (which include home health aides, occupational and physical therapist assistants and others) do not have paid sick days according to authors' calculations from the CDC data.

Paid sick days bring multiple benefits to employers, workers, and their families. The public health benefits of paid sick days coverage are substantial, including safer work environments and reduced spread of illness (especially during pandemics). The U.S. is an outlier in providing paid sick leave, which poses a particular health risk to the nation. Many workers cannot afford to take time off if they become ill; moreover, they may fear losing their jobs if they do so. Consequently, they report to work, which can exacerbate their illness or spread disease to others.

Notably, many of these workers are in rapidly graying crucial care and service professions that involve close contact with others; often, people who are themselves highly vulnerable to illness. Older workers constitute a significant proportion of those working in crucial care and service professions, although 33% of U.S. workers are over age 50. About 29% of workers in healthcare-

Table 1. Many frontline workers (old and young) do not have access to paid sick leave: selected occupations by age and paid sick leave access, 2018.

Select Frontline Occupations	Number of Older Workers (Age 50 and Over)	Share of Older Workers (Age 50 and Over)	Share of Older Workers without Paid Sick Leave	Share of Younger Workers (Age 18–49) without Paid Sick Leave
Healthcare Support Occupations	1,088,156	29%	50%	40%
Building and Grounds Cleaning and Maintenance Occupations	2,107,540	42%	58%	65%
Transportation and Material Moving Occupations	3,294,852	34%	52%	50%
Total Employed	51,393,546	33%	40%	38%

Source: Author's calculations from CDC 2018 National Health Interview Survey (NHIS)
Notes: Sample includes individuals who reported being employed (18 years and older). Access to paid sick leave rates are calculated for employed individuals who responded yes or no to the following question:""Do you have paid sick leave on your main job or business""

support occupations are over 50 years old, as are a large (42%) of building, grounds cleaning, and maintenance workers. Need an Amazon delivery, or a shipment of hospital supplies? Thirty-four percent of transportation and material moving workers are over age 50.

Even more worrisome for our public health infrastructure is the fact that a large proportion of older workers also provides unpaid care to other older individuals. In 2019, 28% of older workers reported that they have provided unpaid care during the past three months (Hofferth et al., 2018), care that can include a broad range of activities, including assistance with activities of daily living such as bathing, dressing, or toileting, or help with tasks such as cooking, shopping, or managing finances. The average age of spousal caregivers is 62.3 (AARP, 2015). In short, older caregivers are taking care of even older people. In light of the current COVID-19 pandemic, that means that high-risk workers are often taking care of even higher-risk individuals.

But the perils of not having access to paid sick leave are not limited to older individuals' own access to sick leave. Many millennials still live with their parents (Vespa, 2017) and do not have access to sick leave. Without paid leave they put their elderly parents and grandparents at risk of getting ill.

We need paid sick leave and earned income tax credit policies to help older workers in the midst of the COVID–19 crisis

Besides maintaining basic hygiene by adequately investing in public health systems, what else can be done to minimize the impact of the virus on older workers in key support jobs? We argue for the following: requiring paid sick leave, using the tax code for progressive stimulus, and providing additional safety net protection.

Require paid sick leave: improve the stimulus package and move on to a permanent fix

The lack of paid sick leave for older workers on the front lines will hurt public health. It is bad for the worker, who may try to work through an illness, and it is bad for any other individuals who contract the illness because a sick person is showing up for work, further spreading disease. Ideally, the COVID-19 response legislation would have permanently required employers to allow every worker to earn paid sick leave of, say, 14 days for any reason, not just due to a particular virus. But the current legislation does not go this far. It expires at the end of 2020 and is limited in scope: it only provides paid sick leave to those who are quarantined or who are seeking a medical diagnosis for COVID-19 symptoms. Moreover, it exempts large employers like Walmart and Amazon, which is a major shortcoming when large employers employ more than half of the workforce, and these large employers are particularly active during the pandemic.

Use the tax code for progressive stimulus

One way of protecting older workers and stimulating the economy is to utilize the Earned Income Tax Credit (EITC), although this would have had limited impact during the early 2020 coronavirus crisis because tax filing was extended only 90 days to accommodate late filers. However, it would not be surprising if expanding the EITC comes back to the table, because the tax code is a great place to embed a stimulus: such an action would be quick, timely, temporary, and targeted. As tax-day looms, the EITC can put money in the pockets of low wage workers who have the highest propensity to spend, helping boost demand and mitigate the coming recession. But the EITC is a mixed bag for older workers. Childless workers above 65 years old or below 25 years of age are ineligible to receive the credit. Thus, the effect of the EITC would differ between two people who do exactly the same work: the ineligible worker would receive less income because they would not qualify for a supplement from the federal government (Farmand, 2019).

Workers also need health and safety protection, especially older workers

The virus–stimulus legislation did not include the protective equipment called for by worker advocates, an outcome that might have been avoided had worker protections been stronger. Historically, the most effective advocates for worker safety have been unions (Weil, 1991). Without unions, older workers are not likely to have the means to require an employer to provide protective gear. Legislation for older worker union representation is needed as one path to ensure the provision of health and safety protection. In the absence of union advocacy, Congress could take steps to impose higher health and safety standards for all workers and bypass the union pathway to provide the large proportion of older workers on the frontlines advocacy for more protection.

Conclusion

Older workers constitute a significant proportion of those working in crucial care and service professions but are much more susceptible than younger workers to becoming seriously ill from COVID-19. Despite this fact, 40% of older workers have no paid sick leave. Moreover, a significant number of older people are unpaid caregivers, thus risking exposing even higher risk individuals to the virus should the worker become sick. Protecting older workers on the job and providing paid sick leave is thus critical to maintaining and improving both their own health and the public health during the coronavirus pandemic. Over the longer run, expanding paid sick leave and worker health and safety protections would work swiftly to mitigate the effects of future pandemics. At the same time, effective wage subsidies and union protection would lessen the impact of future recessions as workers age. Both approaches are needed for an effective economic response to public health disaster and to an ordinary economic recession.

Key Points

- Older workers are at higher risk of contracting the coronavirus; they disproportionately work in areas of high exposure to COVID-19 and over one-fourth provide unpaid eldercare.
- Older workers are more susceptible than younger workers to becoming seriously ill by COVID-19; 40% of older workers do not have access to paid sickleave.
- Federal legislation should mandate paid sick leave for all workers for public health improvement.

Disclosure statement

No potential conflict of interest was reported by the authors.

References

AARP. (2015). *Caregiving in the U.S.* AARP Public Policy Institute. https://www.aarp.org/content/dam/aarp/ppi/2015/caregiving-in-the-united-states-2015-report-revised.pdf.

Blewett, L. A., Rivera Drew, J. A., King, M. L., & Williams, K. C. W. (2019). *IPUMS health surveys: National health interview survey, version 6.4 [dataset].* IPUMS. https://www.nhis.ipums.org.

Coronavirus Preparedness and Response Supplemental Appropriations Act. (2020).

Farmand, A. (2019). *Impacts of the earned income tax credit on wages of ineligible workers.* Schwartz Center for Economic Policy Analysis (SCEPA), The New School.

Flood, S., King, M., Rodgers, R., Ruggles, S., & Warren., J. R. (2020). *Integrated public use microdata series, current population survey: Version 7.0 [dataset].* University of Minnesota.

Ghilarducci, T., & Novello, A. (2017). *The labor consequences of financializing pensions.* Schwartz Center for Economic Policy Analysis (SCEPA), The New School.

Hofferth, S. L., Flood, S. M., & Sobek., M. (2018). *American time use survey data version 2.7 [dataset].* University of Maryland and Minneapolis, MN: IPUMS, 2018.

Riou, J., Hauser, A., Counotte, M. J., & Althaus, C. L. (2020). *Adjusted age-specific case fatality ratio during the COVID-19 epidemic in Hubei, China, January and February 2020.* MedRxiv, 2020.03.04.20031104. https://doi.org/10.1101/2020.03.04.20031104.

Vespa, J. (2017). *The changing economics and demographics of young adulthood: 1975–2016.* U.S. Census Bureau: Current Population Reports. Retrieved from https://www.census.gov/content/dam/Census/library/publications/2017/demo/p20-579.pdf

Weil, D. (1991). Enforcing OSHA: The role of labor unions. *Industrial Relations: A Journal of Economy and Society, 30*(1), 20–36. https://doi.org/10.1111/j.1468-232X.1991.tb00773.x

Older Adults and the Economic Impact of the COVID-19 Pandemic

Yang Li and Jan E Mutchler

ABSTRACT

The COVID-19 pandemic has impacted communities throughout the United States and worldwide. While the implications of the concomitant economic downturn for older adults are just beginning to be recognized, past experience suggests that the consequences could be devastating for many. Analyses indicate that more than one out of five Americans aged 65 years or older live in counties where high infection rates and high economic insecurity risks occur simultaneously. These findings highlight the overlap between current infection patterns and subsequent challenges to economic security that are impacting older people. Strategies and supports for getting people back to work must take into account the large segment of older people who rely on earnings well into later life. Social Security serves as the foundation of economic security for older adults across the income continuum, but it is frequently insufficient in and of itself, let alone during a crisis. Recognizing the importance of cost of living in shaping economic security highlights the need for the federal and state governments and municipalities to take older people into account in the economic recovery effort.

The COVID-19 pandemic is disrupting lives and communities throughout the United States and worldwide. At this writing, it is too early to assess the full impact of the pandemic, yet we recognize that older adults, members of racial and ethnic minority groups, and residents of many urban areas in the United States are experiencing especially high risk of illness and death (Centers for Disease Control and Prevention, 2020; Van Dorn et al., 2020). As impacts of the disease continue, the economic consequences of the pandemic, and the responses to it, are starting to unfold as jobs are lost, businesses close, and financial markets waver. While the implications of the current economic downturn for older adults are just beginning to emerge, past experience suggests that the consequences could be devastating for many.

As communities across the United States respond to the pandemic, considerable overlap between the health and economic impacts on older adults becomes apparent, a reflection of the disproportionate challenges encountered by older adults in some locations. As of this writing, more than a third (36%) of all adults aged 65 years or older in the United States live in a county that is simultaneously among the highest third of counties in terms of COVID-19 prevalence and the highest fifth of counties in terms of cost of living,[1] according to estimates from the Elder Index, a county-level measure of the income needed by older adults to meet basic needs. In these counties, the average annual cost of living in 2019 was 26,615 USD for a single renter, about 20% higher than the national median of 22,368 USD; as well, the average cost of living for single owners with and without a mortgage was about 22% and 12% higher than national median levels, respectively. This overlap reflects the especially heavy impact of COVID-19 on some densely populated urban areas, where the cost of living is typically higher relative to the rest of the country.

This perspective identifies groups within the older population that confront the disproportionate economic impact of the COVID-19 pandemic, highlighting geographic differences related to the cost of living encountered by older adults, as well as the extent to which average living expenses are covered by Social Security benefits at the county level. It also discusses the short- and long-term impacts of the economic downturn on the financial security of older Americans. We focus our discussion on people aged 65 years or older, including those who are still working and are therefore at risk of employment disruption, as well as people who have retired and are relying on non-wage income sources.

Later-life economic security and COVID-19

Many older people struggle to get by even in normal times. Although the official poverty rate for Americans aged 65 years or older has been about 10% in recent years (Semega et al., 2019), analyses based on the Elder Index suggest that far more have incomes falling short of what they need to cover necessary expenses (Mutchler et al., 2019). As many as 25% of adults aged 65 or older depend largely or exclusively on Social Security benefits (Dushi et al., 2017), yet average benefits alone fall short of necessary expenses virtually everywhere in the United States (Mutchler et al., 2018). Economic security, defined as having an income sufficient to cover living costs (Mutchler et al., 2018), has been especially elusive among older women, racial and ethnic minorities, as well as among people in communities with high costs of living (Mutchler et al., 2017).

With COVID-19, we are likely to see a differential economic impact on various types of cost and income across segments of the older population consistent with existing disparities. Our estimates show that high cost-of-living communities are disproportionately impacted by the pandemic. People who are coping with high living expenses in some of these communities are simultaneously exposed to higher rates of infection. For example, in the highest third of counties in terms of COVID-19 prevalence, the average rental cost for a one-bedroom apartment per month was 726 USD in 2019, compared to 602 USD in the lowest third of counties (calculated by the authors based on the Elder Index). Housing affordability has been a challenge for many older adults (Stone, 2018), and an increasing share of older homeowners still have a mortgage (Butrica & Mudrazija, 2016; Collins et al., 2020). As well, many older people still face high out-of-pocket medical expenses due to chronic conditions, the high cost of medications, and gaps in coverage provided by Medicare and supplemental plans (Cubanski et al., 2014). Should high rates of COVID-19 infection also lead to higher prices for food and other services, affordability problems may be exacerbated and some people with limited income may see their resources stretched even further.

Prior evidence suggests that Social Security, a major source of income for many retirees, is tapped more during economic downturns (Rutledge et al., 2012). Yet, the extent to which Social Security benefits cover basic needs is highly variable across locations (Mutchler et al., 2018). As reported earlier, more than a third of adults aged 65 years or older live in counties where both COVID-19 prevalence and cost of living are among the highest in the nation. When Social Security benefit coverage is considered, our estimates further demonstrate that more than one out of five (21%) adults aged 65 years or older in the United States live in counties that are simultaneously among the highest third in terms of COVID-19 prevalence and the lowest quintile for coverage of the cost of living by average Social Security benefits (see Figure 1). In these counties, the average Social Security benefit covers at most two-thirds of the cost of living for a single renter in good health aged 65 years or older. This means that, even with Social Security benefits, many older adults in highly impacted counties need to find additional resources to make ends meet, especially those of lower socioeconomic status, who have fewer resources to rely on (Dushi et al., 2017). Even some older adults with income from savings, investments, or 401(k) accounts may experience financial strain, confronting the risk of falling into economic insecurity if losses in those assets are sizable.

Federal, state, and local governments have been devising ways to offset the financial impact of the COVID-19 crisis on individuals and families. One such mechanism is the economic stimulus sent directly to people, in accordance with the federal CARES Act, which is intended to help those with middle and low incomes during the current downturn. The stimulus, including a one-time payment of 1,200 USD to an eligible person and 2,400 USD to a qualifying

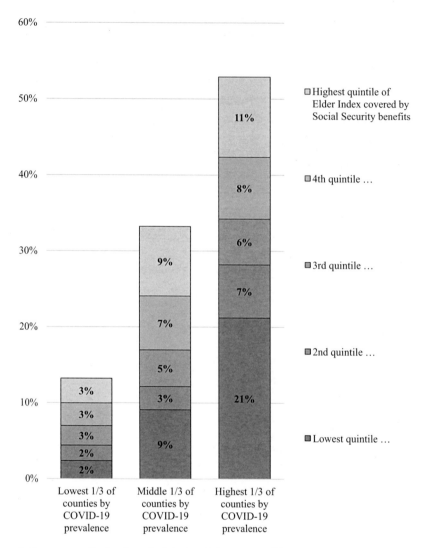

Figure 1. Percentage distribution of adults aged 65 years or older across U.S. counties classified by COVID-19 prevalence and Social Security benefit coverage rate.
Source: authors' calculation based on data from the Johns Hopkins University, American Community Survey, the Elder Index, and the Social Security Administration. Estimates are based on reported COVID-19 cases through May 1, 2020. Prevalence is defined as the number of reported COVID-19 cases per 100,000 residents at the county level. Social Security benefit coverage rate is defined as the percentage of Elder Index covered by the average Social Security benefits per county. Less than 1% of all COVID-19 cases were not included because the counties of these cases were not reported or identifiable. Cases from cruise ships and correctional facilities were excluded. Elder Index values were based on those for single renters in good health in each county.

couple, offers needed financial support valued by residents in every corner of the nation. Yet it does not contribute to basic needs to the same extent for older adults across communities, due in large part to variability in the cost of living. As Table 1 illustrates, across five selected counties with a relatively high

Table 1. Monthly cost of living covered by stimulus for eligible older one-person and two-person households in selected counties.

County	One-person Renter Household			Two-person Renter Household*		
	Elder Index per Month	Stimulus	Monthly Index Covered by Stimulus	Elder Index per Month	Stimulus	Monthly Index Covered by Stimulus
Nassau, New York	$2,945	$1,200	41%	$3,900	$2,400	62%
Bergen, New Jersey	$2,698	$1,200	44%	$3,540	$2,400	68%
Suffolk, Massachusetts	$3,090	$1,200	39%	$4,011	$2,400	60%
Marion, Ohio	$1,794	$1,200	67%	$2,715	$2,400	88%
Orleans, Louisiana	$1,952	$1,200	61%	$2,762	$2,400	87%
US average	$2,118	$1,200	57%	$3,017	$2,400	80%

Source: authors' calculation. *Estimates for two-person households assume that both members qualify for stimulus.

prevalence of the disease at the time of this writing, the stimulus checks cover between 39% (Suffolk, Massachusetts) and 67% (Marion, Ohio) of one month's necessary expenses for a single older adult, and between 60% and 88% of the monthly cost for a two-person household where both members qualify for the stimulus. Like the impact of the economic downturn itself, the benefit realized by older adults from the stimulus is highly variable, based on differences in the cost of living across communities.

A large share of older workers are employed in industries hit especially hard by the pandemic, such as retail trade, and may experience elevated exposure to the risk of unemployment and income loss (Bureau of Labor Statistics [BLS], 2020). In the short term, many older adults who had been working may lose their jobs or have their hours reduced, and these experiences may be more common in areas where COVID-19 is more widespread. Although older adults with multiple sources of income, including pensions, assets, and earnings, have stronger financial protections than those who lack these resources (Social Security Administration, 2016) and therefore may be better positioned to weather financial downturns, a growing share of people approach retirement without financial cushions in the form of savings or assets (Chen et al., 2020).

The economic downturn is likely to impact most types of resources

As in past economic downturns, most types of economic resources are likely to be impacted by the fallout of the COVID-19 crisis, including pensions, savings, assets, and earned income. People in or nearing retirement will be especially hard hit by the COVID-19 crisis, with financial consequences extending far beyond the immediate downturn. Older adults who are already retired may not be as financially affected as those who are still in the labor force: while the former may experience potentially higher costs and lower interest or dividend income, if applicable, the latter may be especially affected through lost wage income. On the whole, impacts associated with the pandemic may worsen the economic outlook for many older adults, especially those with fewer sources and lower levels of income, as some lose wages and others deplete savings in an effort to weather the economic downturn.

Consequences for pensions are expected, as some employers have already suspended their 401(k) match for employees in a number of industries, especially in the travel and retail sectors (Center for Retirement Research, 2020). Even when enrolled, workers may reduce their contributions during downturns, as past evidence shows (Dushi et al., 2013). Participants in defined benefit plans are also at risk, including most federal government workers who are enrolled, 15% of full-time private-sector workers (BLS, 2019a), and 83% of full-time state and local government workers (BLS, 2019b). Historical evidence suggests that many state and local pensions experienced funding shortfalls following the Great Recession (Munnell et al., 2010). As the impact of the current economic downturn unfolds, plan finances may worsen again. Combined, consequences for pensions may affect both current retirees and those who are still working, as the latter will depend on plans that are being impacted when they retire in the coming years.

Many older adults lack resources that could help buffer financial hardship when other income sources decline. A recent study by the Federal Reserve Bank indicates that having liquid assets on hand significantly reduces the risk of all types of hardship, including regular bill, rent or mortgage delinquency, as well as food and medical hardship (Gallagher & Sabat, 2017). Yet, among U.S. adults aged 60 to 79, about half do not have emergency savings and, among those 80 years of age and over, close to 40% are without emergency savings (Harvey, 2019). In one study, it was estimated that among those who are partly or fully retired, just over 20% of non-Hispanic blacks and about 40% of Hispanics have liquid assets compared to about 60% of non-Hispanic whites (Larrimore et al., 2017). The pandemic may have an even greater impact on older workers because they have fewer working years left to pay off debt and rebuild savings as they combat shortfalls in income during the current economic downturn.

Lessons from the past indicate that older workers have limited options in a recession: either saving more, working longer, or living on less in retirement (Munnell & Rutledge, 2013). The Great Recession especially impacted resources of middle-income older people: those in the bottom two quintiles held very few financial assets and were relatively unaffected by market decline, while middle-income individuals saw declines in interest income (Munnell & Rutledge, 2013). As well, the impact on resources among older adults as a result of an economic downturn may affect some segments of the older population more than others. Past evidence shows that the decline in assets as a result of the Great Recession has been disproportionately borne by older women, especially older women of racial minorities whose lifetime financial disadvantage was compounded by macroeconomic instability (Baker et al., 2019). These same groups experience a higher risk of economic insecurity during normal times (Mutchler et al., 2017).

At the current stage of the COVID-19 pandemic, the risk of unemployment is widespread among workers in the United States, including many among the 37 million Americans age 55 years or older who were participating in the labor force as the pandemic began (BLS, 2020). Workers aged 65 years or older are less likely to be able to work from home, compared to their younger counterparts (BLS, 2019c), and thus may be more likely to experience unemployment as a result of the current crisis. Late-career workers are also more likely to suffer job loss when a recession hits around the time of retirement (Coile & Levine, 2011), and typically experience longer spells of unemployment relative to younger workers (Monge-Naranjo & Sohail, 2015). Historical evidence from past downturns suggests that older workers who lose their jobs may never recover their former income levels (Farber, 2017) and that even when reemployed, older workers' new jobs are less likely to offer employer-sponsored pension and health plans (Johnson & Kawachi, 2007). Older workers, especially those who are less educated (Cahill et al., 2015; Coile & Levine, 2011; Munnell, 2019), may find it difficult to work longer as they are seen as expensive and lacking necessary skills, and employers may be reluctant to invest in them given their short remaining time in the labor force. Combined, the long view on jobless late-career workers during economic downturns is not optimistic, as the displacement may lead to lower income, reduced savings and job security (Butrica et al., 2012), loss of health insurance, and potentially long-term impacts on health (Pool et al., 2018; Wilkinson, 2016). Furthermore, some older workers experiencing employment disruption feel compelled to enroll for Social Security benefits earlier than they had planned (Rutledge et al., 2012), with negative implications for the benefits received in the long run.

Conclusion

As the economic consequences following from the COVID-19 crisis unfold, it is expected that older Americans' financial resources will be impacted, as they have been during previous economic downturns. These factors will hit harder in high-cost areas of the country, where economic security is already precarious for many older people. Analyses offered in this paper show that more than one out of five Americans aged 65 years or older live in counties where high infection rates and high economic insecurity risks occur simultaneously. These findings highlight the overlap between current infection patterns and subsequent challenges to economic security that are impacting older people in many areas throughout the United States.

Safeguarding the economic security of older people as we move through and beyond the COVID-19 crisis requires policy effort on many levels. Strategies and supports for getting people back to work must take into account the large segment of older people who rely on earnings well into later life. As well, this crisis is a reminder that Social Security serves as the foundation of economic security for older adults across the income continuum, but it is insufficient in and of itself, let alone during a crisis. Recognizing the importance of cost of living in shaping economic security highlights the critical roles of the federal and state governments and municipalities in taking older people into account in the economic recovery effort.

Note

1. Calculated by the authors based on data from the Johns Hopkins University, American Community Survey, and the Elder Index. Estimates are based on reported COVID-19 cases through May 1, 2020. Prevalence is defined as the number of reported COVID-19 cases per 100,000 residents at the county level. Less than 1% of all COVID-19 cases were not included because the counties of these cases were not reported or identifiable. Cases from cruise ships and correctional facilities were excluded. Elder Index values were based on those for single renters in good health in each county.

Key points

- More than one out of five Americans age 65 years or older live in counties where high infection rates and high economic insecurity risks occur simultaneously.
- Social Security serves as the foundation of economic security for older adults across the income continuum, but it is insufficient in and of itself.
- Older adults in geographic areas with high costs of living may experience greater financial strain due to the pandemic.

Acknowledgments

We thank funders of the Elder Index for their important contributions to our work, including RRF Foundation for Aging, National Council on Aging, The Henry and Marilyn Taub Foundation, The Silver Century Foundation, and Gary and Mary West Foundation.

Disclosure statement

No potential conflict of interest was reported by the authors.

References

Baker, A., West, S., & Wood, A. (2019). Asset depletion, chronic financial stress, and mortgage trouble among older female homeowners. *The Gerontologist*, *59*(2), 230–241. https://doi.org/10.1093/geront/gnx137

Bureau of Labor Statistics. (2019a). *Table 2. Retirement benefits: Access, participation, and take-up rates, private industry workers, March 2019*. https://www.bls.gov/ncs/ebs/benefits/2019/ownership/private/table02a.pdf

Bureau of Labor Statistics. (2019b). *Table 2. Retirement benefits: Access, participation, and take-up rates, state and local government workers, March 2019*. https://www.bls.gov/ncs/ebs/benefits/2019/ownership/govt/table02a.pdf

Bureau of Labor Statistics. (2019c). *Table 1. American time use survey: Workers who could work at home, did work at home, and were paid for work at home, by selected characteristics, averages for the period 2017–2018*. https://www.bls.gov/news.release/flex2.t01.htm

Bureau of Labor Statistics. (2020). *The employment situation – April 2020*. https://www.bls.gov/news.release/pdf/empsit.pdf

Butrica, B. A., Johnson, R. W., & Smith, K. E. (2012). 3. Potential impacts of the great recession on future retirement incomes. In R. Maurer, O. S. Mitchell, & M. J. Warshawsky (Eds.), *Reshaping retirement security: Lessons from the global financial crisis* (pp. 36–63). The Oxford University Press.

Butrica, B. A., & Mudrazija, S. (2016). *Home equity patterns among older American households*. The Urban Institute. https://www.urban.org/sites/default/files/publication/85326/home-equity-patterns-among-older-american-households_0.pdf

Cahill, K. E., Giandrea, M. D., & Quinn, J. F. (2015). Retirement patterns and the macroeconomy, 1992–2010: The prevalence and determinants of bridge jobs, phased retirement, and reentry among three recent cohorts of older Americans. *The Gerontologist, 55*(3), 384–403. https://doi.org/10.1093/geront/gnt146

Center for Retirement Research. (2020). *COVID-19 crisis: Economic data*. https://crr.bc.edu/wp-content/uploads/2020/04/401k-Suspension-Appendix_2020.pdf

Centers for Disease Control and Prevention. (2020). Severe outcomes among patients with coronavirus disease 2019 (COVID-19)—United States, February 12–March 16, 2020. *Morbidity and Mortality Weekly Report, 69*(12), 343–346. https://doi.org/10.15585/mmwr.mm6912e2

Chen, A., Hou, W., & Munnell, A. H. (2020). *Why do late boomers have so little retirement wealth?* (Issue in Brief 20-4). Center for Retirement Research at Boston College. https://crr.bc.edu/wp-content/uploads/2020/02/IB_20-4.pdf

Coile, C. C., & Levine, P. B. (2011). Recessions, retirement, and social security. *American Economic Review, 101*(3), 23–28. https://doi.org/10.1257/aer.101.3.23

Collins, J. M., Hembre, E., & Urban, C. (2020). Exploring the rise of mortgage borrowing among older Americans. *Regional Science and Urban Economics, 83*(July 2020), 103524. https://doi.org/10.1016/j.regsciurbeco.2020.103524

Cubanski, J., Swoope, C., Damico, A., & Neuman, T. (2014). *How much is enough? Out-of-pocket spending among Medicare beneficiaries: A chartbook*. The Henry J. Kaiser Family Foundation. https://www.kff.org/medicare/report/how-much-is-enough-out-of-pocket-spending-among-medicare-beneficiaries-a-chartbook/

Dushi, I., Iams, H. M., & Tamborini, C. R. (2013). Contribution dynamics in defined contribution pension plans during the great recession of 2007–2009. *Social Security Bulletin, 73*(2), 85. https://www.ssa.gov/policy/docs/ssb/v73n2/v73n2p85.html

Dushi, I., Iams, H. M., & Trenkamp, B. (2017). The importance of social security benefits to the income of the aged population. *Social Security Bulletin, 77*(2), 1–12. https://www.ssa.gov/policy/docs/ssb/v77n2/v77n2p1.html

Farber, H. S. (2017). Employment, hours, and earnings consequences of job loss: US evidence from the displaced workers survey. *Journal of Labor Economics, 35*(S1), S235–S272. https://doi.org/10.1086/692353

Gallagher, E., & Sabat, J. (2017, November). Cash on hand is critical for avoiding hardship. *In the Balance: Perspectives on Household Balance Sheets, 18*. Federal Reserve Bank of St. Louis. https://www.stlouisfed.org/~/media/publications/in-the-balance/images/issue_18/itb18_nov_2017.pdf

Harvey, C. S. (2019). *Unlocking the potential of emergency savings accounts*. AARP Public Policy Institute. https://www.aarp.org/content/dam/aarp/ppi/2019/10/unlocking-potential-emergency-savings-accounts.doi.10.26419-2Fppi.00084.001.pdf

Johnson, R. W., & Kawachi, J. (2007, March). *Job changes at older ages: Effects on wages, benefits, and other job attributes*. The Urban Institute. https://www.urban.org/sites/default/files/publication/46226/311435-Job-Changes-at-Older-Ages.PDF

Larrimore, J., Durante, A., Park, C., & Tranfaglia, A. (2017). *Report on the economic well-being of US households in 2016*. Board of Governors of the Federal Reserve System. https://www.federalreserve.gov/publications/files/2017-report-economic-well-being-us-households-201805.pdf

Monge-Naranjo, A., & Sohail, F. (2015). The composition of long-term unemployment is changing toward older workers. *The Regional Economist*. The Federal Reserve Bank of St. Louis. https://www.stlouisfed.org/~/media/publications/regional-economist/2015/october/unemployment.pdf

Munnell, A. H. (2019). Socioeconomic barriers to working longer. *Generations, 43*(3), 42–50. https://www.jstor.org/stable/pdf/26841731.pdf

Munnell, A. H., Aubry, J. P., & Quinby, L. (2010, April). *The funding of state and local pensions, 2009–2013*. Center for Retirement Research at Boston College. https://crr.bc.edu/wp-content/uploads/2010/04/slp_10-508.pdf

Munnell, A. H., & Rutledge, M. S. (2013). The effects of the great recession on the retirement security of older workers. *The Annals of the American Academy of Political and Social Science, 650*(1), 124–142. https://doi.org/10.1177/0002716213499535

Mutchler, J., Li, Y., & Roldan, N. (2019). *Living below the line: Economic insecurity and older Americans, insecurity in the States 2019* (Paper 40). Center for Social and Demographic Research on Aging Publications. https://scholarworks.umb.edu/cgi/viewcontent.cgi?article=1039&context=demographyofaging

Mutchler, J., Li, Y., & Xu, P. (2017). *Living below the line: Economic insecurity and older Americans, racial and ethnic disparities in insecurity, 2016* (Paper 18). Center for Social and Demographic Research on Aging Publications. https://scholarworks.umb.edu/cgi/viewcontent.cgi?article=1017&context=demographyofaging

Mutchler, J., Li, Y., & Xu, P. (2018). How strong is the social security safety net? Using the elder index to assess gaps in economic security. *Journal of Aging & Social Policy, 31*(2), 123–137. https://doi.org/10.1080/08959420.2018.1465798

Pool, L. R., Burgard, S. A., Needham, B. L., Elliott, M. R., Langa, K. M., & De Leon, C. F. M. (2018). Association of a negative wealth shock with all-cause mortality in middle-aged and older adults in the United States. *Journal of the American Medical Association, 319*(13), 1341–1350. https://doi.org/10.1001/jama.2018.2055

Rutledge, M. S., Coe, N. B., & Wong, K. (2012). *Who claimed social security early due to the great recession?* (Issue in Brief 12-14). Center for Retirement Research at Boston College. https://crr.bc.edu/wp-content/uploads/2012/07/IB_12-14-508.pdf

Semega, J., Kollar, M., Creamer, J., & Mohanty, A. (2019, September). *Income and poverty in the United States: 2018* (U.S. Census Bureau, Current Population Reports, P60-266). US Government Printing Office. https://www.census.gov/content/dam/Census/library/publications/2019/demo/p60-266.pdf

Social Security Administration. (2016). *Income of the aged chartbook, 2014* (SSA Publication No. 13-11727). https://www.ssa.gov/policy/docs/chartbooks/income_aged/2014/iac14.pdf

Stone, R. I. (2018). The housing challenges of low-income older adults and the role of federal policy. *Journal of Aging & Social Policy, 30*(3–4), 227–243. https://doi.org/10.1080/08959420.2018.1462679

Van Dorn, A., Cooney, R. E., & Sabin, M. L. (2020). COVID-19 exacerbating inequalities in the US. *The Lancet, 395*(10232), 1243–1244. https://doi.org/10.1016/S0140-6736(20)30893-X

Wilkinson, L. R. (2016). Financial strain and mental health among older adults during the great recession. *Journals of Gerontology Series B: Psychological Sciences and Social Sciences, 71*(4), 745–754. https://doi.org/10.1093/geronb/gbw001

Unclaimed Defined Benefit Pensions Can Help COVID-19 Economic Recovery

Anna-Marie Tabor

ABSTRACT

The COVID-19 economic crisis makes it vitally important that workers who earned defined benefit pensions receive them at retirement. Unfortunately, billions of dollars that could help cushion the financial shock are sitting unclaimed, because the people who they belong to cannot locate the company responsible for paying them. As defined benefit pension plans have been terminated, merged and moved over the years, large numbers of deferred vested participants have not been notified about their benefits. The widespread and growing practice of insurance company pension buy-outs can be especially problematic for participants without notice. Broader use of electronic disclosures for pensions also threatens to make the situation worse. In the wake of COVID-19, policy makers should take steps to ensure that pension benefits are part of the economic recovery.

Defined benefit pension plans guarantee workers a monthly payment for the rest of their lives, once they have worked a certain number of years for their employer. Even after leaving their jobs, they retain the right to claim the pension when they retire. A decreasing, but still significant number of private employers currently provide defined benefit pension plans to their active employees. Defined benefit pensions were an even more common benefit earlier in the working lives of people who are retiring now. Workers who earned defined benefit pensions include a cohort of people in their 60s and 70s who may face involuntary retirement due to COVID-19, or otherwise may need immediate access to retirement funds.

Billions of dollars that could be supporting retirees right now are instead sitting unclaimed (Bruce et al., 2004). People retiring in the wake of COVID-19 may thus be shocked to learn that accessing their retirement savings is not easy. In some cases, they may be cut off from their benefits entirely – not by declining markets, or underfunded pension plans, but simply through a lack of accurate and timely information about how to access their funds after the original plan changes hands, or is terminated.

This essay argues that Congress and the Department of Labor (DOL) should act to ensure that lost pension money is part of rebuilding the economy. Pension reform is one element of discussions in Washington about the post-COVID economic recovery (Bradford, 2020). Addressing lost and unclaimed pension benefits should be included in the discussion. Policy makers should enhance the process of notifying pension plan participants about changes to their plans, should create a public database to share archived information about where pension benefits are located, and should ensure that anticipated revisions to e-disclosures for pension plans do not prevent people from obtaining important information about their plans.

Pensions and COVID-19

According to the Bureau of Labor Statistics (BLS), in 2019, 51% of private employers offered a retirement plan to their employees (Bureau of Labor, 2019). Among private sector employees, just over half participate in an employer-sponsored retirement plan. These plans can be broadly divided into two categories – defined benefit plans, and defined contribution plans. Defined benefit pensions provide a set, monthly benefit to retirees that is guaranteed from the time workers reach retirement age – generally, 65 – until the end of their lives. A worker must meet a number of requirements in order to earn a defined benefit pension, including accumulating enough years of service to earn a "vested" or non-forfeitable benefit. Many employers offer another, different type of retirement plan – defined contribution plans, through which amounts saved grow tax-free in dedicated accounts until retirement, when they may be withdrawn all at once, or over time.

Defined benefit plans can be further divided into two categories: plans sponsored by private employers, and plans sponsored by public entities, such as states and municipalities. Most (86%) state and local government employees have access to a defined benefit plan, versus 16% of private sector employees (Bureau of Labor, 2019). Some state and local pension plans face long-term funding challenges that are being exacerbated by COVID-19 (Oh, 2020). This essay focuses primarily on the specific challenges faced by workers who earned defined benefit pensions with private employers, but have difficulty obtaining them, a potentially devastating challenge for people retiring due to the economic crisis.

Defined benefit pension plans have many positive features for workers planning for their retirement. By guaranteeing a fixed payment each month, they take much of the risk out of retirement planning for individuals. Most pensioners do not have to worry about their pension income falling due to volatile financial markets. When retirees receive their benefit as a monthly payment, they do not need to be concerned about budgeting to make the money last their entire lifetimes.

Workers and retirees with pensions are protected by the federal Employee Retirement Income Security Act (ERISA) of 1974 (Public Law No. 93–406 (1974)). The Internal Revenue Service and the Department of Labor play roles in regulating private pensions. In most instances, defined benefit pension plan benefits are guaranteed by the Pension Benefit Guaranty Corporation (PBGC), which pays benefits in the event that the employer sponsoring the plan files for bankruptcy.

The same defined benefit plan features that offer security to workers also make them costly for employers. Ensuring that payments guaranteed decades ago are paid out in full creates significant risks for pension plans and their sponsors. (Mercer & PBGC, 2017). The plans do offer tax benefits to employers, but along with these tax benefits come extensive compliance costs, including costs associated with premium payments to the PBGC. These costs and risks have led many employers to terminate their defined benefit pension plans in favor of less costly and less risky alternatives (Butrica et al., 2009).

There are millions of current retirees as well as people who are approaching retirement who are counting on these benefits to sustain them for the rest of their lives (Pension Benefit Guaranty Corp, 2019). The PBGC estimates that about 35 million U.S. workers and retirees are currently covered by PBGC-insured plans. If they learn at retirement age that they cannot collect their money after all, their finances are unlikely to have time to recover. This is especially true now, with the additional economic challenges of COVID-19 weighing on people of retirement age.

The impacts of COVID-19 on defined contribution plans underscore the value of a defined benefit pension in weathering the economic downturn. Struggling employers may decide to stop making 401K matching contributions (Groom Law Group, 2020). Workers who are not yet at retirement age may take advantage of emergency tax provisions in the Coronavirus Aid, Relief, and Economic Security, or CARES Act, that allow them to raid their defined contribution accounts to pay for current expenses. Permitting access to retirement accounts may address the immediate emergency, but at the expense of longer term savings for retirement. However, an estimated 40% of public and private sector workers who participate in a defined contribution plan, also participate in a defined benefit pension plan (Pension Rights Center, 2019). For these workers, the security of the defined benefit pension payment can offset reductions in their defined contribution accounts.

Defined benefit plan terminations

Federal law protects pensions that workers have already earned, but it does not require employers to keep offering a defined benefit pension forever. In fiscal 2019 alone, 1,782 defined benefit and defined contribution plans pursued standard termination, affecting about 300,000 participants (PBGC, 2019).

The accumulated number of plan terminations since 1975 exceeds 140,000, affecting millions of individuals (Pension Benefit Guaranty Corp, 2017). In the Great Recession, plan termination activity increased somewhat over prior years. While it is not yet clear whether the COVID-19 crisis will lead to a similar increase, as explained below, terminations that have already occurred will create challenges in accessing pension benefits.

Private employers must follow detailed regulations when terminating a defined benefit pension plan. Once someone has worked long enough to "vest," or earn a right to their pension benefit, that benefit is subject to an extensive set of protections under ERISA. When a pension plan is terminated at a time when it has enough money to pay all promised pensions, vested benefits for participants must be preserved. This can happen in several ways, but under law, participants should receive the full value of their pension. One option for preserving benefits is paying out the full value as a lump sum. Another option is for the pension plan to pay a life insurance company to provide annuities for pension plan participants that pay benefits equivalent to what they would have received under the pension. In some cases, a missing participant's benefit may be deposited with the PBGC prior to termination, so that the participant can claim it at a later date.

Tracking a terminated pension

Retiree benefits easily can fall through the cracks, despite these legal protections. When a pension plan ceases to exist, the responsibility for paying benefits may shift to an entirely different entity with a different name from the original pension plan, or to the Pension Benefit Guaranty Corporation. These transitions necessitate careful record keeping to ensure that no participants are lost in the administrative shuffle. Unfortunately, many pension plan participants do not know about these transactions, or how they will impact pension benefits. This is especially true for "deferred vested participants," who earned a benefit from a former employer, but may have separated from that employer years ago (Advisory Council on Employee Welfare and Pension Benefit Plans, 2013).

In theory, former employees should hear from their pension plan if changes are afoot, so that they know how to protect their pension rights, and where to claim their benefits when they reach retirement age. ERISA and its implementing regulations require notice to the people whose benefits are affected by terminations. In reality, the situation is more complex. The system relies on participants telling their pension plans when their contact information changes. However, workers who move, or who lose or change jobs may not provide updated contact information to their employers (Advisory Council on Employee Welfare and Pension Benefit Plans, 2013). Job tenure has fallen in the years since ERISA was passed in 1974 (Bureau of Labor Statistics, 2018).

Workers who switch jobs multiple times during their careers may find it particularly challenging to update information for multiple retirement benefits. This is a particular concern at this time, when workers who are newly unemployed and preoccupied with concerns related to the pandemic may inadvertently neglect to take the steps necessary to protect their pensions (Miller, 2020). Notably, Hispanic and African American workers – who are also more likely to be negatively impacted by COVID-19 and the economic crisis – tend to have lower job tenure than other U.S. workers (Bureau of Labor Statistics, 2018).

Even when retirees update their information, there are several other reasons why plans may not have accurate information in their files (Harthill et al., 2019). Corrupted records at the pension plan are a prime culprit. Information in electronic databases may be based on historic information that was recorded decades ago. The information may have been recorded inaccurately in the first instance. Or, information may have been omitted, altered, or destroyed over the years. The risk of inaccuracies is higher if a pension plan has been through transitions due to mergers and acquisitions, or due to changes in the entity that administers the plan.

Furthermore, when a plan realizes that it has inaccurate contact information – for example, because mail is returned – the plan may not take sufficient steps to locate the missing participant. There is limited and inconsistent guidance from federal regulatory agencies on what steps plans must take to track down missing participants in order to send important notices.(Harthill et al., 2019). For example, the PBGC indicates that terminating plans must use a commercial tracing service to find a participant, if the amount of a monthly benefit exceeds 50 USD (Pension Benefit Guaranty Corporation, n.d.). The DOL's guidance does not require use of a commercial service to track lost participants (U.S. Department of Labor, 2014).

Recent enforcement activity by the Department of Labor has pressured defined benefit pension plans to do more to find missing participants, and also provides some idea of the scope of the problem. Since 2017, the Labor Department has identified over 2 USD billion in benefits that private pension funds under its jurisdiction failed to pay on time because they made insufficient efforts to track down the owners (Employee Benefits Security Administration, 2018). This number is likely the tip of the iceberg, as the Department's limited enforcement resources are unlikely to cover the full extent of the problem across the market. These enforcement actions are well-timed. Connecting retirees with billions of dollars in pensions that they already have earned is simply good policy at a time when Congress is spending trillions on COVID-19 relief.

As this article goes to press, it is anticipated that DOL soon will promulgate a new, final electronic disclosure regulation (DOL EBSA, 2019). Under the proposed rule, most retirement plan participants would be automatically provided with electronic notifications, unless they affirmatively "opt-out" and request to receive them in paper form. These electronic notifications could be as ephemeral as an e-mail with a link to a website that describes how the change could affect the recipient's retirement account. Under the proposed regulation, a participant scanning e-mails could easily miss important information about a plan termination or other changes in the plan.

Transfers to insurance companies create a regulatory patchwork

When pensions are transferred to insurance companies, participants encounter an even thornier set of problems. Typically, this happens when an employer terminates a fully-funded pension plan, and purchases an annuity contract with a life insurance company to provide individual pension participants with monthly payments that are equivalent to their original pensions (Aon, 2020). In theory, this is a desirable practice because it preserves many of the participant-friendly aspects of a monthly pension that would be lost if the participant instead received the value of the pension in a lump sum payment, or rolled the benefit into a defined contribution account. But when this transaction takes place, it fundamentally changes the underlying financial product from a pension to an insurance contract, and the applicable laws change as well. Protections under the federal pension statutes are lost (Pension Benefit Guaranty Corp, 1991). When something goes wrong in the transaction – such as the employer omitting names from the list of participants, or an error in calculating the amount of the pension – there is no easy recourse with either the terminated pension plan, or with the insurance company that assumed the obligation.

If the pension plan had inaccurate records to begin with, those inaccuracies will be carried over to the new annuity. In particular, if the pension plan's participant contact information is inaccurate, the inaccurate information will be transferred to the insurance company. Under current regulatory guidance, individual participants can obtain information about annuities that were purchased for them from the PBGC (Pension Benefit Guaranty Corporation, n.d.). However, many people do not know to go to the PBGC to seek this important information. If the termination occurred long ago, the details contained in PBGC records may be very limited.

Some retirees may track down the insurance company that currently holds the annuity, despite never having received the required notices (Syre, 2020). The PBGC offers assistance through its Missing Participants Program – but information about this program is not widely known beyond the few attorneys practicing in this niche area (Pension Benefit Guaranty Corp, 2018). Even if the participant learns the name of the insurance company holding the annuity, that company may not retain the annuity until the participant reaches retirement. Pension risk transfers are a multi-billion dollar financial market (Rojas,

2018). There is no guarantee that the insurance company where the pension plan purchases the annuity contract will continue holding the portfolio indefinitely. That company could later sell the pension-based annuities to a different insurance company, creating further confusion for individual participants. The federal pension laws provide no protections requiring notice to pension plan participants about changes that happen when annuities are transferred between insurance companies.

Recent enforcement actions by state regulators and the U.S. Securities and Exchange Commission (SEC) are shining a light on this problem. In 2018 and 2019, insurer Met Life entered into settlement agreements with regulators in Massachusetts and New York related to its failure to pay annuities owed to pensioners (Reinicke, 2019). The SEC entered into a related settlement agreement in 2019 (Securities and Exchange Commission, 2019). These actions involved allegations concerning Met Life's practice of "presuming dead" any annuitants who failed to respond to two letters mailed at age 65 and 70 to the address on file, even if the contact information was out of date. The estimated number of people impacted was over 13,000 (Raymond, 2018).

The current crisis creates an opportunity for action

COVID-19 complicates retirement financial planning in multiple ways that will reverberate across generations. The health and economic impacts of the pandemic may cause workers to retire sooner than they intended (Rampell, 2013). Others will be prevented from growing their retirement savings, due to job losses, volatile markets, and unexpected, COVID-19 related expenses, as well as structural changes made to employer-sponsored retirement plans by companies seeking cost-cutting measures in order to stay afloat.

The last financial crisis taught that people approaching retirement are particularly vulnerable in a recession (Rampell, 2013). They have less time to recover from a shock to their personal finances so soon before they start drawing down savings. If they lose their jobs, they are less likely than younger workers to find reemployment; and if they do return to work, it may be at a lower level of compensation than before the recession. They may decide to claim Social Security early to make up financial shortfalls – a decision that can have a permanent, negative impact on earning power for the remainder of their lives (Singletary, 2020). These effects may be even more pronounced on people of color, for whom these impacts are compounded by systemic inequality and discrimination in housing and hiring (Mather, 2015).

Defined benefit pensions were designed to reduce these risks to retirees, making it especially troubling that retirees might not be able to locate their benefits at this time. A monthly, fixed pension payment is an especially valuable financial asset during a recession. Action is needed to ensure that retirees can get the money they have earned.

Recommendations

Enhancements to existing law and regulations are required to correct the gaps described above. The current system unfairly puts the burden on individual retirees to keep track of the complex financial transactions that have taken place since they left their employment. The following steps are necessary to ensure that retirees are not separated from their money in the current crisis.

Require complete and timely disclosure

Congress should enhance disclosure and notice requirements to ensure that workers and retirees know about the major transactions that impact their pensions, including changes in plan structure or location, terminations, and the related purchases of annuity contracts. When a pension becomes an annuity, impacted consumers should receive multiple notices about the change that include specific information about where they can go to collect their benefits when they retire. The Department of Labor should issue new and more rigorous guidance requiring plan administrators to invest meaningfully in tracking down missing participants when plans are terminated.

Create a national pension database

Congress should create a database to track the location of retirement plans. The registry should include both defined benefit pensions, and defined contribution accounts. It also should include information about pensions that are converted to insurance annuities. Going forward, pension plan administrators should submit information about new transactions to the database. In addition, significant and valuable historic information that currently resides only in US Government archives – including the names of annuity companies tied to terminated pension plans – should be made available to the public. In 2018 Senators Elizabeth Warren and Steve Daines introduced a bill, the "Retirement Savings Lost and Found Act" (S. 2474), which would have created a national pension registry. The legislation did not advance in 2018, and should be reconsidered in the coming months as part of efforts to revive the economy post COVID-19.

Assess the impact of any new e-disclosure regulations

As this article goes to press, the Department of Labor is expected to adopt a final rule that broadens the role of e-mail in providing important disclosures to participants about their plans. The proposed regulation was deeply flawed. Benefit information is simply too important to risk losing in an electronic inbox, especially during the current crisis. Any expansion in the use of electronic notifications should be carefully monitored to evaluate its impact on plan participants, including their ability to track changes in their pension plan.

Conclusion

The existing federal regulatory framework for pensions was created in 1974 – a time when computers still took up entire rooms, and secondary markets for financial products were far less developed than they are today. In the post-COVID-19 months and years ahead, the outdated laws and regulations that govern defined benefit pensions will be taxed as never before. Enhancing disclosure and notice requirements, and making information on current and historic pension plans available to the people who earned benefits, will help.

Key points

- Retirees will need access to earned defined benefit pensions during and after the COVID-19 emergency.
- Pension plan terminations are a common occurrence that present significant obstacles to claiming benefits.
- After a plan termination, many participants may not know where to go to claim their retirement benefits.
- Participants need better notification and information about changes that impact their pensions.

Disclosure statement

No potential conflict of interest was reported by the author.

Funding

The author thanks the RRF Foundation for Aging; and the Administration for Community Living, U.S. Department of Health and Human Services (DHHS) for their support. The points of view and opinions expressed are the author's own.

References

Advisory Council on Employee Welfare and Pension Benefit Plans. (2013, November). *Locating missing and lost participants*. U.S. Department of Labor. https://www.dol.gov/sites/dolgov/files/EBSA/about-ebsa/about-us/erisa-advisory-council/2013-locating-missing-and-lost-participants.pdf

Aon. (2020, March). *2020 U.S. Pension risk transfer annuity settlement market update.* https://retirement-investment-insights.aon.com/defined-benefit/aon-2020-pension-risk-transfer-market-whitepaper

Bradford, H. (2020, May 15). House relief package addresses multiemployer plans. *Pensions & Investments.* Bureau of Labor Statistics. https://www.pionline.com/legislation/house-relief-package-addresses-multiemployer-plans

Bureau of Labor. (2019, March). *National compensation survey: Employee benefits in the United States, March 2019.* Author. https://www.bls.gov/ncs/ebs/benefits/2019/ownership_tab.htm

Bureau of Labor Statistics. (2018, January). *Table 3. Distribution of employed wage and salary workers by tenure with current employer, age, sex, race, and Hispanic or Latino ethnicity.* U.S. Bureau of Labor Statistics Economic News Release. Author. https://www.bls.gov/news.release/tenure.t03.htm

Butrica, B. M., Iams, H. M., Smith, K. E., & Toder, E. J. (2009). *The disappearing defined benefit pension and its potential impact on the retirement incomes of baby boomers.* Social Security Office of Retirement and Disability Policy. https://www.ssa.gov/policy/docs/ssb/v69n3/v69n3p1.html

Employee Benefits Security Administration. (2018). *Fact sheet: EBSA restores over $2.5 billion to employee benefit plans, participants and beneficiaries.* Author. https://www.dol.gov/sites/dolgov/files/EBSA/aboutebsa/our-activities/resource-center/fact-sheets/ebsa-monetaryresults

Groom Law Group. (2020, April 15). *Corporate pensions in turbulent economic times: An overview of key issues and options for plan sponsors.* JD Supra. https://www.jdsupra.com/legalnews/corporate-pensions-in-turbulent-81464/

Harthill, S., Goldberg, E., & Familoni, O. (2019). Chapter 3. missing and unresponsive participants in ERISA plans: Current challenges and recommendations. In *New York University Review of Employee Benefits and Executive Compensation.* Matthew Bender & Company, Inc.

Mather, M. (2015, Nov.) Effects of the Great Recession on Older Americans' Health and Well Being. In Today's Research on Aging. Population Reference Bureau.

Mercer & PBGC. (2017, December 7). *Pension de-risking study analyzing the drivers of pension de-risking activity.* Pension Benefit Guaranty Corporation. https://www.pbgc.gov/sites/default/files/appendix_i_-_de-risking_study.pdf

Miller, M. (2020, May 10). Lost your job but still have a 401(k)? Here's what to do with it. *The New York Times.* https://www.nytimes.com/2020/05/10/business/401k-rollover-faq.html

Oh, S. (2020, March 24). Market rout leaves public pension funds nursing a nearly $1 trillion loss for fiscal 2020: Moody's. *Market Watch.* https://www.marketwatch.com/story/market-rout-leaves-public-pension-funds-nursing-a-nearly-1-trillion-loss-for-fiscal-2020-moodys-2020-03-24

Pension Benefit Guaranty Corp. (1991, January 14). *Opinion letter dated January 14, 1991, 29 CFR part 2613.* Author. https://www.pbgc.gov/sites/default/files/legacy/docs/oplet/91-1.pdf

Pension Benefit Guaranty Corp. (2017). *Data tables, table S-3, PBGC terminations and claims, 1975–2017, single employer program.* Author. https://www.pbgc.gov/sites/default/files/2017_pension_data_tables.pdf

Pension Benefit Guaranty Corp. (2018). *Fiscal year 2018 annual report.* Author. https://www.pbgc.gov/about/annual-reports/pbgc-annual-report-2018

Pension Benefit Guaranty Corp. (2019). *Fiscal year 2019 annual report.* Author. https://www.pbgc.gov/about/annual-reports/pbgc-annual-report-2019

Pension Benefit Guaranty Corporation. (n.d.). *Missing participants program filing instructions for PBGC-insured singled-employer defined benefit plans terminating on or after*

January 1, 2018. Author. https://www.pbgc.gov/sites/default/files/form-mp100-instructions.pdf

Pension Rights Center. (2019, July 15). *How many American workers participate in workplace retirement plans?* http://www.pensionrights.org/publications/statistic/how-many-american-workers-participate-workplace-retirement-plans

Rampell, C. (2013, February 3). In hard economy for all ages, older isn't better … it's brutal. *The New York Times.* https://www.nytimes.com/2013/02/03/business/americans-closest-to-retirement-were-hardest-hit-by-recession.html

Raymond, N. (2018, December 19). MetLife settles Massachusetts case over unpaid pensions. *Reuters.* https://www.reuters.com/article/us-metlife-pension-massachusetts/metlife-settles-massachusetts-case-over-unpaid-pensions-idUSKBN1OI1ML

Reinicke, C. (2019, December 19). MetLife agrees to pay $10 million fine to settle allegations it didn't make pension payments -and even mistakenly declared some workers deceased. Business Insider.

Rojas, W. (2018, December 17). Pension buyouts likely to be bolder, if not bigger, in 2019. *Bloomberg Law.* https://news.bloomberglaw.com/employee-benefits/pension-buyouts-likely-to-be-bolder-if-not-bigger-in-2019

Securities and Exchange Commission. (2019, December 18). *MetLife to pay $10 million for long-standing internal control failures.* Author. https://www.sec.gov/news/press-release/2019-269

Singletary, M. (2020, April 10). Should you take social security early? For some, coronavirus changes the math on waiting until you're 70. *Washington Post Blogs.* https://www.washingtonpost.com/business/personal-finance/should-you-take-social-security-early-for-some-coronavirus-changes-the-math-on-waiting-until-youre-70/2020/04/10/e85486a8-7a6e-11ea-b6ff-597f170df8f8_story.html

Syre, S. (2020, March 18). Tracking down benefit when employer transforms pension into annuity. *The Gerontology Institute Blog.* http://blogs.umb.edu/gerontologyinstitute/2020/03/18/pac-case-study-tracking-down-benefit-when-employer-transforms-pension-into-annuity/

Bruce,E. & Turner, J. (2004) Lost pension money: who is responsible? Who benefits? In John Marshall Law Review (UIC John Marshall Law School).

U.S. Department of Labor. (2014, August 14). *Field assistance bulletin no. 2014-01.* https://www.dol.gov/agencies/ebsa/employers-and-advisers/guidance/field-assistance-bulletins/2014-01

U.S. Department of Labor Employee Benefits Security Administration. (2019, October 23). "Default electronic disclosure by employee pension benefit plans under ERISA," 84 Fed. Reg. 56894. *Federal Register.* https://www.federalregister.gov/documents/2019/10/23/2019-22901/default-electronic-disclosure-by-employee-pension-benefit-plans-under-erisa

Documenting and Combating Ageism

The COVID-19 Pandemic Exposes Limited Understanding of Ageism

Laurinda Reynolds

ABSTRACT

During the COVID-19 pandemic, justification for orders to shelter in place have emphasized the vulnerability of older people. Although other at-risk groups were sometimes mentioned, the emphasis on older people could have effects on attitudes about aging and older people for decades to come. This essay provides a comprehensive biopsychosocial description of ageism and discusses the pandemic as a "focusing event" that exemplifies the extreme social consequence of ageism for the entire older population. It suggests revisions to the Elder Justice Act and utilization of programs such as the Reframing Aging, Age-Friendly University, and Ageism First Aid initiatives to reduce ageism in the wake of the pandemic.

Introduction

The COVID-19 pandemic has exposed ignorance about what ageism is and ageism's potential for direct impact on aging outcomes and death like no other situation could. The ignorance is not isolated to the general public. Despite decades of ageism research across various disciplines, many professionals and academics in the health and helping professions have a superficial understanding of ageism which, in turn, contributes to ageism in measurable ways (Ng et al., 2015). This perspective thus begins with a comprehensive and multidisciplinary description of ageism as a biopsychosocial phenomenon. It then discusses the COVID-19 pandemic as a "focusing event" that exemplifies the extreme social consequence of ageism for the entire older population. How ageism has been manifested during the COVID-19 pandemic, along with resulting moral and ethical dilemmas, are illustrated with comments made by the Lieutenant Governor of Texas. Next, it identifies the relevance of the Elder Justice Act of (2009) for addressing ageism in the wake of the pandemic, as well as various interventions to reduce ageism in society and the health and

Author Affiliation: Primary author of Ageism First Aid, an online course underwritten in part, by the Academy for Gerontology in Higher Education's Founders Innovation Fund, through a grant from the Retirement Research Foundation (now the RRF Foundation for Aging), and supported by the Gerontological Society of America.

helping professions, including the Reframing Aging Initiative, the Age-Friendly University Movement, and the online course, Ageism First Aid.

Ageism, the biopsychosocial phenomenon

Politicians, representatives of government agencies, and professionals in the health and helping professions responding to the COVID-19 pandemic have confirmed the need for a comprehensive description of ageism by placing disproportionate emphasis on the need to shelter in place due to the vulnerability of people ages 60 years and older. As of 2016 there were fewer than 70 million 60+ people in the United States, while the other groups at high risk, including adults with heart disease, diabetes, asthma, and a history of smoking, far exceeds 70 million. In light of these figures, the disproportionate messaging about risk based on age rather than disease or other conditions reflects ageism and sadly, many professionals in the field of aging have not recognized the danger of this emphasis and have thus participated in the messaging. The COVID-19 pandemic confirms that professionals must gain a deeper understanding of ageism and how it is messaged.

The curriculum for Ageism First Aid (Gerontological Society of America [GSA], 2020b), an online course created to reduce ageism among professionals and paraprofessionals working in the health and helping professions, was developed to fully convey what ageism is without the use of scholarly terminology. This synthesis of the curriculum provides a comprehensive descriptive definition of ageism and its related subconstructs. Ageism is a modern biopsychosocial phenomenon that cultivates negative subconscious attitudes (implicit bias) about aging and older people within individuals, groups, and society, while cultivating positive implicit bias for being young and youthful. Individuals develop the negative bias from early childhood into adulthood through repeated exposure (priming) to depictions of aging and older people that evoke negative images (negative aging stereotypes). Until midlife, the priming effects (negative subconscious impressions) manifest in thoughts and behaviors directed at older individuals and groups. Upon reaching midlife, the priming effects influence perceptions and expectations of self during aging (ageism against future-self).

The biopsychosocial nature of ageism is displayed through intersectionality and interactions across the three primary domains. Biologically, observable aging-related changes in appearance and reproduction during midlife trigger recognition of aging in the self and others. The observations trigger implicit psychological and behavioral responses, including the internalization of ageism (negative beliefs about self), the externalization of ageism (negative behaviors toward self and others), and vulnerability to aging stigma (being marked by negativity about aging while aging). In response to observations, individuals may also change social behaviors and activity levels in ways that increase the likelihood of matching internalized negative beliefs; they may also begin to self-monitor function (notice normal errors and attribute them to being older), which decreases self-efficacy (justified belief in the capability to accomplish a task). When individuals begin to match a negative aging stereotype, it anecdotally confirms personal belief in the stereotype, beliefs held by friends and family members, and in some cases, beliefs across all levels of society, e.g., when the aging individual is a public figure. Intrapersonal anecdotal confirmation of a stereotype cultivates acceptance of marginalization (being treated as a second-class citizen) and, for observers, rationalizes personal behaviors and acceptance of social policies that marginalize older people.

Ageism fosters individual and social behaviors toward older people that range from microaggressions (helping behaviors that cultivate or affirm helplessness), to demeaning (patronizing and pejorative) behaviors and physical, emotional, and financial harm (abuse, neglect, and exploitation, respectively). All older people are not equally vulnerable to the harmful behaviors fostered by ageism. An individual's vulnerability to ageism, abuse, neglect, and/or exploitation is influenced by multiple biopsychosocial factors. Biologically, factors such as physiological health, stamina, and ableness guard against or contribute to vulnerability; so too do psychological factors (e.g., personality, mental health, self-perceptions, self-efficacy) and sociological factors (e.g., access to resources and support systems). Consider the example of a self-reliant person being told "you are too old to do that." The person may ignore the statement or react strongly and reject the judgment. On the other hand, if a person who relies on others for care is told they are too old, the statement can add to the aging stigma and if coupled with intimidation, the statement and behavior could constitute psychological abuse.

Ageism messages are generated at all levels of society, by government, institutions, media, businesses, organizations, local communities, cultures, religions, and family groups, as well as by individuals in positions of authority, family members, friends, and even strangers. Ageism messages are conveyed in the content and by the omission of content in policies, physical environments, entertainment and news media, advertisements, non-verbal gestures and behaviors, and other sources. Within the health and helping professions, messages about aging that fail to differentiate aging from the effects of diseases, disorders, chronic illness, and the social determinants of health, and messages that fail to differentiate aging from the effects of injuries, excessive wear and tear, and sensory damage that progress over time contribute to ageism. Depending on the source, format, and situation, an ageism message can impact an older person or group, and in some situations negatively impact the entire older population. Messages range from obvious (overt and intentional) to insidious (neither the source nor target recognize the ageism). The messages can be unintentional and implicit, e.g., microaggressions, or the inadvertent result of compassionate ageism (well-intentioned advocacy for a subgroup of older people that results in a negative generalization to the entire older population).

The COVID-19 pandemic: an ageism-related focusing event

The COVID-19 pandemic is a "focusing event" that exemplifies the extreme social consequences of unintentional and compassionate ageism for the entire older population. How ageism has manifested during the pandemic, along with resulting moral and ethical dilemmas, is illustrated in comments made by the Lieutenant Governor of Texas, Dan Patrick. In an appearance on FOX News, the Lieutenant Governor explained that he and other grandparents would be willing to die to save the economy for the sake of their grandchildren (JJ Knows the Way, 2020). Like most other politicians and leaders, his focus was on older people as a risk group, rather than on subgroups of adults with health risks. The message had individual and social implications and since the broadcast, there has been an extensive backlash. However, in this article the purpose of identifying this comment is to point out how the major subconstructs of ageism, internalization, externalization, and politicization, have manifested during the pandemic.

If Patrick's statement was sincere, *then* it provides an example of internalized ageism, Patrick's believes that his life is less important than the economy and that this is wisdom that comes with age (a positive aging stereotype). *If* sincere, *then* it also provides an example of externalized ageism, both because Patrick was imposing his internalized beliefs about the lesser value of older people on other older people and because the message drew on the positive aging stereotype to pressure older people into an agreement and to increase acceptance of the idea across all age groups.

Regardless of sincerity, as statements made by a person of authority in state government, *there was* a devaluing of being older and an increased value placed on being younger, which sent a powerful ageism message to both older and younger people in the state. Furthermore, as a person with financial means and access to the best health care Patrick is more likely to survive the virus than the average older person, making his statement an example of privilege as well. *Sincere or not*, because Patrick is a politician concerned with gaining the favor of higher-ranking politicians and constituents, *this is* an example of how aging and ageism becomes politicized.

Patrick's statement also presents a new version of the Trolley Problem originally posed by Philippa Foot (1967). The Trolley Problem was a simple ethical dilemma that forced a choice between allowing one person to die to save five other people. The COVID-19 *Pandemic Problem*, as posed by the Lt. Governor and other high-ranking politicians and pundits, is a scenario forcing a choice between the lives of older people and a healthy economy. Compounding this problem is a second ethical and moral dilemma. When beds and equipment are in short supply, physicians are forced to choose who to provide with hospital care and treatment. There are many factors that contribute to the risk for and survival of COVID-19; however, age seems to dominate messages to the public. This raises a question about how choices to hospitalize and provide care have been made when physicians must make a choice between a healthy older person and a younger person with risk factors such as heart disease, asthma, and tobacco use. We may never know.

The Elder Justice Act and the COVID-19 response

The words of Dr. Paul Batalden, "every system is perfectly designed to get the results it gets," were first uttered decades ago and they have application now, during the pandemic (Carr, 2008). Which social policies could be improved to reduce the opportunity for aging to be politicized and for ageism to influence decisions during the COVID-19 pandemic? A notable example is the Elder Justice Act (EJA) of 2009, a federal policy that was reauthorized in 2017. The EJA a) defines elder abuse, neglect, and exploitation in terms of individual behaviors directed at older individuals; b) provides federal resources to prevent, detect, intervene in, and treat elder abuse, neglect, and exploitation; and c) when appropriate, authorizes prosecution of elder abuse, neglect, and exploitation.

The EJA did not anticipate the possibility of societal neglect of the entire older population; however, the definition of individual neglect, "the failure of a caregiver or fiduciary to provide the goods or services that are necessary to maintain health and safety of an elder" (Elder Justice Act of 2009), can be applied to an analogous if-then social scenario. *If*, it would be neglect for a fiduciary to withhold lifesaving treatment for an older person to increase a beneficiary's inheritance; *then*, ending social distancing prematurely and increasing deaths among older people to preserve the economy for future generations could also constitute neglect. The COVID-19 pandemic, as a *focusing event, may well* open a *policy window* that allows advocates to revise the EJA to address abuse, neglect, and exploitation at a societal level and minimize opportunities for situations like the pandemic to be politicized.

Likewise, the EJA could provide explicit guidance around choices to deny hospitalization or treatment and, at minimum, make clear that these decisions cannot be based solely on age under any circumstances. The EJA should clarify that all risk and risk mediating factors for patients of any age be considered in decisions about who to hospitalize or treat when there is a shortage of resources. The revisions should also prevent insurers from withholding authorizations for treatment based solely on age.

Interventions to reduce ageism

There are a variety of strategies and resources that have been developed in recent years and, if widely implemented, could help to reduce ageism both during and after the COVID-19 pandemic. The **Reframing Aging Initiative** is a long-term educational campaign that utilizes positive images of aging and metaphors to positively prime younger people for aging and to reverse the decades of negative images impressed upon the minds of adults and people who are currently aging. The Initiative is developing materials to directly address ageism during the COVID-19 pandemic (GSA, 2020c). A major investment of capital to fund a nationwide campaign as the pandemic continues to unfold could yield short-term benefits and reduce the impact of the ageism messages during the first wave of the pandemic.

The **Age Friendly University (AFU) Movement** is a grassroots effort that employs a variety of strategies, including networking, professional development training, collaboration, intergenerational projects, and educational interventions. Each constituent is a strategy that can have a measurable positive impact on attitudes about aging over the short and long-term for younger and older students, faculty, and administrators, as well as in the community surrounding the institution (GSA, 2020a). Faculty leading the AFU Movement have developed tools and strategies that support faculty interested in making their institution more age friendly. In the wake of the pandemic, joining the AFU Movement can help reduce the impact of the ageism messages expressed during the pandemic within institutions and reduce their impact on the older people living in nearby communities.

The online course **Ageism First Aid (AFA)** is a scalable educational intervention for people currently working in entry-level to executive positions in the field of aging and for students and workers preparing to enter the field. The implementation of AFA within the Aging Network and institutions can immediately reduce ageism manifesting in settings where older people receive services and support (GSA, 2020b). COVID-19 has exposed a limited understanding of ageism and ageism awareness among leaders in positions of authority and among professionals in the health and helping professions. Reducing ageism's influence and impact as the pandemic continues to unfold is critical. Taking AFA is a convenient and time efficient way to gain the knowledge and awareness needed to reduce the post-pandemic ageism effects.

Conclusion

There is little that can be done to reduce the short-term effects of the ageism messages of the COVID-19 pandemic will have. We can only look forward and implement effective strategies that will help everyone in the field of aging gain a shared and comprehensive biopsychosocial understanding of ageism. Practitioners in the field of aging need to learn how to avoid ageism messages in their speech, writing, and behavior in curriculum, articles, classrooms, housing, long-term support and service settings, and government agencies. Advocacy efforts must be accomplished without inadvertently contributing to ageism, and efforts to renegotiate and revise social policies and implement initiatives to address and prevent ageism must become a priority.

Key Points

- COVID-19 has exposed a lack of understanding about what ageism is.
- The case of the Lt. Gov. of Texas illustrates dimensions and constructs of ageism in the context of COVID-19.
- Social policy revisions and initiatives are needed to reduce the prevalence of ageism exemplified by COVID-19.

Disclosure statement

No potential conflict of interest was reported by the author.

Funding

No funding was received for this work.

References

Carr, S. (2008, August 1). *A quotation with a life of its own*. Patient Safety & Quality Healthcare. https://www.psqh.com/julaug08/editor.html

Elder Justice Act of 2009 Title XX, Social Security Administration, Subtitle A Sec. 2001. [42 U.S. C. 1397] Subtitle B Sec. 2011. [42 U.S.C. 1397j] 2020.

Foot, P. (1967). *The problem of abortion and the doctrine of the double effect*. Virtues and Vices. Basil Blackwell, 1978. http://www2.econ.iastate.edu/classes/econ362/hallam/Readings/FootDoubleEffect.pdf

Gerontological Society of America. (2020a, April 30). *Age-Friendly University (AFU) global network*. https://www.geron.org/programs-services/education-center/age-friendly-university-afu-global-network

Gerontological Society of America. (2020b, April 30). *Ageism first aid*. https://www.geron.org/programs-services/education-center/ageism-first-aid

Gerontological Society of America. (2020c, April 30). *Reframing aging initiative*. https://www.geron.org/programs-services/reframing-aging-initiative

JJ Knows the Way. (2020, March 24). *TX Lt Gov Dan Patrick suggests grandparents willing to die for US economy in Fox News Interview*. https://www.youtube.com/watch?v=IGmy3exFvvI

Ng, R., Allore, H. G., Trentalange, M., Monin, J. K., & Levy, B. R. (2015). Increasing negativity of age stereotypes across 200 years: Evidence from a database of 400 million words. *Plos One*, *10*(2), 1–6. http://doi.org/10.1371/journal.pone.0117086

Not Only Virus Spread: The Diffusion of Ageism during the Outbreak of COVID-19

Federica Previtali ⓘ, Laura D. Allen ⓘ*, and Maria Varlamova ⓘ*

ABSTRACT
During the COVID-19 pandemic, we face an exacerbation of ageism as well as a flourish of intergenerational solidarity. The use of chronological age is an unjustified threshold for the creation of public policies to control the spreading of the virus; doing so reinforces intrapersonal and interpersonal negative age stereotypes and violates older persons' human rights to autonomy, proper care treatment, work, and equality. By overlooking differences within age groups, measures formulated solely on the basis of age are unable to target beneficiaries' needs. Concurrently, several initiatives are trying to overcome ageist practices by providing different types of assistance to older adults on the basis of need rather than chronological age. The Marie Skłodowska-Curie Innovative Training Network EuroAgeism calls on policymakers to refrain from ageist practices and language, as they exacerbate our ability to meet the COVID-19 crisis and future emergencies.

Introduction

The outbreak of the novel coronavirus, COVID-19, impacts our daily lives and the lives of all the people around us, regardless of their age, in unprecedented ways. Many governments set up measures and policies to slow the spread of the COVID-19 pandemic to protect people and to reduce expected negative health and socio-economic consequences. Taking into consideration that testing protocols vary between countries, it is reported that older adults constitute a higher percentage of confirmed COVID-19 cases and deaths (NYC Health, 2020). Older adults are at a significantly increased risk of developing severe and debilitating illness from COVID-19 (World Health Organisation, 2020a), because of the physiological changes associated with aging, decreased immune function and multimorbidity, as well as the co-existence of various risk factors (health, psychosocial and economic).

---

*Both these authors contributed equally.

Although people of all ages may be severely affected, it is older adults who are at the center of the news media and political discussion and regulations.

This perspective reflects on the policies developed to stop the pandemic that might increase ageism and therefore be harmful to older persons as well as the whole society. The following discussion focuses on the arbitrary use of chronological age, the related outcomes of targeting older persons as vulnerable and the consequences of overlooking differences within age groups. It highlights the importance of refraining from ageist attitudes and behaviors that exacerbate a phenomenon that might impair individuals' rights as well as intergroup relations in the long term.

Ageism and the use of chronological age

Ageism is not a new phenomenon. Observations of ageism can be traced at least as far back as to the coinage of the term by Robert Butler in 1969 (Butler, 1969). Numerous studies demonstrate how ageism has become reified (e.g., Ayalon & Tesch-Römer, 2018), infiltrating all aspects of society, from working life to healthcare and access to services (Officer & de la Fuente-núñez, 2018). In this respect, ageist attitudes, as other forms of discrimination, have become institutionalized in public policies (Butler, 1980). In the last 50 years, the acknowledgment of the aging of the population and the related expenses for pensions and health care by governments has contributed to the notion that older people are a burden for national economies (Walker, 2012). At the extreme, this opinion has led some politicians to hope for a "killer flu epidemic … which disproportionately affects elderly" to solve the fiscal problems attributed to population aging (Walker, 2012, p. 814). Examples, like this one, of overtly, though typically less extreme, ageist accounts are visible throughout society. Even more so than usual, ageist policy proposals have been put forward during the COVID-19 pandemic.

Chronological age has frequently been used as a foundation for various policies promulgated in light of COVID-19, even though no international agreement exists on which age cutoff to use (such as, 60, 65, 70 or 75), thereby demonstrating the arbitrariness of the threshold. The unquestioned idea that chronological age objectively defines groups, overlooking their inner differences, is an ageist assumption, as it supports prejudice, stereotypes, and discrimination on the basis of age. Our claim is that although the connection between the presence of chronic illnesses and age is observed, being chronologically old does not equal being at once vulnerable, in a precarious state of health, or less valuable. Hence, we, the undersigned researchers of the Marie Skłodowska-Curie Innovative TrainingNetwork EuroAgeism,[1] dismiss the notion that policies should be created on the basis of mere chronological age: this is an example of ageism and reflects harmful ageist attitudes and behaviors within our society.

We recognize that older adults are at a higher risk of violation of human rights during the outbreak, as stated by United Nations human rights experts (United Nations Human Rights Office of the Commissioner, 2020). In this regard, we stand against the policy of performing triage based solely on chronological age (e.g., Baker & Fink, 2020; Popescu & Marcoci, 2020). Older individuals should not suddenly lose the right to autonomy and agency of choice. Every life matters, therefore triage protocol should be case-specific, approached through discussion, and based on scientific evidence and medical needs.

Ageism is harmful and has deleterious consequences for people of all ages. Policies and measures based merely on chronological age fail to consider the individual differences and the intersection of different social, economic and health factors that instigate vulnerability and the need for support. For example, age-based confinement policies developed to limit the transmission of COVID-19 create a double pitfall. First, they free the younger population from responsibility, creating an illusion that young persons are not affected, are invincible, and do not have a role to play in the containment. The initial portrayal of the pandemic as affecting only older adults has exposed society to a higher spread of the contagious disease. It has led, for example, to younger persons partying during the American Spring Break (Miller, 2020), gathering in college fraternities (Silva, 2020), attending parties in Japan after being in high-risk European countries (Takashima, 2020), and moving from the red zone in North Italy to the South where the virus had heretofore been less prevalent (Di Marino, 2020).

Second, chronologically-based policies and official statements reinforce old age as vulnerable and dependent, thereby sustaining ageism. Ayalon and colleagues discuss how media communication and public measures based on chronological age reinforce negative age stereotypes during the COVID-19 outbreak (Ayalon et al., 2020), citing reports that urged folks over 70 years of age to stay indoors or news articles that criticized the decision of providing intensive care to those over 90 years old. The idea that overtly ageist attitudes should not be condemned seems accepted in this difficult time: public discussion using the hashtag #BoomerRemover has praised the virus for helping us reduce the public expense devoted to older persons (Morrow-Howell et al., 2020). Similarly, in the US, the Texas Lt. Governor stated that grandparents should consider sacrificing themselves for the greater good of their children's future (Coughlin & Yoquinto, 2020); and in the UK, the death of older persons due to COVID-19 was reported to be beneficial for the economy, as "culling elderly dependents" (Warner, 2020 as cited in Human Rights Watch, 2020) echoing the sentiments of nearly 10 years ago that a pandemic affecting older persons would be beneficial (Walker, 2012). These ageist assumptions accentuate the intergenerational anger and the use of hate speech in pitting young against old, especially when institutions reinforce this narrative. Individuals may internalize these messages, and thus a vicious cycle of ageism develops.

Moreover, ageism could prevent older adults from acknowledging their physiological and immunological risk and needs because of a desire to avoid association with the stigmatized and stereotyped group of older persons (Aronson, 2020). Each of us – decision-makers, policymakers, healthcare professionals, and news reporters – should be aware of problems of ageism and its pernicious societal and individual effects. We should be more cautious to actively refrain from ageist language, recognizing that older adults are a heterogeneous group that continue to make valuable contributions to society (The Framework Institute, 2020).

Ageism and physical distancing

Social isolation measures vary between countries, some are age-based, and some are universal; however, the key issue is how such measures are communicated and applied and whether they reinforce negative age stereotypes. The belief that society does not need older adults and will not miss them if they self-isolate during this time (e.g., Coughlin & Yoquinto, 2020) denies the importance of their participation in the community.

Older adults continuously and actively contribute to society with paid and unpaid work (United Nations Economic Commission for Europe, 2019a); they constitute a great bulk of informal care for partners, grandchildren and others (United Nations Economic Commission for Europe, 2019b); they are a vital part of voluntary and civic society (Principi et al., 2014); they support intergenerational transfers (Silverstein, 2006); and they secure the continuity of our identity, heritage, and memories. Moreover, older adults are assisting others during this crisis; for example, those who are retired healthcare professionals answered the call and returned to work, in Canada (Lowrie, 2020), the US (Simmons-Duffin, 2020), the UK (British Medical Association, 2020), and Italy (Ministry of Health, 2020).

The ability to cope with social isolation does not depend just on age, but also on other factors such as the availability of social support, the size of the household, the urban or rural location, the attainability of technology, the accessibility of services, and even psychological factors and regular lifestyle. For example, access to digital technology, as well as digital literacy, has proved to be a key element in the ability to cope with quarantine requirements; it allows people to work from home, order groceries and medicine, or stay socially connected (Friemel, 2016). We encourage policymakers to acknowledge the digital divide as a potential barrier and to make an extra effort in ensuring that persons of all ages have access to technologies that influence their ability to realize their basic rights.

Ageism and inequalities

The current pandemic is also highlighting the inequalities that the intersection of various socio-demographic factors creates. For example, refugees, migrants, prisoners, people experiencing homelessness, those living in rural or deprived areas, or persons without social support may face additional challenges. Folks living in congregated settings, such as residential care, are more exposed to risks of contagion, and the lack of resources and personal protective equipment in this setting exacerbates the issue. According to the New York Times, in the US, at least 28,000 residents and workers died from the novel coronavirus in nursing homes, amounting to one-third of the total deaths as of May 11 (Yourish et al., 2020). The same situation can be seen in Italy, where 6,773 persons have died in nursing homes. Of the total, 40% have been related to COVID-19, and the evaluation is based only on one-third of the residential care structure of the country (Caccia et al., 2020). The cases in nursing homes are aggravated by complicated initial conditions, such as questionable care standards (Cenziper et al., 2020) or understaffing in healthcare facilities that increase the risk of inappropriate care (World Health Organisation, 2020b). We encourage policymakers to give more attention to persons in vulnerable situations. This should be done regardless of their date of birth, including those with preconditions, already socially excluded, having financial difficulties, and with limited access to healthcare and other services. Especially in an emergency situation, there is a need for creative and alternative policies and actions that increase social connections, social protection, and accessible solutions.

The relationship between age and gender is also notable during the outbreak. Even though data (Data2x, 2020) for COVID-19 so far show the same number of cases between men and women, men are more susceptible to enter a critical condition and are more likely to die. Moreover, women, especially older and migrant women, represent the majority of caregivers. Traditional roles require women to look after children, grandchildren, and those in vulnerable situations. This limits their work and economic opportunities while close contact increases their exposure to infectious diseases. The problem of abuse and domestic violence (Kingkade, 2020) has also come to the forefront.

Conclusion

The deleterious practices described so far exist alongside positive actions, which should also be acknowledged. At the local as well as national and international levels, intergenerational support has increased. Authorities and volunteers are helping older adults and persons in vulnerable situations in running errands; psychological support is offered over the telephone through help lines; online courses and activities are available; and financial aid is provided to respond to job loss or to purchase technological equipment (Age Platform Europe, 2020). We want to spotlight the collective effort, from the governments that are protecting older adults from possible harm, to the hard work of the healthcare professionals who are working under extreme pressure and daily risk. We applaud the intergenerational solidarity that has spontaneously spread. Helping by picking up groceries, going to the pharmacy, paying the bills, or teaching how to use video chat is an admirable way of strengthening connections across generations while maintaining physical distance.

Still, ageism and ageist practice have been harmful during the outbreak of COVID-19 when a collective effort is needed. They hinder the ability of policies to target the population in the most vulnerable situations and to recognize the diversity within age groups, therefore violating individual rights. We encourage everyone to be sensitive toward ageism during this critical time and to let intergenerational help and solidarity prevail.

Key points

- Ageism has harmful consequences, and the pandemic has further increased its incidence.
- Ageism hinders policies to target populations in vulnerable situations.
- Policies based on mere chronological age endanger intergenerational solidarity.
- During the emergency, policymakers should refrain from ageist language and challenge age stereotypes to abstain from ageist practices.

Note

1. The MSCA-ITN EuroAgeism, funded under Horizon 2020 and Marie Sklodowska-Curie Actions, is a multi-disciplinary, multi-sectoral, science-policy international network of researchers, policymakers and social and health care professionals. The aim of the network is to tackle ageism and raise awareness of ageist practices and policies in clinical, social and everyday settings. Senior and early-stage researchers explore the ways to promote inclusive and age-friendly societies, to improve labor market conditions for all ages, and to ensure that access to goods and services is not limited by one's age. Please refer to our website (https://euroageism.eu/policy_projects/perspective-on-ageism-and-covid-19-upcoming-publication/) for the list of signatories to the MSCA-ITN Innovative Training Network EuroAgeism.

Disclosure statement

No potential conflict of interest was reported by the authors.

Funding

This project has received funding from the European Union's Horizon 2020 research and innovation progamme under the Marie Skłodowska-Curie grant agreement No 764632.

ORCID

Federica Previtali ⓘ http://orcid.org/0000-0002-4918-1522
Laura D. Allen ⓘ http://orcid.org/0000-0002-5251-5677
Maria Varlamova ⓘ http://orcid.org/0000-0001-9104-8103

References

Age Platform Europe. (2020, April 2). *COVID-19: Good practices/initiatives.* Retrieved May 15, 2020, from https://www.age-platform.eu/age-news/covid-19-good-practices-initiatives

Aronson, L. (2020, March 28). Ageism is making the pandemic worse. *The Atlantic.* https://www.theatlantic.com/culture/archive/2020/03/americas-ageism-crisis-is-helping-the-coronavirus/608905/

Ayalon, L., Chasteen, A., Diehl, M., Levy, B. R., Neupert, S. D., Rothermund, K., Tesh-Römer, C., & Wahl, H. (2020). Aging in times of the COVID-19 pandemic: Avoiding ageism and fostering intergenerational solidarity. *The Journals of Gerontology: Series B,* (20), 1–4. https://doi.org/10.1093/geronb/gbaa051

Ayalon, L., & Tesch-Römer, C. (Eds.). (2018). *Contemporary perspectives on ageism. International perspectives on aging 19.* Springer Open.

Baker, M., & Fink, S. (2020, March 31). At the top of the Covid-19 curve, how do hospitals decide who gets treatment? *The New York Times.* https://www.nytimes.com/2020/03/31/us/coronavirus-covid-triage-rationing-ventilators.html

British Medical Association. (2020, May 12). *COVID-19: Retired doctors returning to work.* Retrieved May 15, 2020, from https://www.bma.org.uk/advice-and-support/covid-19/practical-guidance/covid-19-retired-doctors-returning-to-work

Butler, R. N. (1969). Age-ism: Another form of bigotry. *The Gerontologist, 9*(4 part 1), 243–246. https://doi.org/10.1093/geront/9.4_Part_1.243

Butler, R. N. (1980). Ageism: A foreword. *Journal of Social Issues, 36*(2), 8–11. https://doi.org/10.1111/j.1540-4560.1980.tb02018.x

Caccia, F., Moro, N. M., Massenzio, M., Pinna Roat, D., & Testa, A. (2020, April 19). Coronavirus, Iss: «Dal 1° febbraio morti 6773 anziani nelle Rsa, il 40% per Covid-19». *Corriere della Sera.* https://www.corriere.it/cronache/20_aprile_19/coronavirus-strage-silenziosa-nonni-deceduti-rsa-a0580548-81b0-11ea-b7e0-dce1b61a80bf.shtml?refresh_cecp

Cenziper, D., Jacobs, J., & Mulcahy, S. (2020, April 17). Hundreds of nursing homes with cases of coronavirus have violated federal infection-control rules in recent years. *The Washington Post.* https://www.washingtonpost.com/business/2020/04/17/nursing-home-coronavirus-deaths/?arc404=true

Coughlin, J., & Yoquinto, L. B. (2020, April 13). Many parts of america have already decided to sacrifice the elderly. *The Washington Post.* https://www.washingtonpost.com/outlook/2020/04/13/many-parts-america-have-already-decided-sacrifice-elderly/

Data2x. (2020). *Gender data and resources related to COVID-19.* United Nation Foundation. https://data2x.org/resource-center/gender-and-data-resources-related-to-covid-19/

Di Marino, A. (2020, February 25). Al Sud i Danni Collaterali Dell'emergenza. Sindaci Spiazzati Dai Ritorni Rorzati. *La Stampa*. https://www.lastampa.it/cronaca/2020/02/25/news/al-sud-i-danni-collaterali-dell-emergenza-sindaci-spiazzati-dai-ritorni-forzati-1.38512545

The Framework Institute. (2020, May 8). *Framing C19: We're in this together*. http://www.frameworksinstitute.org/assets/files/COVID19/framing-c19_-were-in-this-together_2.pdf

Friemel, T. N. (2016). The digital divide has grown old: Determinants of a digital divide among seniors. *New Media & Society, 18*(2), 313–331. https://doi.org/10.1177/1461444814538648

Human Rights Watch. (2020, April 7). *Rights risks to older people in COVID-19 response*. https://www.hrw.org/news/2020/04/07/rights-risks-older-people-covid-19-response

Kingkade, T. (2020, April 5). Police see rise in domestic violence calls amid Coronavirus lockdown. *The NBC News*. https://www.nbcnews.com/news/us-news/police-see-rise-domestic-violence-calls-amid-coronavirus-lockdown-n1176151

Lowrie, M. (2020, March 17). COVID-19: Thousands of doctors, nurses rally to government call to fight Coronavirus. *The National Post*. https://nationalpost.com/news/thousands-of-doctors-nurses-answer-call-to-help-with-covid-19-effort

Miller, R. W. (2020, March 21). 'If I get corona, I get corona': Coronavirus pandemic doesn't slow spring breakers' party. *The USA Today*. https://eu.usatoday.com/story/travel/destinations/2020/03/19/spring-break-beaches-florida-look-packed-despite-coronavirus-spread/2873248001/

Ministry of Health. (2020). *Covid-19, in Gazzetta Ufficiale Il Decreto Per Il Potenziamento del Ssn*. http://www.salute.gov.it/portale/nuovocoronavirus/dettaglioNotizieNuovoCoronavirus.jsp?lingua=italiano&id=4188

Morrow-Howell, N., Galucia, N., & Swinford, E. (2020). Recovering from the COVID-19 Pandemic: A focus on older adults. *Journal of Aging & Social Policy*. https://doi.org/10.1080/08959420.2020.1759758

NYC Health. (2020). Coronavirus Disease 2019 (COVID-19). *Daily Data Summary*. https://www1.nyc.gov/assets/doh/downloads/pdf/imm/covid-19-daily-data-summary-deaths-04152020-1.pdf

Officer, A., & de la Fuente-núñez, V. (2018). A global campaign to combat ageism. *Bulletin of the World Health Organisation, 96*, 299–300. https://doi.org/10.2471/BLT.17.202424

Popescu, D., & Marcoci, A. (2020, April 22). Coronavirus: Allocating ICU beds and ventilators based on age is discriminatory. *The Conversation*. https://theconversation.com/coronavirus-allocating-icu-beds-and-ventilators-based-on-age-is-discriminatory-136459

Principi, A., Jensen, P., & Lamura, G. (Eds.). (2014). *Active ageing: Voluntary work by older people in Europe*. Bristol University Press. https://doi.org/10.2307/j.ctt1ggjk6v

Silva, C. (2020, March 18). Fraternities reprimanded for hosting parties amid COVID-19 scare. *The Emory Wheel*. https://emorywheel.com/fraternities-reprimanded-amid-covid-19-scare-for-hosting-parties/

Silverstein, M. (2006). Ten - Intergenerational family transfers in social context. In R. H. Binstock, L. K. George, S. J. Cutler, J. Hendricks, & J. H. Schulz (Eds.), *Handbook of aging and the social sciences* (6th ed., pp. 165–180). Academic Press.

Simmons-Duffin, S. (2020, March 25). States get creative to find and deploy more health workers in COVID-19 fight. *The National Public Radio*. https://www.npr.org/sections/health-shots/2020/03/25/820706226/states-get-creative-to-find-and-deploy-more-health-workers-in-covid-19-fight?t=1587739313901

Takashima, M. (2020, March. 31). Officials plead with young people to stop partying during pandemic. *The Asahi Shimbun*. http://www.asahi.com/ajw/articles/13260124

United Nations Economic Commission for Europe. (2019a). *Active ageing index. Analytical report*. United Nations. https://www.unece.org/fileadmin/DAM/pau/age/Active_Ageing_Index/ECE-WG-33.pdf

United Nations Economic Commission for Europe. (2019b). *The challenging roles of informal carers* (UNECE Policy Brief on Ageing No. 22). United Nations. https://www.unece.org/fileadmin/DAM/pau/age/Policy_briefs/ECE_WG1_31.pdf

United Nations Human Rights Office of the Commissioner. (2020). *No exceptions with COVID-19: "Everyone has the right to life-saving interventions" – UN experts say*. Office of the United Nations High Commissioner for Human Rights. https://www.ohchr.org/EN/NewsEvents/Pages/DisplayNews.aspx?NewsID=25746&LangID=E

Walker, A. (2012). The new ageism. *The Political Quarterly, 23*(4), 812–819. https://doi.org/10.1111/j.1467-923X.2012.02360.x

Warner, J. (2020, March 3). Does the fed know something the rest of us do not with its panicked interest rate cut? *The Telegraph*. https://www.telegraph.co.uk/business/2020/03/03/does-fed-know-something-rest-us-do-not-panicked-interest-rate/.

World Health Organisation. (2020a). *Older people are at highest risk from COVID-19, but all must act to prevent community spread*. http://www.euro.who.int/en/health-topics/health-emergencies/coronavirus-covid-19/statements/statement-older-people-are-at-highest-risk-from-covid-19,-but-all-must-act-to-prevent-community-spread

World Health Organisation. (2020b). *WHO and partners call for urgent investment in nurses*. https://www.who.int/news-room/detail/07-04-2020-who-and-partners-call-for-urgent-investment-in-nurses

Yourish, K., Lai, R. K. K., Ivory, D., & Smith, M. (2020, May 11). One-third of all U.S. coronavirus deaths are nursing home residents or workers. *The New York Times*. https://www.nytimes.com/interactive/2020/05/09/us/coronavirus-cases-nursing-homes-us.html

Six Propositions against Ageism in the COVID-19 Pandemic

Hans-Joerg Ehni and Hans-Werner Wahl

ABSTRACT

The risk of developing severe illness from COVID-19 and of dying from it increases with age. This statistical association has led to numerous highly problematic policy suggestions and comments revealing underlying ageist attitudes and promoting age discrimination. Such attitudes are based on negative stereotypes on the health and functioning of older adults. As a result, the lives of older people are disvalued, including in possible triage situations and in the potential limitation of some measures against the spread of the pandemic to older adults. These outcomes are unjustified and unethical. We develop six propositions against the ageism underlying these suggestions to spur a more adequate response to the current pandemic in which the needs and dignity of older people are respected.

The risk of developing severe illness from COVID-19 and of dying from it increases with age (Grasselli et al., 2020; Richardson et al., 2020). This statistical association has led to numerous highly problematic policy suggestions and comments revealing underlying ageist attitudes and promoting age discrimination. Such attitudes are based on negative stereotypes of the health and functioning of older adults. As a result, the lives of older people are disvalued. Doubts are raised if the costs of isolation measures are worthwhile just to protect older people who are allegedly at the fringe of death anyway. Age limits are proposed to restrict access to intensive care. It is suggested that older people should isolate themselves instead of requiring widely implemented social distancing measures (see also Brooke & Jackson, 2020).

Due to constant repetition and consistency with ongoing negative age stereotyping (Ayalon et al., 2020; Ng et al., 2015), ageist suggestions have become prominent, taken-for-granted, and rarely questioned statements in the pandemic communication. The needs of older people remain largely unaddressed – for instance, how to reduce the burden of social isolation. Against this backdrop we offer six propositions on the basis of gerontological knowledge and an ethics of aging against the ageism which is present in the current reactions to the COVID-19 pandemic.

Proposition 1: older adults are highly heterogeneous – their health and functioning is better than negative stereotypes suggest

Older people aged 65 years and older remain the most heterogeneous group in society as reflected in thousands of studies documenting inter-individual variability in psychological performance, social needs, and personality characteristics, as well as key health and medical indicators such as somatic functioning, chronic conditions, self-perceived health, cognitive health, and impairment in activities of daily living functioning (Lindenberger & Reischies, 1999; Lowsky et al., 2014; Steinhagen-Thiessen & Borchelt, 1993). Even amongst the very old, over 80 years of age, the significant biological processes of change do not lead to a leveling of this heterogeneity, both overall and in specific areas such as gait function (Callisaya et al., 2010; Mitnitski et al., 2017; Nelson & Dannefer, 1992). In other words, chronological age is an "empty variable" and an extremely poor guide for accurately predicting behavior, needs, performance, loss of function, illness, and comorbidity (Birren & Schroots, 1996; Lowsky et al., 2014; Settersten & Mayer, 1997; Steinhagen-Thiessen & Borchelt, 1993). Therefore, chronological age alone is also in no way suitable for allocating medical and care resources, seen in the current pandemic most prominently by introducing age limits for intensive care in triage decisions, which has been suggested in Italy (Vergano et al., 2020) and in Switzerland (Scheidegger et al., 2020), as we will discuss in more detail in the next section.

Instead, we expect all actors to align their statements regarding older adults and COVID-19 with the recognition that older people are an extremely diverse group with great importance to our community; they are active in voluntary work, provide a lot of instrumental help as grandparents, and are also important consumers (see findings on "productive aging", summarized by Diehl & Wahl, 2020). Yes, they are also more at risk for severe illness from COVID-19, but by no means does this apply equally to everyone above a specific chronological age. Those with preexisting conditions and significant multimorbidity are particularly at risk. This subgroup is probably approximately 20% of the age group over 65 years of age (Sheehan et al., 2019). Although a highly significant group in the crisis (Béland & Marie, 2020), only a relatively small proportion of those 65 years and older live in institutions (e.g., 4% in Germany) where the effects of COVID-19 have been especially devastating (Comas-Herrera et al., 2020).

Proposition 2: age limits for intensive care and other forms of medical care are inappropriate and unethical

The exponential increase of COVID-19 with severe disease progression is currently leading to dramatic shortages in intensive care in many countries.

For such situations of scarcity and the tragic decisions to which they lead, there are often no binding guidelines and regulations currently in place. The physicians, who treat patients under severe psychological strain, are forced to decide who is to receive artificial ventilation and whose lives should be saved if there are no longer enough beds available in intensive care. Based on the traditional triage in war-zone situations, expert committees around the world are currently developing recommendations.

The Italian Society for Anesthesia, Analgesia, Resuscitation and Intensive Care Medicine (Vergano et al., 2020) recommends that age limits should be a direct criterion for access to intensive care treatment due to the current scarcity of resources. In addition, the Society recommends that resources should be used in such a way as to maximize the years of life gained, which also means giving priority to younger people. Such considerations presuppose that an alleged longer life span of a younger person can be weighed against the shorter life span of an older person. This supposition is flawed, in part, due to the diversity of older people, whose life expectancy may show significant variation even at more advanced ages. More importantly, however, dignity requires that the same value should be attributed to human lives without regard to age, gender, ethnicity, or impairments.

In Germany, the German Ethics Council has emphasized this latter point in its ad hoc statement (Deutscher Ethikrat, 2020); so too have seven German medical societies together with the Academy for Ethics in Medicine in recommendations for dealing with situations of scarcity (Deutsche Interdisziplinäre Vereinigung für Intensiv- und Notfallmedizin (DIVI) et al., 2020). These recommendations are essentially based on the prospects of individual patient success, which is based on their state of health. In this way, as many human lives as possible can be saved while respecting the rights of individuals. Age as a criterion for intensive medical treatment is explicitly rejected. However, caution is required to ensure that chronological age is not reintroduced through the back door as a placeholder for supposed chances of success. Here, too, the diversity of older people should be emphasized. Health and functioning of each patient should be considered carefully in decisions about medical care and its limitations. Simplistic uses of chronological age to deny care should be avoided and a societal debate on these issues is urgently needed to avoid implicit rationing on an arbitrary basis.

Proposition 3: mass deficit views of old age are dangerous to older citizens and societies at large – intergenerational solidarity must be strengthened

We believe that negative age stereotyping is currently taking place on a massive scale in light of COVID-19. Statements are common in which older people are uniformly categorized as "at risk" and that the reduction of this risk is also the main reason for the current measures to limit the spread of the pandemic. This view is simply inaccurate since not all older people may be at elevated risk, and not all those who are at risk are simply above a certain age. Male gender and obesity seems as well to facilitate severe cases of COVID-19. Other risk factors such as pollution, mutations of the virus, and genetic dispositions are discussed and remain unclear. Therefore, highlighting advanced age may not only raise unjustified worries among older adults, but may also lead to feelings of false safety among other age groups.

Moreover, public debates in which the lives of older people are disvalued and considered expendable could have hugely detrimental effects on the physical and mental health of older adults (see also B. R. Levy et al., 2020). Stereotype research on aging has clearly shown that negative age stereotypes can be quickly triggered in older people (Diehl et al., 2020; Wurm et al., 2017) and that they are three times more powerful in their unpleasant effects than positive stereotypes (e.g., all older people are wise) in their positive effects (Meisner, 2012). Many findings suggest that negative age stereotypes can be expressed in somatic illnesses and functional health, and not only on the psychological level (Westerhof et al., 2014; Wurm et al., 2017). We also know that negative age self-stereotyping is indicated in inflammatory processes, for example, by C-reactive protein, and leads to reinforced and raised cortisol secretions (B. R. Levy et al., 2000, 2016; Stephan et al., 2015). These are all physiological pathways that are closely related to cardio-vascular disease and severe loss of cognitive performance, among other conditions.

It may be that the consequences of negative age attributions could even increase the susceptibility to COVID-19, say, through its effects on enhanced inflammatory responses, though, of course, nobody knows. At the very least we must investigate. We hope for a hypothesis that is partially recognized and supported by existing findings and arguments to render it plausible – and that this plausibility, in turn, mitigates the use of such ageist arguments going forward.

In light of negative age stereotyping, older people could also feel pressured to refuse medical care in connection with a potential scarcity of medical resources. Also, the internalized disvalue of their own lives could lead to corresponding advance directives that prematurely close off avenues to potentially beneficial interventions. It is important that nobody receives unwanted burdensome end-of-life care, and this must be addressed as well in the current situation; yet it is still more important that older people are not pressured into writing statements in which they "voluntarily" renounce appropriate treatment.

Negative stereotypes and expressions of disvalue may have huge and unforeseeable negative effects on older people and the health system at large (B. R. Levy et al., 2020). Negative stereotypes of old age undermine intergenerational solidarity as part of the general camaraderie, cooperation, and social cohesion now needed as a common reaction to prevent unnecessary harm in the current pandemic. Thus, it is crucial to raise public awareness among experts, policy makers, and the media to avoid such stereotypes in the communication about the disease and the reactions to it.

Proposition 4: resisting the assumption of a paternalistic attitude toward older adults in the crisis is important

We must avoid treating older people with a paternalistic attitude and telling them what they can and cannot do (Ayalon et al., 2020; Fingerman & Trevino, 2020; Morrow-Howell et al., 2020). They are the group in our community with the greatest amount of life experience. For the most part, they act reasonably and in accordance with the needs of the situation without being told by others to do so. So, extending "social distancing" only above chronological age limits is unnecessary as well as discriminatory. Current older adults are historically the generation highest in physical capacity, cognitive functioning, and educational level ever (Carstensen, 2011; Diehl & Wahl, 2020). This capability is the best prerequisite for cooperative communication; there is no need to target them separately from other age groups.

By contrast, we could listen and learn from our older adults, who could act as advisors during this crisis. As mentioned before, they have by far the most life experience and they know about privations from previous situations and experiences. But nobody seems to want to give them a voice. Why not?

Proposition 5: the COVID-19 crisis demands fostering the use of modern information and communication technologies among older adults

At the present moment, information and communication media holds a crucial place in our society. Please do not say that they, older adults, are not capable. For example, around 77% of over 65-year-olds in Germany today have a conventional personal computer and 52% have a notebook (Doh, 2019). Tablet computers are (also) becoming increasingly popular among older people, and already account for 28%. Smartphones are being used by older people at around 46%, meaning that almost half of the people over the age of 65 can potentially use all the functions that smartphones offer today. The number of internet users over the age of 65 now amounts to 75%. In other countries (e.g., Denmark), emerging trends are even more promising. Thus, older people are far from starting from scratch where the use of information and communication technologies are concerned.

The digitalization of learning and schooling is currently promoted and accelerated during the COVID-19 crisis through the provision of the necessary technological equipment and infrastructure. In the same way, we propose to provide free tablet computers and support to the thousands of older people in need, for instance in nursing homes, which we know are suffering from social withdrawal symptoms (Berg-Weger & Morley, 2020; Marston et al., 2020). In addition, we would suggest the organization of nationwide conversations and exchange networks to maintain social participation of older adults (see also Czaja, 2017; Czaja et al., 2018). Physical and mental fitness training can also be offered efficiently in this way. Even if the evidence on mental fitness training ("Brain Games") is not fully convincing (Simons et al., 2016): the same principle applies as with physical fitness training: use it or lose it. We know that forms of engagement and new stimuli are generally beneficial to older people; because of the current restrictions, older people have a higher risk of worsening relatively quickly through "disuse" in basic functional-motor-cognitive skills. This deterioration is completely unnecessary if we act now to prevent long-term negative effects.

Proposition 6: the COVID-19 crisis not only demands the best of virology but also the best of gerontology for policy guidance and understanding the consequences of the crisis at large

Virology has been placed center-stage in Germany and other countries. Virologists have provided valuable expertise, professional recommendations, and orientation in the current situation. Other scientific disciplines are also in demand. Gerontology is particularly important when it comes to giving equal and appropriate consideration to the health and well-being of all citizens in the current crisis. Gerontologists have thus been called upon to share their knowledge and expertise in contributing to the development of policies addressing the specific needs of older people. We estimate, for example, that approximately 15–25% of older people aged 80 years and older cannot easily cope with a strategy of social isolation and contact exclusion (DeJong Gierveld & van Tilburg, 2010) – and by no means only in nursing homes! Here, policy makers need the immediate proactive advice and suggestions for support programs that gerontologists can provide.

The crisis is also likely to change the way many older people experience their own aging. Many opportunities for social interaction and participation are currently not existing. New ways to create such opportunities have to be found and supported. Here, gerontology is now called upon to better understand what is happening psychologically to older people by utilizing targeted research in the field. The participation of older adults in myriad gerontological studies proves that they have no problem when research is conducted with them, compared to when research is conducted on them, and they can always say no, as is the ethical standard. Then, of course, translation is necessary. As human beings, older adults have the right to have the best research generated not only by virologists, but also by gerontologists to support their quality of life and prevent permanent damage.

Conclusion

This crisis provides an opportunity to learn and improve upon past practice. This opportunity includes better understanding the living situations of older people and how to counteract the problems affecting them. Older adults have a lot of strengths and many are functionally well in physical and mental terms. We doubt our readers have frequently encountered such characterizations of older individuals in the recent debate linked to COVID-19, although the evidence available in contemporary gerontology clearly supports such a statement (e.g., Diehl & Wahl, 2020). Now is the moment to create a broader awareness both about negative stereotypes against older people and their harmful impact, and the strengths of older adults, their valuable contributions to society, and their potential.

We are currently experiencing a situation in which numerous moral dilemmas and conflicts are arising. It is difficult to find the best course of action. It is tempting to fall into a crude utilitarianism that values lives differently, where we pit one group against another and give lower priority to those who have a lower value attributed to them. Too often, the lives of older people are weighed less than others: they should simply be isolated because they are the most vulnerable; they have lived their lives and have had their chance at living a fulfilling life; they are, in any case, amongst those who are going to die soon. These and similar arguments can be found in everyday discussions as well as in the opinions of experts and ethicists. At the extreme, such views might contribute to breaks in civilization, as in Spain, where the residents of a nursing home were left to their own devices and ultimately died (Rada, 2020). These views contradict the basic values of our society as expressed in the idea of human rights. Importantly, this refers to equal value and respect of each human being and the right to nondiscrimination on the basis of traits such as age, gender, race, or disability (Gosepath, 2011; Nickel, 2019). Such arguments undermine attitudes such as being happy about the rescue of a 95-year-old patient or sacrificing oneself for the care of residents suffering from dementia in nursing homes. Especially in a crisis, it is important to preserve the basic values of our society and to protect the rights of individuals, especially the weakest. We must all be reminded of our basic human vulnerability, which requires mutual protection, care and solidarity in the midst of this pandemic.

Key Points

- Some measures suggested as reactions to the COVID-19 pandemic demonstrate underlying ageist attitudes.
- We develop six propositions against this ageism to illustrate what more adequate responses to the pandemic would look like.
- We outline what lessons can be learned to improve the situation of older adults after the pandemic

Disclosure statement

There are no conflicts of interest to report.

References

Ayalon, L., Chasteen, A., Diehl, M., Levy, B., Neupert, S. D., Rothermund, K., Tesch-Römer, C., & Wahl, H.-W. (2020). Aging in times of the COVID-19 pandemic: Avoiding ageism and fostering intergenerational solidarity. *Journal of Gerontology: Psychological Sciences*. Editorial (Online only). https://doi.org/10.1093/geronb/gbaa051

Béland, D., & Marie, P. (2020). COVID-19 and long-term care policy for older people in Canada. *Journal of Aging & Social Policy*. https://doi.org/10.1080/08959420.2020.1764319

Berg-Weger, M., & Morley, J. E. (2020). Loneliness and social isolation in older adults during the COVID-19 pandemic: Implications for gerontological social work. *The Journal of Nutrition, Health & Aging*, 24(5), 456–458. Published online. https://doi.org/10.1007/s12603-020-1366-8

Birren, J. E., & Schroots, J. J. F. (1996). History, concepts, and theory in the psychology of aging. In J. E. Birren & K. W. Schaie (Eds.), *Handbook of the psychology of aging* (4th ed., pp. 3–23). Academic Press.

Brooke, J., & Jackson, D. (2020). Older people and COVID-19: Isolation, risk and ageism. *Journal of Clinical Nursing*. https://doi.org/10.1111/jocn.15274

Callisaya, M. L., Blizzard, L., Schmidt, M. D., McGinley, J. L., & Srikanth, V. K. (2010). Ageing and gait variability–a population-based study of older people. *Age & Ageing*, 39(2), 191–197. https://doi.org/10.1093/ageing/afp250

Carstensen, L. L. (2011). *A long and bright future. Happiness, health, and financial security in an age of increased longevity*. Broadway Books.

Comas-Herrera, A., Zalakain, J., Litwin, C., Hsu, A. T., Lane, N., & Fernandez, J.-L. (2020, May 6). *Mortality associated with Covid-19 outbreaks in care homes: Early international evidence*. Article in LTCcovid.org, International Long-Term Care Policy Network, CPEC-LSE, 3 May 2020. https://ltccovid.org/wp-content/uploads/2020/05/Mortality-associated-with-COVID-3-May-final-5.pdf.

Czaja, S. J. (2017). The role of technology in supporting social engagement among older adults. *Public Policy & Aging Report*, 27(4), 145–148. https://doi.org/10.1093/ppar/prx034

Czaja, S. J., Boot, W. R., Charness, N., Rogers, W. A., & Sharit, J. (2018). Improving social support for older adults through technology: Findings from the PRISM randomized controlled trial. *The Gerontologist*, 58(3), 467–477. https://doi.org/10.1093/geront/gnw249

DeJong Gierveld, J., & van Tilburg, T. (2010). The De Jong Gierveld short scales for emotional and social loneliness: Tested on data from 7 countries in the UN generations and gender surveys. *European Journal of Ageing, 7*(2), 121–130. https://doi.org/10.1007/s10433-010-0144-6

Deutsche Interdisziplinäre Vereinigung für Intensiv- und Notfallmedizin (DIVI), Deutsche Gesellschaft für Interdisziplinäre Notfall- und Akutmedizin (DGINA), Deutsche Gesellschaft für Anästhesiologie und Intensivmedizin (DGAI), Deutsche Gesellschaft für Internistische Intensivmedizin und Notfallmedizin (DGIIN), Deutsche Gesellschaft für Pneumologie und Beatmungsmedizin (DGP), der Deutschen Gesellschaft für Palliativmedizin (DGP), & und der Akademie für Ethik in der Medizin (AEM). (2020). *Entscheidungen über die Zuteilung von Ressourcen in der Notfall und der Intensivmedizin im Kontext der COVID-19-Pandemie Klinisch-ethische Empfehlungen.* https://www.aem-online.de/fileadmin/user_upload/COVID-19_Ethik_Empfehlung-v2.pdf

Deutscher Ethikrat. (2020). *Solidarität und Verantwortung in der Corona-Krise.* Ad hoc Empfehlung. https://www.aem-online.de/fileadmin/user_upload/DER_ad-hoc-empfehlung-corona-krise.pdf

Diehl, M., Brothers, A. F., & Wahl, H.-W. (2020). Self-perceptions and awareness of aging: Past, present, and future. In K. W. Schaie & S. L. Willis (Eds.), *Handbook of the psychology of aging* (8th ed.). Elsevier (will be published in the second half of 2020).

Diehl, M. K., & Wahl, H.-W. (2020). *The psychology of later life: A contextual perspective.* American Psychological Association Books.

Doh, M. (2019). *Auswertung von empirischen Studien zur Nutzung von Internet, digitalen Medien und Informations- und Kommunikations-Technologien bei älteren Menschen* [Review of empirical studies on the use of information and communication technology in older adults]. Expert statement for the eighth report on old age of the German Government. German Centre of Gerontology.

Fingerman & Trevino. (2020, April 7). Don't lump seniors together on coronavirus. Older people aren't all the same. *USA Today.* https://eu.usatoday.com/story/opinion/2020/04/07/coronavirus-seniors-lead-diverse-lives-death-rate-varies-column/2954897001/

Gosepath, S. (2011). *Equality.* Stanford Encyclopedia of Philosophy. https://plato.stanford.edu/archives/spr2011/entries/equality/

Grasselli, G., Zangrillo, A., Zanella, A., Antonelli, M., Cabrini, L., Castelli, A., Coluccello, A., Foti, G., Fumagalli, R., Iotti, G., Latronico, N., Lorini, L., Merler, S., Natalini, G., Piatti, A., Ranieri, M. V., Scandroglio, A. M., Storti, E., Cecconi, M., Pesenti, A., & Cereda, D. (2020). Baseline characteristics and outcomes of 1591 patients infected with SARS-CoV-2 admitted to ICUs of the Lombardy Region, Italy. *JAMA, 323*(16), 1574. http://dx.doi.10.1001/jama.2020.5394

Levy, B. R., Hausdorff, J. M., Hencke, R., & Wei, J. Y. (2000). Reducing cardiovascular stress with positive self-stereotypes on aging. *Journals of Gerontology: Psychological Sciences, 55B* (4), P205–P213. http://dx.doi.10.1093/geronb/55.4.P205

Levy, B. R., Moffat, S., Resnick, S. M., Slade, M. D., & Ferrucci, L. (2016). Buffer against cumulative stress: Positive age self-stereotypes predict lower cortisol across 30 years. *GeroPsych: The Journal of Gerontopsychology and Geriatric Psychiatry, 29*(3), 141–146. http://dx.doi.10.1024/1662-9647/a000149

Levy, B. R., Slade, M. D., Chang, E., Kannoth, S., & Wang, S. (2020). Ageism amplifies cost and prevalence of health conditions. *The Gerontologist, 60*(1), 174–181. http://dx.doi.10.1093/geront/gny131

Lindenberger, U., & Reischies, F. (1999). Limits and potential of intellectual functioning in old age. In P. B. Baltes & K. U. Mayer (Eds.), *The Berlin aging study: Aging from 70 to 100* (pp. 329–359). Cambridge University Press.

Lowsky, D. J., Olshansky, S. J., Bhattacharya, J., & Goldman, D. P. (2014). Heterogeneity in healthy aging. *Journal of Gerontology: Biological and Medical Sciences, 69*(1), 640–649. http://dx.doi.10.1093/gerona/glt162

Marston, H. R., Musselwhite, C., & Robin Hadley, R. (2020, May 6). *COVID-19 vs social isolation: The impact technology can have on communities, social connections and citizens.* https://ageingissues.wordpress.com/2020/03/18/covid-19-vs-social-isolation-the-impact-technology-can-have-on-communities-social-connections-and-citizens/?fbclid= IwAR1sUsffKNd_G5u6d_oc0Z56u4Es7HyoCJYKr0qSnqFxX68pD3PY5JaSl7g:.

Meisner, B. A. (2012). A meta-analysis of positive and negative age stereotype priming effects on behavior among older adults. *The Journals of Gerontology, Series B: Psychological Sciences and Social Sciences, 67*(1), 13–17. http://dx.doi.10.1093/geronb/gbr062

Mitnitski, A., Howlett, S. E., & Rockwood, K. (2017). Heterogeneity of human aging and its assessment. *The Journals of Gerontology: Series A, 72*(7), 877–884. http://dx.doi.10.1093/gerona/glw089

Morrow-Howell, N., Galucia, N., & Swinford, E. (2020). Recovering from the COVID-19 pandemic: A focus on older adults. *Journal of Aging & Social Policy*, 1–9. Online published. http://dx.doi.10.1080/08959420.2020.1759758

Nelson, E. A., & Dannefer, D. (1992). Aged heterogeneity: Fact or fiction? The fate of diversity in gerontological research. *The Gerontologist, 32*(1), 17–23. http://dx.doi.10.1093/geront/32.1.17

Ng, R., Allore, H. G., Trentalange, M., Monin, J. K., & Levy, B. R. (2015). Increasing negativity of age stereotypes across 200 years: Evidence from a database of 400 million words. *Plos One, 10*(2), e0117086. Published online. http://dx.doi.10.1371/journal.pone.0117086

Nickel, J. (2019). Human rights. *The Stanford Encyclopedia of Philosophy*. https://plato.stanford.edu/archives/sum2019/entries/rights-human/

Rada, A. G. (2020). Covid-19: The precarious position of Spain's nursing homes. *British Medical Journal, 369*, m1554. http://dx.doi.10.1136/bmj.m1554

Richardson, S., Hirsch, J. S., Narasimhan, M., Crawford, J. M., McGinn, T., Davidson, K. W., Barnaby, D. P., Becker, L. B., Chelico, J. D., Cohen, S. L., Cookingham, J., Coppa, K., Diefenbach, M. A., Dominello, A. J., Duer-Hefele, J., Falzon, L., Gitlin, J., Hajizadeh, N., Harvin, T. G., Kim, E. J., ... Zanos, T. P. (2020). Presenting characteristics, comorbidities, and outcomes among 5700 patients hospitalized with COVID-19 in the New York City Area. *JAMA*. http://dx.doi.10.1001/jama.2020.6775

Scheidegger, D., Fumeaux, T., Hurst, S., & Salathé, M. (2020). *Covid-19-Pandemie: Triage von intensivmedizinischen Behandlungen bei Ressourcenknappheit.* Retrieved from Bern: https://www.samw.ch/de/Ethik/Themen-A-bis-Z/Intensivmedizin.html

Settersten, R. A., & Mayer, K.-U. (1997). The measurement of age, age structuring, and the life course. *Annual Review of Sociology, 23*(1), 233–261. http://dx.doi.10.2307/2952551

Sheehan, C., Domingue, B. W., & Crimmins, E. (2019). Cohort trends in the gender distribution of household tasks in the United States and the implications for understanding disability. *Journal of Aging and Health, 31*(10), 1748–1769. Online-Published. http://dx.doi.10.1177/0898264318793469

Simons, D. J., Boot, W. R., Charness, N., Gathercole, S. E., Chabris, C. F., Hambrick, D. Z., & Stine-Morrow, E. A. L. (2016). Do "brain-training" programs work? *Psychological Science in the Public Interest, 17*(3), 103–186. http://dx.doi.10.1177/1529100616661983

Steinhagen-Thiessen, E., & Borchelt, M. (1993). Health differences in advanced old age. *Ageing & Society, 27*(4), 619–655. http://dx.doi.10.1093/ppar/prx034

Stephan, Y., Sutin, A. R., & Terracciano, A. (2015). Younger subjective age is associated with lower C-reactive protein among older adults. *Brain, Behavior, and Immunity, 43*, 33–36. http://dx.doi.10.1016/j.bbi.2014.07.019

Vergano, M., Bertolini, G., Giannini, A., Gristina, G., Livigni, S., Mistraletti, G., & Petrini, F. (2020). Clinical ethics recommendations for the allocation of intensive care treatments in exceptional, resource-limited circumstances: the Italian perspective during the COVID-19 epidemic. *Critical Care, 24*(1). http://dx.doi.10.1186/s13054-020-02891-w.

Westerhof, G. J., Miche, M., Brothers, A. F., Barrett, A. E., Diehl, M., Montepare, J. M., Wahl, H.-W., & Wurm, S. (2014). The influence of subjective aging on health and longevity: A meta-analysis of longitudinal data. *Psychology and Aging, 29*(4), 793–802. http://dx.doi.10.1037/a0038016

Wurm, S., Diehl, M., Kornadt, A. E., Westerhof, G. J., & Wahl, H.-W. (2017). How do views on aging affect health outcomes in adulthood and late life? Explanations for an established connection. *Developmental Review, 46*, 27–43. http://dx.doi.10.1016/j.dr.2017.08.002

Recovery

Recovering from the COVID-19 Pandemic: A Focus on Older Adults

Nancy Morrow-Howell, Natalie Galuci, and Emma Swinford

ABSTRACT

As we look toward recovery from the COVID-19 pandemic, we overview challenges to be minimized, including economic setbacks, health and well-being effects, and highlighted ageism, racism, and classism. We articulate opportunities to be seized, including increased comfort with technology and online platforms; stronger family and intergenerational connections, renewed energy to combat social isolation; more respect for self-care and time management; increased awareness about the importance of advance directives; and, potentially, increased interest across disciplines to work on issues of aging society. Ongoing efforts to improve policies and programs for longer, healthier lives might now be more productive, as we communicate to consumers, public officials, and everyday citizens who may be more aware of what isn't working, what is at stake, and what might be improved.

Although it is not clear what our lives will look like over the next few months, we can anticipate what challenges and opportunities are emerging as a result of this pandemic. If we articulate these challenges and opportunities, we might move more quickly to minimize the negative outcomes of the spread of COVID-19 and maximize positive changes that might be possible. In that spirit, we identify and discuss challenges and opportunities arising from the COVID-19 pandemic with hopes that all of us – researchers, educators, practitioners, advocates, providers, government bureaucrats, and elected officials – will redouble our engagement in research, advocacy, policy, and program development to improve our aging society in ways that benefit people across the life course.

This article has been republished with minor changes. These changes do not impact the academic content of the article.

Challenges to be mitigated

A series of challenges have arisen in the wake of the COVID-19 pandemic, including economic setbacks and adverse health and well-being effects. At the same time, the COVID-19 pandemic has placed a spotlight on the deleterious effects of deep-seated ageism, sexism, and racism on older Americans.

Economic setbacks

Older adults will have a harder time reentering the workforce
People of all ages are currently affected by the record-breaking unemployment rates brought on by COVID-19-related business closures. Unemployment rates are projected to reach a high of 32.1% by the end of the second quarter, according to the St. Louis Federal Reserve Bank, with about 50 million Americans being unemployed. This is higher than the unemployment rate during the Great Depression (Faria-e-Castro, 2020). When the unemployment situation stabilizes, we expect to see what we have seen in the past: that although younger workers might fare worse with initial job loss, older workers will fare worse in reentering the workforce. In fact, after the recession in 2008, adults age 62 years and older were the least likely age group to become reemployed once they lost their jobs; and they were also more likely to retire earlier than planned and quit their job search within 9 months of becoming unemployed (Johnson & Butrica, 2012). Age discrimination plays a role here because in the face of large numbers of job applicants, employers can apply more arbitrary selection criteria when making hiring decisions and may be more influenced by negative age stereotypes (Neumark & Button, 2014).

Older adults have lost retirement savings
The effects of income loss and financial market declines on retirement savings are yet unknown, but it is clear at this moment that retirement savings accounts have taken a hit (Singletary, 2020). Older workers may be reconsidering when they will retire, and some people in retirement may feel the need to reenter the workforce. Before the pandemic, the trends toward later retirement, transitional work, and encore careers were underway, and people were working longer – both because they wanted to and because they needed to. But now, more of us will "need to" to make up for lost income and savings. Efforts to modify workplace environments, policies, and practices to support longer working lives will be more important than ever.

Just as older workers may need to work longer, organizations may need to cut budgets to survive and regain financial footing in the recovery period. Older workers have been and will continue to be at risk for age discrimination in the workplace. Older workers experience bias in training and advancement opportunities; and given higher salaries and health insurance costs, they often experience pressure to retire early (Olson, 2017). Thus, workplace solutions must address the age discrimination that puts older workers at higher risk of depression, health declines, and job dissatisfaction (Marchiondo et al., 2019).

Health and wellbeing effects

Older adults have experienced disruption in usual services

During this crisis, shelter-in-place orders and the closing of organizations have prevented many people from having their preexisting physical, emotional, and social needs met through aging network services and the health-care system. Many of the agencies that "serve vulnerable seniors are scrambling to adjust and minimize potential damage" (Graham, 2020). For example, Area Agencies on Aging and home-delivered meals programs are working to fill the gaps created when senior centers and congregate meal programs shuttered. At the same time, volunteer drivers, many of whom are older adults, cannot fulfill their assignments because they are self-isolating. These changes to nutrition programs can cause older adults with a limited budget to rely on processed foods, making it difficult to achieve adequate nutrition. Alterations in diet can lead to complications with underlying health conditions (Goger, 2020). As another example, home care agencies are struggling to retain clients and workers because both groups are opting out of routine care arrangements in fear of contracting the virus. This lack of attention to personal care, medication management, and nutrition will lead to deterioration of health and the need for more supportive services in the long term (Kwiatkowski & Nadolny, 2020).

At the same time, support services are jeopardized, the health-care system has narrowed its focus to managing COVID-19 cases, meaning other health-care appointments and procedures are being delayed. Regular checkups, non-urgent provider visits, and elective procedures are being canceled, putting older patients at higher risk of worsening health deterioration (Graham, 2020). Compounding this situation are concerns that when medical care is more readily available, there will be backlogs of needed surgeries, screenings, checkups, and appointments, further straining the system and delaying routine care.

Older adults may have lasting emotional effects from increased isolation and anxiety

Social isolation and loneliness have been linked to negative physical and mental health outcomes, such as increased depression and anxiety symptoms (National Academies of Sciences, Engineering and Medicine, 2020) and increased risk of hypertension, cardiovascular disease, obesity, cognitive decline, and death (National Institute on Aging, 2019). Even before this period of sustained social distancing, social isolation was disproportionately affecting older adults because of diminished social networks, living arrangements, and transportation limitations (National Academies of Sciences, Engineering and Medicine, 2020). During this pandemic, older adults have received stricter directives on social distancing, as they were one of the first groups encouraged to stay home. Older adults who have experienced a prolonged period of isolation may encounter health effects that long outlast their time in quarantine. The impact of this period of isolation on future physical and emotional well-being of older adults is yet to be determined.

Older adults who have contracted the coronavirus may have increased health vulnerabilities

Currently, data indicate that most people who contract COVID-19 will see a full recovery, but the long-term effects of the illness are not fully understood, particularly for patients who need more intensive care (Schumaker, 2020). It is probable that these ongoing complications will disproportionately affect older people who have been sicker and more likely to die from virus-related complications. People who require the use of ventilators are more likely to experience damage to the lungs or a longer recovery period – and not all will return to full functionality. Additionally, researchers are concerned that COVID-19 may be associated with cardiac injury, as preliminary data indicate that COVID-19 may cause heart damage in patients with and without previous heart problems (Shi, 2020).

Ageism, racism, and classism

Older adults may experience stronger internal and external ageism

The crisis has revealed engrained ageism and age-stereotyping in this society. Attitudes and actions in response to this pandemic have been attributed to reduced *concern about* and *value attributed to* older people: countries were slow to respond because ONLY old people were at risk; treatment and mitigation protocols have been more adequately developed for children and youth in certain hospitals; and saving the economy may be more important than saving these older lives. We have heard an old phrase "thinning the herd" and the new phrase "#boomerremover." Fears of the need to ration resources in hospitals led the Office for Civil Rights to issue a statement to prevent lifesaving medical care from being administered on the basis of age (Fink, 2020).

There has been an outcry by aging advocates about this ageism and concerns that we will experience setbacks in efforts to confront the image of old age as a state of frailty, vulnerability, and less value. Dr. Louise Aronson also points out internalized ageism may be strengthened because some older adults themselves have resisted identifying as at-risk because it means they are acknowledging the reality of their age (Aronson, 2020). We will have to regain any hard-won advances in reducing the external and internal ageism exacerbated in this pandemic.

Older adults of color and those with lower socioeconomic status are at increased risk for physical and economic challenges caused by COVID-19

As we enumerate these challenges, we are aware of not only the ageism, but also the racism and classism that is highlighted by this pandemic. Older African-Americans, with higher rates of morbidity and less access to health care going into this crisis, are dying at higher rates when they contract the illness (Evelyn, 2020). Less well-educated older workers are less likely to be able to work from home and their paycheck may depend on them being in service jobs with increased exposure to the virus (Goldbaum, 2020). Low-income older adults have less access to computers and online technologies that have eased the burden of isolation for so many people (Choi, 2013). Intergenerational living arrangements undertaken for economic survival might present solutions for childcare during this period of homeschooling, yet grandparents do not have options to social distance and self-care in these circumstances.

Opportunities to be seized

Despite challenges stemming from the COVID-19 pandemic, opportunities for improving the lives of older adults may arise from this crisis. These opportunities pertain to increased connectivity through technology, family, and intergenerational relationships and to improved quality of life by reducing social isolation, increasing self-care and management, and improving awareness of advanced directives and other legal documents. Finally, there may be opportunities to address the shortage of professionals specializing in the field of aging.

Increased connectivity

Older adults have improved their technology skills and gained experience using online platforms

Before this pandemic, there was a steady growth in the number of tech-savvy older people. It was documented that 75% of people over 65 years of age go online every day; between 2013–2017, smartphone ownership increased by 24% in adults over 65 (Nash, 2019). Motivation and opportunities to learn were growing and then social distancing and sheltering in place created a "sink or swim" moment for many reluctant or unskilled users. Research has shown that older adults are eager to learn technology skills and are particularly motivated to use these skills when they see a need for it (Boulton-Lewis, 2006). We saw the need: video-conferencing to carry on our work, ordering groceries, taking exercise classes online, and talking to family members and health-care providers. This has been an opportunity for older adults to get more comfortable using technology and for community and health-care providers to offer remote programming. We are in a better position for programs and people alike to connect online even after social distancing measures are lifted (Finn, 2020).

Familial and intergenerational connections have grown stronger

Many families are finding that the pandemic has encouraged them to more regularly communicate. In the absence of regular family dinners and celebrations, we are missing these interactions and appreciating their importance. There are numerous stories of family and neighbors connecting. For example, *The New York Times* recently published a story about a grandmother speaking with her grandson more and two grandparents recording their voices reading bedtime stories to their young grandchildren (Conger, 2020). Although there is a concern that younger adults may harbor resentment to older adults whose vulnerability led to social distancing, sheltering in place, and economic decline, it is common to see younger people creating opportunities to help older adults in need of ongoing social contact or grocery shopping. Numerous intergenerational programs have emerged, like *Students to Seniors*, a program where students and older adults engage in virtual conversations, or *Zoomers to Boomers*, an intergenerational grocery delivery service.

Improved quality of life

There may be renewed energy to combat social isolation

We entered this pandemic with respect to the negative effects of social isolation and with the emergence of programs to increase social connections (National Academies of Sciences, 2020). The coronavirus pandemic has increased momentum in this arena. Numerous news and resource sites focus on the risks and consequences of social disconnection and present strategies for combatting isolation. The coronavirus has shed light on this longstanding concern with a new sense of urgency, and there seems to be a sincere investment in decreasing isolation and loneliness moving forward.

Older adults are gaining more respect for self-care and time management

The outbreak may be changing how we think and act toward our own physical and mental health. Multiple sources are calling attention to the importance of schedules, sleep, diet, exercise, and social connection, and self-care skills are surfacing as truly important on a daily basis. Further, we are learning firsthand about what gives us meaning and purposeful engagement. Separated from jobs, professional connections, volunteer and grandparent roles, and routine social gathering, we are learning how to use time; according to Joe Coughlin, this is a "fire drill," a trial run for how we might spend our time in retirement (Coughlin, 2020).

There is increased awareness about the importance of advance directives and other legal documents

Despite pleas from legal and health-care professionals, we entered this pandemic with only about half of Americans having had end of life conversations with loved ones, and only 27% with formal documentation (Hamel, 2017; Newcomb, 2020). In March, the requests for a common advance planning tool called "Five Wishes" saw a tenfold increase (Aleccia, 2020). In addition, there are a number of general and COVID-19 specific end-of-life planning resources that were developed and can be accessed for free through sites like Respecting Choices and The Conversation Project. Many people now have a better understanding of the importance of clearly communicating preferences and decisions and are taking steps to start this process. We can find ways to sustain this movement.

Expanded workforce specializing in aging

There may be an upswing in interest among professionals across disciplines to work with older adults and issues of public health

COVID-19 has highlighted both the resiliency of the older adult population and the challenge to ensure that this large and diverse population can access the resources, information, and services they need. We may have the opportunity to address the long-standing problem that not enough people are coming into professions that serve older adults and address issues of an aging society (Foley, 2018). Because of the range of career options and capacity to make an impact, students and professionals across multiple disciplines (physicians, nurses, psychologists, social workers, health administrators, public health professionals, nonprofit managers, etc.) may express more interest in working on issues of an aging society.

Conclusion

The challenges we are facing can be expected, and in fact, none of them are new. Our state and regional agencies on aging, private and nonprofit agencies, advocacy organizations, and universities have been grappling with these issues in one form or another for years. But now, it seems our efforts to improve policies and programs for longer, healthier lives might be more productive, as we communicate to consumers, public officials, and everyday citizens who may be more aware of what isn't working, what is at stake, and what might be improved. Further, we can hope that the spotlight thrown on the inequalities experienced by disadvantaged people during this crisis will bring a stronger commitment to working toward social justice and health equity.

Key points

- We must minimize negative outcomes of COVID-19 and maximize positive changes that might be possible.
- Older adults have lost retirement savings and reentering the job market will be difficult.
- Physical and mental health may be compromised even after the pandemic is over.
- This crisis has spotlighted engrained ageism, racism, and classism.
- Positive changes can come from increased levels of technology use, self-care, and time management.

Disclosure statement

No potential conflict of interest was reported by the authors.

References

Aleccia, J. (2020, March 31). *Sheltered at home, families broach end-of-life planning*. Kaiser Health News. Retrieved from: https://khn.org/news/coronavirus-medical-directives-end-of-life-planning/

Aronson, L. (2020) Ageism is making the pandemic worse. *The Atlantic*, March 28, 2020.

Boulton-Lewis, G. (2006). Learning and active aging. *Educational Gerontology*, *32*(4), 271–282. https://doi.org/10.1080/03601270500494030

Choi, N. (2013). The digital divide among low-income homebound older adults: Internet use patterns, ehealth literacy, and attitudes towards computer/internet use. *Journal of Medical Internet Research*, *15*(5), e93. https://doi.org/10.2196/jmir.2645

Conger, E. (2020, March 27). *As life moves online, an older generation faces a digital divide*. The New York Times. Retrieved from: https://www.nytimes.com/2020/03/27/technology/virus-older-generation-digital-divide.html?action=click&module=RelatedLinks&pgtype=Article

Coughlin, J. (2020, March 29). *Here's why COVID-19 is your retirement fire drill*. Forbes. Retrieved from: https://www.forbes.com/sites/josephcoughlin/2020/03/29/heres-why-covid-19-is-your-retirement-fire-drill/#4b105afb52aa

Evelyn, K. (2020, April 8). *'It's a racial justice issue': Black Americans are dying in greater numbers from COVID-19*. The Guardian. Retrieved from: https://www.theguardian.com/world/2020/apr/08/its-a-racial-justice-issue-black-americans-are-dying-in-greater-numbers-from-covid-19

Faria-e-Castro, M. (2020, March 24). *Back-of-the-envelope estimates of next quarter's unemployment rate [Blog Post]*. Federal Reserve Bank of St. Louis. Retrieved from: https://www.stlouisfed.org/on-the-economy/2020/march/back-envelope-estimates-next-quarters-unemployment-rate.

Fink, S. (2020, March 28). *U.S. civil rights office rejects rationing medical care based on disability, age*. The New York Times. Retrieved from: https://www.nytimes.com/2020/03/28/us/coronavirus-disabilities-rationing-ventilators-triage.html

Finn, C. (2020, April 6). *How tech is helping elderly fight coronavirus lockdown loneliness*. Al Jazeera. Retrieved from: https://www.aljazeera.com/news/2020/04/tech-helping-elderly-fight-coronavirus-lockdown-loneliness-200402185238544.html

Foley, K. (2018). *Workforce updates 2018. Presentation at the American Geriatrics Society (AGS) 2018 Annual Scientific Meeting*, Orlando, FL.

Goger, A. (2020, March 16). *For millions of low-income seniors, coronavirus is a food security issue*. The Brookings Institution. Retrieved from: https://www.brookings.edu/blog/the-avenue/2020/03/16/for-millions-of-low-income-seniors-coronavirus-is-a-food-security-issue/

Goldbaum, C. (2020, March 30). *They can't afford to quarantine. So they brave the subway*. The New York Times. Retrieved from: https://www.nytimes.com/2020/03/30/nyregion/coronavirus-mta-subway-riders.html

Graham, J. (2020, March 18). *Amid pandemic, programs struggle to reach vulnerable seniors living at home*. Kaiser Health News. Retrieved from: https://khn.org/news/as-coronavirus-surges-programs-struggle-to-reach-vulnerable-seniors-living-at-home/

Hamel, L. W. (2017, April 27). *Views and experiences with end-of-life medical care in the U.S.* Kaiser Family Foundation. Retrieved from: https://www.kff.org/other/report/views-and-experiences-with-end-of-life-medical-care-in-the-u-s/

Johnson, R. W., & Butrica, B. A. (2012, May). *Age disparities in unemployment and reemployment during the great recession and recovery [Online Brief]*. The Urban Institute. Retrieved from: https://www.urban.org/sites/default/files/publication/25431/412574-age-disparities-in-unemployment-and-reemployment-during-the-great-recession-and-recovery.pdf.

Kwiatkowski, M., & Nadolny, T. L. (2020, March 26). 'We want to live.' At-risk adults, home health care workers fear coronavirus. USA Today. Retrieved from: https://www.usatoday.com/story/news/investigations/2020/03/26/coronavirus-strains-home-health-care-putting-vulnerable-risk/5083219002/

Marchiondo, L., Gonzales, E., & Williams, L. (2019). Workplace age discrimination: Long-term relationships with health and retirement intentions. *Journal of Gerontology: Social Sciences, 74*(4), 655–663. https://doi.org/10.1093/geronb/gbx095

Nash, S. (2019, April 13). *Older adults and technology: Moving beyond the stereotypes*. Stanford Center of Longevity. Retrieved from: http://longevity.stanford.edu/2019/05/30/older-adults-and-technology-moving-beyond-the-stereotypes/

National Academies of Sciences, Engineering, and Medicine. (2020). *Social isolation and loneliness in older adults: Opportunities for the health care system*. The National Academies Press.

National Institute on Aging. (2019, April 23). *Social isolation, loneliness in older people pose health risks*. National Institute of Health. Retrieved from: https://www.nia.nih.gov/news/social-isolation-loneliness-older-people-pose-health-risks

Neumark, D., & Button, P. (2014, April 7). *Age discrimination and the great recession [Blog Post]*. Federal Reserve Bank of San Francisco. Retrieved from: https://www.frbsf.org/economic-research/publications/economic-letter/2014/april/age-discrimination-older-workers-great-recession/.

Newcomb, B. (2020, April 3). *COVID-19: Why it's time to talk about advance directives*. Leonard Davis School of Gerontology. Retrieved from: https://gero.usc.edu/2020/04/03/covid-19-and-advance-directives/

Olson, E. (2017, August 7). Shown the door, older works find bias hard to prove. The New York Times. Retrieved from: https://www.nytimes.com/2017/08/07/business/dealbook/shown-the-door-older-workers-find-bias-hard-to-prove.html

Schumaker, E. (2020, April 10). *What we know about coronavirus' long-term effects.* ABC News. Retrieved from: https://abcnews.go.com/Health/coronavirus-long-term-effects /story?id=69811566

Shi, S. Q. (2020). Association of cardiac injury with mortality in hospitalized patients with COVID-19 in Wuhan, China. *Journal of American Medical Association Cardiology.* https:// doi.org/10.1001/jamacardio.2020.0950

Singletary, M. (2020, April 13). Investors may be scared, but they are holding tight. Many see recent stock market drops as a sign to buy, not sell. The Washington Post. Retrieved from: https://www.washingtonpost.com/business/2020/04/13/investors-may-be-scared-they-are-holding-tight-many-see-recent-stock-market-drops-signal-buy-not-sell/

Index

Note: **Bold** page numbers refer to tables; *italic* page numbers refer to figures and page numbers followed by "n" denote endnotes.